THE SKIN
AND
SYSTEMIC DISEASE
IN CHILDREN

The Skin
and
Systemic Disease
in Children

SIDNEY HURWITZ, M.D.

Clinical Professor
Pediatrics and Dermatology
Yale University School of Medicine
New Haven, Connecticut

YEAR BOOK MEDICAL PUBLISHERS, INC.
CHICAGO

0   9   8   7   6   5   4   3   2   1

Library of Congress Cataloging in Publication Data
Hurwitz, Sidney, 1925–
   The skin and systemic disease in children.

   Includes bibliographies and index.
   1. Cutaneous manifestations of general diseases.
2. Children—Diseases—Diagnosis.   3. Pediatric
dermatology.   I. Title.   [DNLM: 1. Skin Diseases—in
infancy & childhood.   2. Skin Manifestations—in
infancy & childhood.   WS 260 H967s]
RJ51.C87H87   1985   618.92′5   85–3130
ISBN 0–8151–4784–8

Sponsoring Editor: Diana L. McAninch
Editing Supervisor: Frances M. Perveiler
Copyeditor: Francis A. Byrne
Production Project Manager: R. Allen Reedtz
Proofroom Supervisor: Shirley E. Taylor

To my wife
TEDDY
and my daughters
WENDY, LAURIE, *and* ALISON
*whose continuing support and encouragement
have brought this book to fruition*

Preface

THE UTILIZATION OF CUTANEOUS SIGNS to identify systemic disease has become an invaluable tool in the recognition and management of internal disorders of childhood and adolescence. As interest in pediatric dermatology expands, the need for an up-to-date text which focuses upon the skin and its relation to systemic disease in the young has become increasingly apparent. With this understanding and with the encouragement of many colleagues in pediatrics and dermatology, this book has been written.

The text is designed to provide clinicians with information that will enable them to recognize dermatologic signs and their significance in the diagnosis and treatment of internal disease in the pediatric age group. Emphasis is placed upon pathogenesis and morphology of skin lesions which can serve in the recognition of the new and uncommon as well as the common disorders of childhood. Cutaneous lesions are described in detail both in words and pictures; histopathology and pathogenesis have been included in an effort to enable nondermatologists to recognize cutaneous features and their clinical significance; and tables are utilized to assist in the diagnosis and management of the various disorders.

I am indebted to numerous medical colleagues for their assistance and suggestions and in particular, I wish to express my sincere gratitude to Drs. Irwin M. Braverman and Anthony P. Cipriano for their advice and guidance. Appreciation is also expressed to Sandra Walsh of my office staff for her typing of the manuscript.

The most important persons involved with the preparation of this book have been my wife Teddy and our three daughters, Wendy, Laurie, and Alison. Two years ago, after returning to the United States from a lecture tour of Egypt, I was hospitalized with legionnaires' disease. It was during my long recuperation at home that my wife encouraged me to begin the writing of this text which served to fill my hours with interest and challenge. Without the sustained encouragement and devotion of my wife and the support of my children during this difficult time, this book would not have come to fruition.

My hope is that those who utilize this text will benefit as much from the reading of it as I have from its research and writing.

SIDNEY HURWITZ, M.D.

vii

Contents

Preface vii

1 /**The Hypersensitivity Syndromes** 1
  Urticaria 1
  Serum Sickness 8
  Hereditary Angioneurotic Edema 9
  Annular Erythemas 11
  Erythema Nodosum 17
  Erythema Multiforme 19
  Hypereosinophilic Syndrome 28

2 /**Vasculitic Syndromes** **35**
  Henoch-Schönlein (Anaphylactoid) Purpura 35
  Acute Febrile Neutrophilic Dermatosis (Sweet's Syndrome) 39
  Allergic Granulomatoses 42
  Kawasaki Disease (Mucocutaneous Lymph Node Syndrome) 45
  Periarteritis Nodosa 55
  The Behçet Syndrome 57

3 /**Infectious Diseases With Systemic Manifestations** **65**
  Staphylococcal Scalded Skin Syndrome 65
  Toxic Shock Syndrome 68
  Lyme Disease 72
  Gianotti-Crosti Syndrome (Papular Acrodermatitis of Childhood) 75
  Infectious Mononucleosis 78
  Rickettsial Diseases 81
  Systemic Candidiasis 85
  Chronic Granulomatous Disease of Childhood 88
  Job Syndrome 89

4 /**Disorders of Connective Tissues** **96**
  Disorders of Collagen 96
  Disorders of Elastin 108

5 /**The Collagen Vascular Disorders** **119**
  Lupus Erythematosus 119
  Neonatal Lupus Erythematosus 128
  Dermatomyositis 131

Scleroderma 136
Eosinophilic Fasciitis 140
Juvenile Rheumatoid Arthritis 142
Sjögren's Syndrome 146
Mixed Connective Tissue Disease 148

6 / Endocrine Disorders **157**
Thyroid Disorders 157
Multiple Endocrine Adenomatosis Syndromes 166
Parathyroid Disorders and the Skin 169
Disorders of the Adrenal Glands 174
Pituitary Disorders 179
Disorders Associated with Diabetes 181

7 / Errors of Metabolism **189**
Phenylketonuria 189
Homocystinuria 192
Alkaptonuria (Ochronosis) 193
Hepatolenticular Degeneration (Wilson's Disease) 195
Menkes' Kinky Hair Syndrome 196
The Lesch-Nyhan Syndrome 197
Biotin Deficiency 198
The Hyperlipidemias 203
Tangier Disease 209
The Mucolipidoses 215
"Stiff Skin" Syndrome 216

8 / Neurocutaneous Disorders **220**
Neurofibromatosis 220
Tuberous Sclerosis 227
Incontinentia Pigmenti 233
Hypomelanosis of Ito (Incontinentia Pigmenti Achromians) 237
Nevus Achromicus 238
The Waardenburg Syndrome 239
Vogt-Koyanagi-Harada Syndrome 239
The Alezzandrini Syndrome 240
Multiple Lentigines Syndrome (Leopard Syndrome) 240
The NAME (LAMB) Syndrome 241
The Basal Cell Nevus Syndrome 242
Epidermal Nevus Syndrome 244

9 / The Skin and the Gastrointestinal Tract **250**
Acrodermatitis Enteropathica 250
Dermatitis Herpetiformis 253

Epidermolysis Bullosa 257

Peutz-Jeghers Syndrome 268

Dyskeratosis Congenita 270

Pyoderma Gangrenosum. 272

Gardner's Syndrome 274

Familial Mediterranean Fever 275

10 / Vascular Lesions With Systemic Significance. 283

Cutaneous Hemangiomas 283

Angiokeratomas 294

Disorders Associated With Vascular Dilatation 299

Purpura Fulminans. 306

11 / Photosensitivity Disorders and Systemic Disease in Children 312

Xeroderma Pigmentosum 312

Bloom Syndrome (Congenital Telangiectatic Erythema). 315

Rothmund-Thomson Syndrome (Poikiloderma Congenitale) 317

Cockayne Syndrome 318

Hartnup Disease. 319

Pellagra 321

Kwashiorkor 323

The Porphyrias 325

Erythropoietic Porphyrias 325

Hepatic Porphyrias. 329

12 / The Reticuloendothelial Disorders 336

Histiocytosis 336

Xanthoma Disseminatum 342

Malignant Histiocytosis 343

Juvenile Xanthogranuloma 343

Sarcoidosis 354

Mycosis Fungoides. 358

Subject Index 364

1 / The Hypersensitivity Syndromes

THE ABILITY TO DIAGNOSE internal disease by means of cutaneous signs is a challenging aspect of clinical diagnosis in children as well as adults. Important aspects of systemic disease in children are the disorders of hypersensitivity and their association with precipitating factors and, at times, their possible connection to systemic disease. Hypersensitivity syndromes are based on immunologic or hypersensitivity reactions to foreign proteins such as foods or drugs; to infectious agents, immunizations, malignancies; and, in some instances, to other dermatologic conditions. Although diagnosis of these disorders by detailed history, careful evaluation of clinical features, and appropriate laboratory procedures is usually simple, difficulties frequently arise in determining the etiology because each entity may be associated with numerous underlying factors.[1, 2]

Urticaria

Urticaria, a systemic disease with cutaneous manifestations, is a common condition. Fifteen per cent of the population experiences this disorder at least once during their lifetime.[3, 4] It is characterized by transient, well-circumscribed wheals that are seen as erythematous, intensely pruritic, elevated recurrent swellings of the skin (Fig 1–1) or mucous membranes.

The etiology of urticaria is often misunderstood and may be related to a multitude of factors. It can be thought of as a symptom complex, caused and perpetuated by multiple factors. Individual lesions are caused by extravasation of fluid from small blood vessels—a reflection of increased permeability of capillaries and small venules. Various pharmacologically activate agents appear to be capable of mediating these changes (kinins, prostaglandins, serotonin, and histamine). Type I hypersensitivity reactions associated with IgE antibodies account for the majority of acute immunologically mediated urticarias[5] and appear to be related to intracellular activity of cyclic AMP (adenosine-3′, 5′-monophosphate). Type III reactions mediated by circulating immune complexes are the second most common type of urticaria; they produce serum sickness-type reactions. Type II reactions mediated by cytotoxic antibodies are rarely a problem and Type IV (delayed or cellular hypersensitivity-type reactions) are not a cause of urticaria.[6, 7]

CLINICAL MANIFESTATIONS.—Typical lesions have a white palpable center of edema with a variable halo of erythema. They vary in size from

1

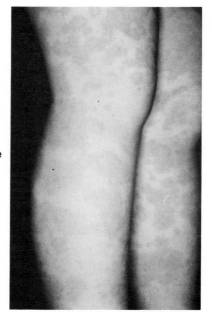

Fig 1–1.—Urticaria. Transient well-circumscribed erythematous wheals on the legs of a 3-year-old child.

pinpoint papules to large lesions several centimeters in diameter. Central clearing, peripheral extension, and coalescence of individual lesions result in a clinical picture of oval, annular, or bizarre serpiginous configurations. They may be localized to one small area or may become so generalized as to cover almost the entire skin surface. Subcutaneous extension may result in large giant wheals. In infants and young children, swelling of the distal extremities with acrocyanosis may be a prominent feature of the urticarial reactions. Occasionally, particularly in infants and young children, bullae may form in the center of the wheal, usually on the legs and buttocks.[6] Individual wheals rarely persist longer than 12 to 24 hours. Those lasting more than 24 hours are probably not true urticaria and may represent another vascular pattern, such as vasculitis or erythema multiforme.

Angioedema, giant urticaria, and Quincke's edema are terms sometimes used to describe large giant wheals and diffuse swelling of the eyelids, hands, genitalia, and mucous membranes (the lips and tongue). Although angioedema may occur on its own, it often accompanies and shares a common etiology with ordinary urticaria.

For convenience, urticaria of less than six weeks' duration is considered acute. Acute urticaria due to food or drugs is generally brief (a few days to weeks). Urticaria that recurs frequently and lasts longer than six weeks is termed chronic. About one-third of cases are of the acute variety.[8] Although the chronic type appears to be more common in middle-aged women, acute urticaria is the most common form seen in young patients.[4] The exact etiology in a particular patient is often unknown and may be associated with hypersensitivity to several possible agents such as foods, drugs, infections, serum injections, insect bites, inhalant or contact allergens, and psychogenic factors. Many physicians still regard urticaria as characteristically and almost invariably allergic in origin.[3] Although an allergic cause can be determined in many cases, in 70% to 80% of patients, particularly those with chronic urticaria, no definite etiology can be established.[3]

Although seldom life-threatening, chronic urticaria has been noted to be an important sign of underlying disease. It may occur in association with malignancy or may be an important sign of connective tissue disease. It can be the first sign of Still's disease (juvenile rheumatoid arthritis) in 7% to 23% of cases of lupus erythematosus[9] and in 10% of patients with acute rheumatic fever. When observed in a patient with arthralgia and fever of unknown origin, it should alert the physician to a possibility of serum hepatitis.[10, 11] Diagnosis and treatment of a patient with chronic urticaria require a complete history and physical examination, appropriate laboratory evaluation, and an awareness of possible underlying disease.

DIAGNOSIS.—It is seldom difficult to make a diagnosis of urticaria, even in the absence of a visible eruption at the time of examination. However, many patients may confuse wheals with blisters or insect bites with hives. Other reaction patterns may also be confused with urticaria. The differential diagnosis of urticaria should include dermographism, arthropod bites, papular urticaria, atopic dermatitis, contact dermatitis, cutaneous mastocytosis, erythema multiforme and other forms of allergic vasculitis.

Histopathologic examination of urticarial lesions reveals dilatation and engorgement of venules and capillaries, edema, and a perivascular lymphocytic infiltrate that is usually sparse but may be dense and intermingled with polymorphonuclear leukocytes and a variable number of eosinophils. Urticarial wheals are characterized by edema of the dermis; in lesions of angioneurotic edema, the edema extends into the subcutaneous and submucosal tissue without infiltrating inflammatory cells.

TREATMENT.—Effective treatment of urticaria depends on the identification of the etiologic factor and its elimination, whenever possible. Symptomatic treatment consists of antihistamines, of which hydroxyzine (Atarax or Vistaril) appears to be the most effective and the drug of choice. When antihistamines are used, they provide symptomatic relief in about 80% of patients, but should not be stopped prematurely. In an effort to prevent recurrences and the development of chronic urticaria, continuing antihistamines for one to two weeks after all signs of urticaria have cleared is recommended.

Antihistamines may be divided into six pharmacologic groups, all having somewhat similar properties. Histamine produces its various effects through receptors on the cell membranes and blood vessels containing H_1 and H_2 receptors.[12] H_1 receptors are blocked by classic antihistamines and H_2 receptors are blocked by cimetidine (Tagamet; Smith Kline and French).[13] When one antihistamine proves ineffective or causes undesirable side effects, an agent from another subgroup should be administered. In cases where an H_1 antihistamine is ineffective, a combination of an H_1 and H_2 antagonist may be effective. Cimetidine, currently the only H_2 antagonist in clinical use,[14] may be useful in combination with an H_1 antihistamine. However, cimetidine probably should not be used alone since it may actually aggravate the urticarial problem.[15]

The subcutaneous administration of 0.1 to 0.5 ml of epinephrine (1:1000) or 0.1 to 0.3 mm of Sus-Phrine (1:200) is also effective and particularly beneficial for patients with angioedema and acute or severe urticaria. Although frequently effective in patients with severe or persistent urticaria, because of potential side effects associated with prolonged steroid therapy, the administration of systemic steroids should be reserved for those patients who are unresponsive to other modes of therapy.

The Physical Urticarias

The physical urticarias are a group of disorders in which wheals occur in response to various physical stimuli. These include dermographism (factitious urticaria), pressure urticaria, cholinergic urticaria, aquagenic urticaria, solar urticaria and cold urticaria. Of these, dermographism and cholinergic urticaria are quite common; cold urticaria is less common; other patterns of physical urticaria are relatively rare.[6]

Dermographism is a sharply localized edematous or wheal reaction with a surrounding zone of erythema that occurs locally within seconds after stroking of the skin. Although its incidence in the normal population is uncertain, firm stroking of the skin induces a whealing reaction in approximately 5% of the normal population.[16] More vigorous or repeated stroking will produce the response in 25% to 50% of normal subjects.

Pressure urticaria is a related disorder characterized by the development of hives or a deeper swelling simulating angioedema, often painful, immediately or after a four- to six-hour delay following local pressure produced by clothing, jewelry, or weight bearing. Because of this delay in appearance, patients frequently fail to appreciate the cause of the disorder.[2]

Cholinergic urticaria (micropapular urticaria) is a very distinctive type of urticaria. It usually starts in adolescence and is associated with heat, exertion, or emotional stress. Seen in 5% to 7% of urticaria cases, it is considered a physical allergy and not a sign of systemic disease.[6] Cholinergic urticaria is characterized by a generalized eruption, usually on the trunk and arms, which consists of discrete, papular wheals, 1 to 2 mm in diameter with or without a surrounding area of erythema[3] (Fig 1–2). The duration of the eruption varies from 30 minutes to several hours.

Acetylcholine, released through some unknown mechanism (perhaps liberated when sweat glands are stimulated by heat, exertion, emotional, or taste stimuli), may stimulate histamine release, thus causing the lesions.[3, 10] The diagnosis is made on the basis of history and the appearance of the eruption several minutes after exercise. Once cholinergic urticaria occurs, the condition may recur for periods of months to years, and then tends toward spontaneous improvement and resolution.

Treatment of cholinergic urticaria consists of systemic antihistamines, particularly cyproheptadine (Periactin) or hydroxyzine (Atarax or Vistaril), awareness of potential precipitating factors, avoidance of heat, excessive exertion, and excitement whenever possible. After a severe attack of cholinergic urticaria, further exertion frequently fails to cause urticaria for periods of 24 hours or more. Some patients find that they can induce attacks by exercise or hot showers. In this way, they achieve freedom from symptoms for varying periods of time.

Aquagenic urticaria, a disorder that resembles but is not identical to cholinergic urticaria, occurs most frequently in adolescence and is characterized by small, intensely pruritic, perifollicular papular wheals with sur-

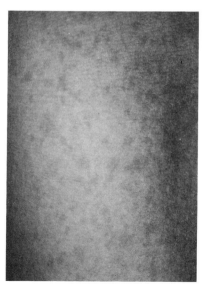

Fig 1–2.—Cholinergic urticaria (induced by heat exertion or emotional stress) on the arm of a 15-year-old girl. Discrete micropapular wheals and a wide area of surrounding erythema.

rounding axon reflex erythema (with sparing of the palms and soles). The disorder is precipitated by contact with water or perspiration (irrespective of temperature). Exercise and other cholinergic factors do not precipitate this disorder, and patients can drink water without adverse reaction.[17] Although the etiology remains unknown, aquagenic urticaria may be related to a toxic substance created by a combination of water and sebum, resulting in local histamine release from the perifollicular mast cells.[18] The administration of antihistamines by mouth seems to reduce the whealing tendency and lessen the severity of the disorder.

Solar urticaria is a rare disorder in which minimal exposure to sunlight at different wavelengths in the visible or ultraviolet light range provokes an almost immediate localized urticarial reaction, with "burning" followed by erythema, wheal, and flare sharply confined to light-exposed sites. Urticaria is usually seen within a few minutes of exposure to sunlight. Although the reaction generally fades within 15 or 30 minutes to an hour or two, scratching and rubbing may lead to secondary eczematization with persisting cutaneous changes.[3]

Solar urticaria is a chronic disease and may appear in individuals from 3 to 52 years of age. It appears to be a disorder of multiple etiologies. The cause is unknown, and the wavelength of light causing the urticarial response (290 to 700 nm) varies considerably from person to person.[19] Although therapy generally is unsatisfactory, oral antihistamines occasionally may be helpful for individuals with this disorder. Repeated gradual exposure to artificial radiation (fluorescent lamps) or sunlight may produce tolerance in some patients.[20, 21] Measures should be directed toward diminishing exposure to sunlight. Chloraquine has been reported to relieve symptoms in a few patients[22] and sunscreen preparations are occasionally beneficial when the precipitating wavelengths are in the sunburn range. Sunscreens appear to be the most consistently helpful form of therapy now available.

Cold urticaria is a disorder characterized by localized or generalized urticaria that develops within a few minutes or hours of exposure to cold air or water. In highly sensitive persons, in whom whealing may be widespread or severe, cold showers or swimming in cold water may produce hypotension and, on occasion, syncope, loss of consciousness, and drowning.[22] If the cold extends to the mucous membranes, respiratory symptoms such as nasal stuffiness, cough, dyspnea, and gastrointestinal symptoms such as swelling of the lips, swelling of the oral mucous membranes, dysphagia, and abdominal cramps may occur.

Cold urticaria can be divided into two forms: a rare congenital or familial type inherited on an autosomal dominant basis and a more common acquired form. Although not sex-linked, familial cold urticaria is more common in females. The disorder may be present at birth or may occur during infancy, and usually develops in early childhood. It is characterized by an urticarial or papular eruption, fever, chills, arthralgia, headache, malaise, muscle tenderness, and, at times, a significant leukocytosis.[24] Although the tendency to familial cold urticaria generally persists for life, the severity of symptoms may decrease with age. The urticarial reaction is usually induced by a generalized body cooling, more often in cold air than cold water. It generally develops after a latent period of several hours and may persist for up to 48 hours.

The acquired form of cold urticaria often appears suddenly, usually in children, but may occur at any age and has an equal incidence in both sexes. Once symptoms develop, they are generally short-lived and, although they may persist indefinitely, usually disappear after a few months or years.

Secondary forms of cold urticaria may also be associated with cold hemolysin and cold agglutinin syndromes. These forms, generally seen in adults, cause Raynaud's phenomenon, acrocyanosis, and cutaneous ulcers. Some cases of cold urticaria manifested by itching, erythema, purpura, atypical Raynaud's phenomenon, and ulceration due to cryoglobulins may also be associated with multiple myeloma, leukemia, kala-azar, systemic lupus erythematosus, and melanoma.

The diagnosis of cold urticaria requires a careful history and investigation for other possible etiologic factors. When the diagnosis remains in doubt, patients should be evaluated for other systemic diseases, particularly lupus erythematosus, cryoglobulinemia, and hereditary angioneurotic edema. Diagnosis of cold urticaria may frequently be assisted by reproduction of symptoms by local applications of an ice cube for periods of two to ten minutes. The best areas for this testing are the face, neck, and in particular the arms. Patients who fail to respond to ice may respond to cold water or generalized cooling of the body.[25]

Patients with severe or widespread cold urticarial reactions should be forewarned of the risk of drowning after loss of consciousness when swimming or bathing in cold water. The treatment of cold urticaria is aided by oral administration of antihistamines, particularly cyproheptadine (Periactin).[26] For those unresponsive to systemic antihistamines, desensitization to cold may be attempted by gradually cooling an extremity in cold water for five to ten minutes a day with a gradual increase in the time of exposure and decrease of the temperature over a period of weeks or months. This treatment is not regularly effective and must be done cautiously in an effort to minimize the risk of systemic reaction.[6]

Serum Sickness

Serum sickness is an allergic reaction characterized by urticaria, malaise, fever, lymphadenopathy, splenomegaly, and swollen and tender joints. The syndrome, originally noted and most commonly seen following the administration of antiserum of horse or rabbit origin, is now most frequently encountered following treatment with drugs. Although penicillin accounts for most cases of serum sickness reactions, other antibiotics, thiouracils, para-aminosalicylic acid, hydralazine, phenylbutazone, sulphonamides, salicylates, and a wide variety of other drugs may be responsible for this disorder. Serum sickness develops gradually, generally within a period of 8 to 14 days following antigenic exposure of nonsensitive individuals, with shorter latent periods when presensitization exists. It is believed to be mediated largely by circulating antigen-antibody complexes (a Type III Arthus reaction), of which gamma G-globulin is the predominant immunoglobulin.

CLINICAL MANIFESTATIONS.—The clinical manifestations of serum sickness are urticaria, malaise, fever, lymphadenopathy, splenomegaly, and swollen and tender joints (Fig 1–3). Localized or generalized edema is common. Although temperatures up to 105° F may occur, the fever is usually slight or moderate. Skin eruptions, the most common and characteristic feature, are present in over 80% of cases. In 90% the rash is urticarial. Morbilliform and scarlatiniform eruptions are less common and erythema multiforme, erythema nodosum, and vasculitic purpura are rarely seen. Lymphadenopathy, the second most common manifestation, often appears initially in the epitrochlear region, but may be generalized or regional. The

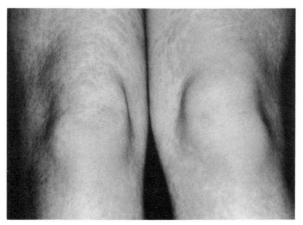

Fig 1–3.—Serum sickness. Urticaria and swollen tender knees in a 16-year-old girl.

latter is particularly common when the allergic reaction is secondary to an injection.

Joint symptoms occur in about 50% of patients and vary in severity from a mild arthralgia to severe polyarthritis. Neurologic manifestations, when present, include peripheral neuritis, radiculitis, optic neuritis, and cerebral edema.[27] A more severe form of serum sickness-like reaction is associated with glomerulonephritis caused by the deposition of antigen-antibody complexes in the kidney. In other instances, serum sickness can result in hypersensitivity angiitis involving multiple organ systems.

TREATMENT.—Serum sickness is generally a self-limiting disease that subsides within two to three weeks. Although rarely fatal, death may occur as a consequence of coronary artery vasculitis or severe neuropathy. Treatment consists of ephedrine, antihistamines, and analgesics. Hydroxyzine appears to be the most effective antihistaminic and antipruritic agent, and may be administered in dosages of 2 mg/kg/24 hour in four divided doses; this amount may be increased twofold for severe cases. If this fails to make the patient more comfortable, systemic corticosteroids are effective, and in severe cases and for individuals with facial or epiglottal edema, epinephrine is indicated. In cases where glottal edema is severe, tracheostomy may be life-saving.[28]

Hereditary Angioneurotic Edema

Hereditary angioneurotic edema (HANE, hereditary angioedema) is a serious but rare form of urticaria characterized by recurrent episodes of edema of the subcutaneous tissue, particularly the hands, feet, and face and of the gastrointestinal or upper respiratory tracts.

An autosomal dominant disorder, the defect is due to a deficiency of the alpha-2 globulin inhibitor of the first component of complement (C_1-esterase inhibitor), which results in transient episodes of increased vascular permeability.[29, 30] Although the pathogenesis of this disorder is not fully understood, it appears that a kinin-like permeability factor generated by the action of C_1-esterase inhibitor on C_4 and C_2, the episodic activation of Hageman factor working through a kinin-forming system of plasma or plasmin, and an elevated capillary filtration rate in affected areas may be the physiologic mediators of attacks.

Two genetic variants of hereditary angioneurotic edema have been described. In the more common type, seen in an estimated 85% of those affected, serum levels of C_1-esterase inhibitor are extremely low because of decreased synthesis in the liver.[31] In its variant form, normal or elevated levels of C_1-esterase inhibitor are present, but the C_1-esterase inhibitor appear to be nonfunctional.[32] Trauma, a major known precipitating factor in many attacks, induces activation of factor XII (the Hageman factor). At-

TABLE 1–1. HEREDITARY ANGIONEUROTIC EDEMA

1. Earliest symptoms often in infancy or early childhood
   a. Usually before age 10
   b. Rarely as late as third decade
2. Mottling of skin may be first sign
3. Sudden attacks of circumscribed subcutaneous edema
   a. Precipitated by minor trauma, infection, extremes of temperature, exercise, or emotional excitement
   b. Usually on the face or an extremity.
4. Depressed serum levels of C_4 and C_2, and demonstration of a functional lack of C_1–esterase inhibitor
5. Asphyxiation in up to 25% of patients

tacks of hereditary angioedema, therefore, may be the result of malfunction of both the contact phase of coagulation and the complement system dysfunction.[29, 33]

CLINICAL MANIFESTATIONS.—The earliest symptoms of hereditary angioneurotic edema (Table 1–1) often begin in infancy or early childhood, usually before the age of 10, rarely as late as the third decade of life. The frequency and severity of attacks are typically exacerbated during adolescence and subside in the fifth decade.[34] Mottling of the skin often occurs early in life and may be the first evidence of the disorder. Affected individuals are prone to sudden attacks of circumscribed subcutaneous edema. The swelling evolves very quickly. It usually affects the face or an extremity, may be severe enough to cause remarkable disfiguration of the affected parts, and generally subsides within one to five days. The skin and mucosal lesions may appear spontaneously or may be precipitated by minor trauma, especially extraction of teeth, strenuous exercise, infection, menses, extremes of temperature, psychic disturbances, or emotional excitement.[35] There is no pitting, discoloration, redness, pain, or itching associated with the edema, and a rash similar to erythema marginatum is noted in some patients, particularly children.

Gastrointestinal involvement, second in order of frequency, is marked by nausea, vomiting, or diarrhea, sometimes with recurrent colic and severe abdominal pain simulating a surgical emergency. Involvement of the mucous membranes of the hypopharynx and larynx, although seen less often, may be particularly severe and result in asphyxiation, the leading cause of death in patients with this disorder. This complication, usually seen in the third decade of life, may occur in 25% of patients.

DIAGNOSIS.—Diagnosis of hereditary angioneurotic edema can be established by the finding of reduced serum levels of C_4 or C_1-esterase inhibitor, or both. The finding of reduced serum levels of C_4 and/or C_2 is a reliable, indirect way of screening patients for the possibility of HANES. However, if these levels are reduced in the presence of normal levels of C_1 inhibitor protein, confirmation must rely on demonstration of a functional lack of C_1-esterase inhibitor by hemolytic or biochemical assay.[36, 37]

TREATMENT.—Although 25% of patients with HANES may die of suffocation during attacks of laryngeal edema, the development of effective therapy now augers a more favorable prognosis.[38] Since clinical manifestations may appear after reproductive capability is reached, all family members should be tested for the presence of functional C_1 inhibitor, not only for therapeutic consideration but also for genetic counseling.[39] Antihistamines and corticosteroids have not been effective in the management of patients, and epinephrine is beneficial in the control of swelling in only a few patients. Intravenous administration of diuretics such as meralluride (Mercuhydrine) or ethacrynic acid is helpful in halting the progression of severe angioedema, and tracheostomy frequently is life-saving in patients with laryngeal obstruction. Although methyltestosterone linguets (in dosages of 10 to 25 mg once daily) may prevent attacks in one-third to one-half of patients, it can produce masculinization in women patients; it is not recommended for children.

Epsilon aminocaproic acid (EACA) inhibits the conversion of plasminogen to plasmin (a known C_1 activator).[40] Its safety in long-term therapy, however, has not been established. In short-term use, its major side effect has been muscle weakness with associated elevation of creatine phosphokinase and aldolase and an increased predisposition to thrombosis and phlebitis. However, its analogue, tranexamic acid, in doses of 1 to 3 gm orally per day, has been effective in aborting attacks of angioedema and has relatively few side effects.

Danazol (Danocrine, Winthrop), in dosages of 200 mg two or three times a day, appears to act on the disease by inducing synthesis of C_1-esterase inhibitor. This accordingly represents one of the first examples of correction of an inherited abnormality by drug therapy. It has fewer androgenic side effects than methyltestosterone, but cannot be used in children and should not be administered to pregnant women.[41]

Annular Erythemas

The annular erythemas (erythema marginatum, erythema annulare centrifugum, and erythema chronicum migrans) represent a group of oval, annular, arcuate, or polycyclic lesions with individual characteristics that allow differentiation into distinct clinical categories. Although not yet proved, it appears that these disorders may be related to cell-mediated urticarial reactions. Their individual appearances and behaviors are characteristic and, therefore, frequently helpful in the clinical diagnosis of various systemic disorders.

Erythema Marginatum and Rheumatic Fever

Erythema marginatum is a distinctive variant of erythema annulare that occurs on the trunk (especially on the abdomen) and the proximal extremities in about 10% of patients with active rheumatic fever and occasionally in patients with juvenile rheumatoid arthritis (Table 1–2). Lesions appear as evanescent pink macules or papules that fade centrally (leaving a pale or sometimes pigmented center), and rapidly expand to form nonpruritic, delicate, reddish-purple rings or segments of rings with flat or elevated reticular, polycyclic, or serpiginous borders (Fig 1–4).

Easily overlooked, erythema marginatum is generally associated with active carditis or arthritis. It is seen more frequently in children than adults with rheumatic fever, frequently follows the onset of migratory arthritis by a few days, but can also occur months after the carditis.[42–44] Lesions are evanescent (fading in a few hours to several days), spread rapidly, and may recur in crops in different areas. Unlike the characteristic rash of juvenile rheumatoid arthritis, lesions of erythema marginatum are larger, spread centrifugally with central clearing, and are limited to the trunk and proximal limbs. Individual lesions may persist for a few hours or for a period of two or three days, and characteristically develop in crops. Although the eruption seldom lasts more than several weeks, it may occasionally recur at sporadic intervals for several months to years, and at times may persist for two years without evidence of rheumatic activity.[2]

Erythema marginatum presents a clinical picture that characteristically resembles a variety of dermatoses, including urticaria, erythema multiforme, and other transient figurate erythemas. Frequently seen more easily in the afternoon, coalescence of polycyclic lesions often result in a characteristic chickenwire-like appearance. Believed to represent a vascular reaction to a preceding streptococcal infection, gentle warming of the skin often enhances visualization of pale or barely perceptible lesions. Histologic features consist of a perivascular infiltrate of neutrophils in the papillary dermis. These findings are helpful and frequently will enable the physician to rule out or suspect a diagnosis of rheumatic fever, often before

TABLE 1–2.—ERYTHEMA MARGINATUM

---

1. Pink macules or papules that fade centrally and expand to form rings or segments of rings
2. Limited to proximal limbs and trunk
3. Lesions are evanescent (fading in a few hours to several days), spread rapidly, and may recur in crops in different areas
4. Associated with fever and active carditis in 10% to 15% of children with acute rheumatic fever, occasionally in patients with juvenile rheumatoid arthritis

---

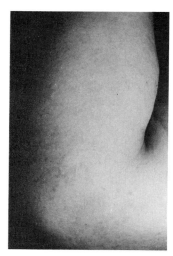

Fig 1–4.—Erythema marginatum. Delicate pink segments of rings with reticular, polycyclic or serpiginous borders on the arm of a 15-year-old girl with rheumatic fever.

other clinical and/or laboratory features of the disease become evident.[45]

Another type of erythema seen in rheumatic fever consists of small 2 to 5 mm dull red macules and urticarial papules that occur on the arms and elbows, buttocks, and knees. Seen in 2% to 3% of patients with rheumatic fever, these lesions do not form rings or develop in crops, are less transient than lesions of erythema marginatum, and last from hours to days.

Seen in from 20% to less than 2% (in more recent series), subcutaneous nodules present another characteristic cutaneous manifestation of rheumatic fever[44, 45] (Table 1–3). Most prevalent in children with extensive cardiac involvement, subcutaneous nodules can coexist with erythema marginatum and are a late manifestation of rheumatic fever. They usually portend serious disease and are observed in no other diseases except granuloma annulare and rheumatoid arthritis. The nodules of rheumatic fever are smaller than those seen in rheumatoid arthritis and last for shorter periods of time, usually less than a month. They tend to occur in crops and often appear in a symmetrical distribution on extensor tendons of the hands,

TABLE 1–3.—SUBCUTANEOUS NODULES IN RHEUMATIC FEVER

1. Seen in up to 20% of patients with rheumatic fever
2. Occur in crops (often in a symmetrical distribution) on extensor tendons of hands, feet, knees, and scapulae, and on the occiput and spinous processes of the vertebrae
3. Lesions are small and last for shorter periods of time than those of juvenile rheumatoid arthritis
   a. 2 mm to 2 cm in diameter
   b. Usually last less than one month

feet, knees, and scapulae, on the occiput, and on the spinous processes of the vertebrae. They are never painful and vary in size from 2 mm to 2 cm in diameter. Lying deep in the connective tissue over bony prominences with freely movable skin over them, they are more readily felt than seen, and, unless a careful search is made, are frequently overlooked. The differentiation of subcutaneous nodules of rheumatic fever from rheumatoid nodules and granuloma annulare is not possible on clinical or histologic grounds alone. The diagnosis of rheumatoid nodules, however, can usually be established if the patient has other cutaneous and systemic features of rheumatic fever.

Erythema Chronicum Migrans

Erythema chronicum migrans is a cutaneous reaction to a tick bite characterized by single or multiple raised erythematous expanding lesions with advancing indurated borders and central clearing (Table 1–4) (Fig 1–5). Although common in Europe, only one case had been reported in the United States by 1970.[48] Since 1972, however, this disorder has now been seen in the northeastern, midwestern, and western United States, most commonly in the summer and early fall, and has been associated with a new syndrome called "Lyme disease" after the community in southeastern Connecticut where the initial cases were first noted[49, 50] (see Chapter 3).

Until 1982, the mechanism of formation of lesions of erythema chronicum migrans remained unknown, but recent studies show that the disorder is mediated by an immunologic reaction associated with a spirochetal infection transmitted by an arthropod vector (a tick of the genus *Ixodes*). In the United States, the disorder has recently been associated with a spirochetal infection (the *Ixodes dammini* spirochete) which has been classified as *Borrelia*[51] (*Borrelia burgdorferi*) (see Chapter 3). The vector responsible for erythema chronicum migrans in Europe is a tick, *Ixodes ricinus*. In the northeast and midwestern United States it is *Ixodes dammini*, and on the west coast (Oregon and California) it has been identified as *Ixodes pacificus*, and in Georgia it is *I. scapularis*.[52]

TABLE 1–4.—ERYTHEMA CHRONICUM MIGRANS

1. Raised erythematous expanding lesions with central clearing and advancing indurated borders
2. 4 to 20 days after a tick bite; rings may reach 20 to 30 cm in diameter and clear within 3 days to 2 weeks
3. Symptoms include local itching, stinging, or burning (may be accompanied by headache, fever, vomiting, fatigue, and regional adenopathy)
4. Histopathology consistent with an arthropod bite

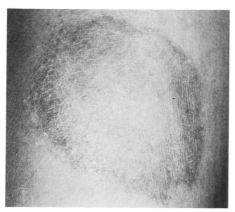

Fig 1–5.—Erythema chronicum migrans. An expanding ringed lesion with central clearing (From Hurwitz S.[1] Used by permission.)

Lesions of erythema chronicum migrans begin as erythematous macules or papules that occur 4 to 20 days after the tick bite and clear in three days to eight weeks. The borders of the lesions then expand to form red rings as great as 20 to 30 cm in diameter, with central clearing. The lesions often itch, sting, or burn, and may be accompanied by fever, headache, vomiting, fatigue, and regional adenopathy.[1] They can be differentiated from those of erythema annulare centrifugum and tinea corporis by rapid peripheral expansion, lack of vesiculation and scaling along the peripheral border, microscopic examination of skin scrapings, and fungal culture. Histologically the lesions are consistent with an arthropod bite and reveal a primarily lymphocytic infiltration, occasionally with some eosinophils. They differ from lesions of erythema annulare centrifugum in which the infiltrate tends to be organized around blood vessels and, unlike vasculitides, they lack prominent polymorphonuclear leukocytes, dermal hemorrhage, or fibrinoid necrosis.[53]

Systemic penicillin, tetracycline, and erythromycin have now been shown to shorten the duration of erythema chronicum migrans and may prevent or attenuate the subsequent arthritis seen in patients with Lyme disease[54, 55] (see Chapter 3). In a study of 157 patients with early Lyme disease, none of those treated with tetracycline developed major complications (meningoencephalitis, myocarditis or recurrent attacks of arthritis). Nearly one-third of those treated, however, had minor late symptoms such as headache, lethargy and musculoskeletal pain. This study also demonstrated tetracycline to be the most effective (penicillin was slightly less effective and erythromycin was least effective of the three antibiotics).[55]

Erythema Annulare Centrifugum

Erythema annulare centrifugum (EAC) is an eruption characterized by persistent, occasionally pruritic, erythematous annular lesions, each with a clear center and a raised, thin, wall-like border, which slowly enlarges centrifugally (Table 1–5) (Fig 1–6). At times the palpable border may be topped by microvesicles or may show a fine collarette scale on its trailing edge, suggesting a diagnosis of tinea corporis.

The etiology of erythema annulare centrifugum is unknown. Although it often occurs without apparent cause, most cases appear to be related to hypersensitivity to an underlying inflammatory or neoplastic disease. In infants, it may be associated with an autoimmune disorder in their mothers.[56] In such instances, the possibility of neonatal lupus erythematosus must be considered. Erythema annulare centrifugum may occur as a cutaneous sign of hypersensitivity to drugs, molds, foods, fungus infection, blood dyscrasia, immunologic disorders, or neoplastic disease.

CLINICAL MANIFESTATIONS.—Erythema annulare centrifugum rarely begins at birth but has been seen in infants as well as older children and adults. Most lesions occur in individuals between 30 and 50 years of age.[57] Primary lesions tend to be single or multiple erythematous edematous papules with a predilection for the trunk, buttocks, thighs, and legs. They are asymptomatic except for occasionally mild pruritus. The rings extend peripherally, usually slowly, 1 to 3 mm per day, sometimes up to 4 cm in a week. As the edematous border moves outward, a desquamating scale is often seen on its trailing edge. New lesions may form within the original circle. The resulting overall shape may be irregular, oval, circinate, semiannular, target-like, or polycyclic. The borders may eventually reach a size of 10 cm or more in diameter. The duration of the disease is extremely variable and may go on for weeks or months and, with new lesions appearing in successive crops, frequently for years.

TABLE 1–5.—ERYTHEMA ANNULARE CENTRIFUGUM

1. Erythematous annular lesions with a clear center and a raised, thin, wall-like border
2. A sign of hypersensitivity to drugs, molds, foods, fungus infection, blood dyscrasia, immunologic disorder, or neoplastic disease
3. Duration varies from weeks to months (new crops may appear for years)
4. Histopathology: focal infiltration of lymphocytes around blood vessels and dermal appendages in a "coat-sleeve" arrangement

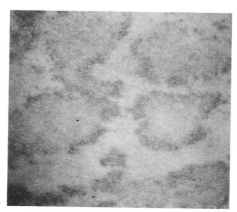

Fig 1–6.—Erythema annulare centrifugum. Slowly expanding annular lesions with dusky centers and palpable scaly erythematous borders. (From Hurwitz S.[1] Used by permission.)

DIAGNOSIS.—Erythema annulare centrifugum must be differentiated from pityriasis rosea, erythema multiforme, tinea corporis, early lesions of lupus erythematosus, granuloma annulare, and erythema chronicum migrans. Fungal infections can be distinguished by their more pronounced epidermal changes, with vesiculation or scaling or both at the edge of the lesions, by microscopic examination of skin scrapings and fungal culture. When the diagnosis is indeterminate, histopathologic examination of cutaneous lesions showing focal infiltration of lymphocytes around the blood vessels and dermal appendages in a "coat-sleeve" arrangement may help establish the true nature of the disorder.

TREATMENT.—Since erythema annulare centrifugum represents a hypersensitivity reaction, treatment depends upon the determination and removal of the underlying cause. Antihistamines produce variable and usually incomplete relief. Although systemic steroids may aid the temporary resolution of lesions, unless the underlying cause is removed, the disorder frequently recurs as soon as medication is discontinued.

Erythema Nodosum

Erythema nodosum represents a delayed cell-mediated hypersensitivity syndrome characterized by red tender nodular lesions, usually on the pretibial surface of the legs (Fig 1–7), and occasionally on other areas of the skin where subcutaneous fat is present (Table 1–6). Although etiologic causes are numerous, the most common are beta streptococcal infections,

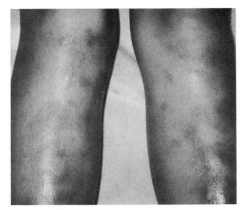

Fig 1–7.—Erythema nodosum. Tender red oval nodules on the pretibial aspect of the leg.

sarcoidosis, and tuberculosis. In children, streptococcal and other respiratory infections and primary tuberculosis are the most common causes of erythema nodosum. Although tuberculosis is an uncommon cause of this disorder today, any child under the age of 5 years with a positive tuberculin test and no evidence of streptococcal infection or other respiratory illness should be considered to have tuberculosis until proved otherwise.[2] Other disorders that may cause erythema nodosum include leprosy, coccidioidomycosis, histoplasmosis, leishmaniasis, cat scratch fever, and fungal infection.[1, 58] Noninfectious disorders that cause erythema nodosum are sarcoidosis, ulcerative colitis, regional ileitis, and reactions to various drugs, particularly sulfonamides, diphenylhydantoin (Dilantin), and contraceptive pills containing ethinyl estradiol and norethynodrel.[59]

Clinical manifestations.—The disease has its greatest incidence in the spring and fall, and is less common in summer. Although most cases

TABLE 1–6.—Erythema Nodosum

1. Red tender nodular lesions on the pretibial surface of the legs
   a. A delayed cell-mediated hypersensitivity
   b. Respiratory infection the most common cause in children
2. Ten per cent of cases are recurrent
3. Histopathologic features:
   a. Lymphocytic perivascular infiltrate in the dermis
   b. Lymphocytes and neutrophils (with histiocytes, giant cells, and at times plasma cells) in the fibrous septa in the subcutaneous fat

occur in the third decade of life, the disorder is frequently seen in children, particularly those above 10 years of age.[60] During childhood, girls are affected slightly more than boys, but in adult life women are affected three to four times as often as men.[2] Lesions, 1 to 5 cm in diameter, occur symmetrically, usually on the pretibial areas, occasionally the knees, ankles, thighs, extensor aspects of the arms, the face, and neck. Initially they appear as bright to deep red, warm and tender, oval, slightly elevated nodules. After a few days they develop a brownish-red or purplish bruise-like appearance (this has been termed *erythema contusiformis*). The eruption usually lasts three to six weeks but may recede earlier if the patient remains in bed. Recrudescences may occur over a period of weeks to months, but attacks are seldom recurrent,[61] and arthralgias may precede, coincide with, or follow the eruption in as many as 90% of cases. In the 10% of patients where the condition may present as a recurring disorder, recurrences are frequently associated with repeated streptococcal infection.[2]

DIAGNOSIS.—Erythema nodosum has a characteristic clinical picture, and diagnosis can generally be made on the basis of physical examination alone. Although diagnosis is usually not difficult, bruises, cellulitis or erysipelas, deep fungal infections (such as Majocchi's granuloma or sporotrichosis), insect bites, deep thrombophlebitis, angiitis, erythema induratum, and fat-destructive panniculitides can be confused with this disorder. When the diagnosis is in doubt, bacterial and fungal cultures and histologic examination of skin biopsies generally will help to clarify the diagnosis.

The principal histologic changes of erythema nodosum are located in the deep dermis and subcutaneous tissue. They consist primarily of lymphocytes and neutrophils (with histiocytes, giant cells, and at times plasma cells) in the fibrous septa between fat lobules as well as in individual fat cells. The dermis shows a moderate degree of perivascular infiltrate composed primarily of lymphocytes.[62]

TREATMENT.—The treatment of erythema nodosum is directed at identification and treatment of the underlying cause. Bed rest, with elevation of patient's legs, helps reduce pain and edema. When pain, inflammation, or arthralgia are prominent, salicylates may be helpful. In chronic or recurrent cases, detailed investigations are necessary to uncover the underlying cause. Intralesional corticosteroids frequently cause rapid involution of individual lesions and in persistent or recurrent eruptions oral corticosteroids may be beneficial.

Erythema Multiforme

Erythema multiforme is a distinctive hypersensitivity reaction characterized by skin and mucous membrane lesions and, in its more severe form, mucosal lesions, constitutional symptoms, and, at times, visceral involvement (Table 1–7). Although usually considered acute and self-limiting, recent observations indicate that erythema multiforme may behave as a chronic recurrent disorder in many people.[2, 63]

Although its pathogenesis remains unknown, erythema multiforme appears to represent the end result of a hypersensitivity reaction to a number of etiologies: viral, bacterial, protozoal, fungal or *Mycoplasma pneumoniae* (Eaton agent) infection; sensitivity to food or drugs; immunizations; and a wide variety of other systemic diseases and physical agents. Whereas drug reactions and malignancies are important causes of erythema multiforme in older persons, infectious diseases are the most prominent precipitants in children and young adults.[1] The most common cause of erythema multiforme appears to be the virus of herpes simplex, with a history of cold sores preceding the development of other lesions by about 3 to 14 days. Recurrences are particularly common in this form of erythema multiforme.[64]

CLINICAL MANIFESTATIONS.—The clinical spectrum of erythema multiforme ranges from a localized eruption of the skin and mucous membranes (erythema multiforme minor) to a severe multisystem disorder (erythema multiforme major) with widespread blisters and severe erosions of the mucous membranes (Stevens-Johnson syndrome). Some authors place a more generalized loss of the epidermis, Lyell's disease (toxic epidermal necrolysis) under the classification of erythema multiforme major. Until more is known about the pathogenesis of both toxic epidermal necrolysis and erythema multiforme, this categorization should remain conjectural[65] (Table 1–8). Toxic epidermal necrolysis, as originally described by Lyell in 1956,[66] actually comprised two entirely different disorders: the subcorneal exfoliative disorder (staphylococcal scalded skin syndrome) and a subepidermal dermatosis (toxic epidermal necrolysis).[67] Staphylococcal scalded skin syndrome is discussed in Chapter 3.

TABLE 1–7.—ERYTHEMA MULTIFORME

1. A distinctive acute hypersensitivity syndrome
   a. Viral, bacterial, protozoal, fungal, or *M. pneumoniae* infection
   b. Food or drugs, immunizations, systemic disease
2. A symmetrical eruption with predilection for the palms, soles, extensor surfaces of arms and legs, and backs of hands and feet
3. Macular, urticarial, and vesiculobullous (the predominant lesions are dull red to dusky flat macules or sharply marginated wheals)
4. Target lesions (the hallmark of the disorder)

TABLE 1–8.—CLASSIFICATION OF
ERYTHEMA MULTIFORME

1. Erythema multiforme minor
   a. Erythematous macules, papules, urticarial, and target lesions
   b. Mucous membrane involvement limited to one surface (usually mouth)
   c. A relatively benign illness with no significant complications
   d. Mortality low
2. Erythema multiforme major (Stevens-Johnson disease)
   a. Starts abruptly with high fever, prostration, extensive eruption, and widespread bullae
   b. Severe involvement of mucous membranes (at least two surfaces)
   c. Mortality 5% to 10%
3. Erythema multiforme major (Lyell's, TEN type)?

Erythema multiforme occurs at any age, with the most severe forms occurring in children and young adults. The disorder may occur at any time of year, but is most common in the spring and fall. The eruption is symmetrical and may occur on any part of the body, with a predilection for the palms and soles (Fig 1–8), backs of the hands and feet, and extensor surfaces of the arms and legs. As the disorder progresses, lesions often extend to the trunk, face, and neck. Oral lesions may occur alone or in conjunction with cutaneous lesions. Seen in 25% of cases of erythema multiforme, they first appear as bullae (that break soon after formation), with swelling and crusting of the lips and development of erosions of the buccal mucosa, gums, and tongue (Fig 1–9).

The term *erythema multiforme* is often confusing to nondermatologists, and should not be applied indiscriminately to any polymorphic eruption. The disorder is a specific hypersensitivity syndrome with a distinctive clinical pattern, the hallmark of which is an erythematous ring (the so-called iris or target lesion). Although a single type of lesion might predominate during a particular attack, the basic lesions are macular, urticarial, and vesiculobullous; the clinical diagnosis can be made readily in most instances if these characteristics are kept in mind.[2] The evolution and resolution of individual lesions last about a week, but the eruption may continue to appear in crops for as long as two or three weeks, thus contributing to the multiforme appearance of the eruption.

The primary lesion of erythema multiforme is a dull red to dusky flat macule, or a sharply marginated wheal, in the center of which a papule or

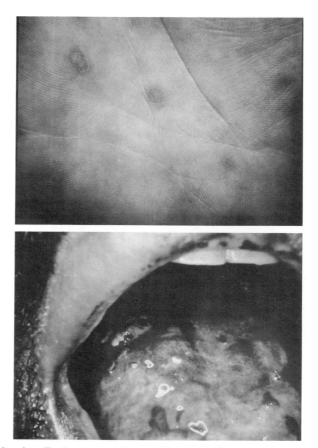

Fig 1–8 (top).—Erythema multiforme. Palmar lesions are highly characteristic of this disorder. (From Hurwitz S.[1] Used by permission.)

Fig 1–9 (bottom).—Erythema multiforme. Blisters, crusting, swelling of the lips and erosions of the tongue.

vesicle develops, thus creating the multiformity of lesions (Fig 1–10). The central area then flattens and develops clearing. As a result, it is not unusual to see iris or target lesions consisting of concentric circles whose bright red rings alternate with cyanotic or violaceous ones. Although occasionally seen in erythema annulare centrifugum, target lesions are highly characteristic of erythema multiforme. Careful inspection of the eruption in erythema multiforme may disclose fine petechiae, the clinical feature that distinguishes lesions of erythema multiforme from those of urticaria and erythema annulare centrifugum.

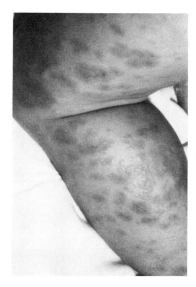

Fig 1–10.—Target lesions and marginated wheals with central vesicles in an infant with erythema multiforme.

STEVENS-JOHNSON DISEASE (ERYTHEMA MULTIFORME MAJOR).

Systemic manifestations of erythema multiforme minor, when present, are mild and consist of low-grade fever, malaise, and myalgia. Severe forms of bullous erythema multiforme with mucocutaneous involvement have been labeled *Stevens-Johnson disease,* after the two physicians who first described this variant of the disorder.[68] Stevens-Johnson disease is an extremely severe form of bullous erythema multiforme (Figs 1–11, 1–12), with high fever, pronounced constitutional symptoms, and widespread bullae, which involve the mucous membranes, conjunctivae, and anogenital areas. The disorder is characterized by a sudden onset and a prodromal period of 1 to 14 days, which can consist of fever, malaise, cough, coryza, sore throat, vomiting, diarrhea, chest pain, myalgia, and arthralgias. Recurrent herpes simplex infection appears to be an important etiologic factor in the milder form of erythema multiforme (EM minor); in the more severe form (Stevens-Johnson syndrome, EM major), mycoplasma infections and drugs appear to be common causes of the disorder.[63]

In the Stevens-Johnson variant, the mucous membranes of the lips, eyes, nasal mucosa, genitalia, and rectum show extensive bullae with a grayish-white membrane, characteristic hemorrhagic crusts, and superficial erosions and ulcerations. The eye changes may be particularly serious, with severe conjunctivitis, corneal ulcerations, keratitis, uveitis, or panophthalmitis. Sequelae may be grave, with a possibility of corneal ulceration and partial or even complete blindness. Pulmonary involvement may occur as

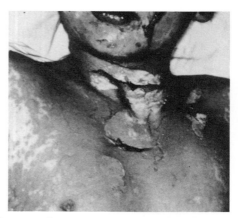

Fig 1–11.—Bullous erythema multiforme (Stevens-Johnson syndrome, erythema multiforme major). Confluent erythema, target lesions, blisters and exfoliation of the epidermis. (From Hurwitz S.[1] Used by permission.)

an extension from the oropharynx and tracheobronchial tree, or may be due to pneumonitis associated with an initiating viral infection or secondary infection. In extreme cases, renal involvement with hematuria, nephritis and, in some cases, progressive renal failure may result. In other instances, esophageal or tracheal ulceration, pyoderma, and/or septicemia may complicate the disorder.

DIAGNOSIS.—Typical cases of simple erythema multiforme (erythema multiforme minor) with symmetrical involvement of the extensor surface of the extremities, involvement of the palms and soles, and the characteristic iris lesions generally offer few problems in diagnosis. The more severe syndrome with marked mucosal damage (Stevens-Johnson disease, erythema multiforme major) is characterized by systemic toxicity, a vesiculobullous erythema multiforme eruption, and mucous membrane involvement affecting two or more mucous membranes.

The cutaneous lesions of erythema multiforme appear in various forms but all have an identical histologic picture; the severity of the histologic reaction determines the clinical appearance of lesions. Microscopic examination of skin lesions reveals edema just below the epidermis, which when mild and moderate, produces urticarial lesions; when the edema is severe, bullae are formed.[69] Other histologic features consist of dilatation of blood vessels, accompanied by a perivascular infiltration composed mainly of lymphocytes, nuclear dust resulting from disintegration of neutrophils and eosinophils (leukocytoclasis), edema, and extravasation of erythrocytes. Whereas previous immunofluorescent examinations of erythema multi-

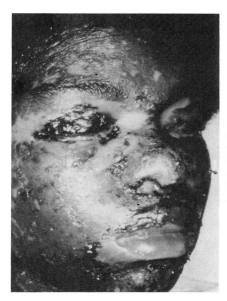

Fig 1–12.—Stevens-Johnson form of erythema multiforme (Stevens-Johnson syndrome). Hemorrhagic crusts of the mucous membranes, extensive bullae, and severe ophthalmic involvement in an adolescent black girl with erythema multiforme major.

forme lesions have been uniformly negative, current studies reveal deposition of C_3, alone or associated with IgM, in the vessels of the papillary dermis when biopsies are obtained early in the course of the lesions. These findings appear to confirm the theory of immune complexes in the etiology of erythema multiforme.[70]

TREATMENT.—The management of erythema multiforme depends upon the clinical status of the patient. A thorough search for the identification and elimination of the underlying cause is imperative. If a drug is suspected, it should be discontinued. Mild cases resolve spontaneously, generally within 5 to 15 days, or may respond to antihistamines, and the mortality is low. Local therapy depends on the type and extent of the lesions. Simple erythema usually requires no treatment. Vesicular, bullous, or erosive lesions may be treated with wet compresses. Colloidal oatmeal baths may also be helpful.

Patients with severe systemic toxicity and widespread bullous involvement (Stevens-Johnson disease, erythema multiforme major) are more difficult. They frequently require hospitalization and have a mortality ranging from 5% to 10% (75). Severe oropharyngeal involvement often necessitates frequent mouthwashes, local application of diphenhydramine (elixir of Benadryl), or topical use of lidocaine (Xylocaine 2% Viscous Solution; Astra) as a topical anesthetic. When ocular involvement is present, ophthalmologic consultation should be obtained. The eyes should be cleansed frequently with separation of the eyelids, and topical antibacterial agents should be utilized to prevent secondary infection. Topical corticosteroids, however, are contraindicated in this area, as they may produce thinning of the cornea and eventual ulceration or perforation.

Liquid diet and replacement intravenous therapy may be required in extreme cases. Fluid lost through the skin must be considered and, when extensive, should be handled in a manner similar to that of patients with extensive burns. Dehydration and shock, electrolyte imbalance, and pulmonary, ocular, and renal involvement should be carefully monitored.

Many authors feel that, despite their controversy, steroids in high dosages are indicated in cases with severe skin or mucous membrane involvement, or when there is evidence of appreciable systemic toxicity. The possibility of secondary infection, however, must be considered, and appropriate antibiotics initiated when indicated. Recent studies, however, suggest that the use of systemic corticosteroids in Stevens-Johnson syndrome may actually increase morbidity and cause prolongation of hospital stay.[76] Since erythema multiforme major can progress to a widespread epidermal necrosis (TEN) with a mortality of 25% to 50% (67), many authorities still favor early use of systemic corticosteroids (1 to 2 mgm of prednisone or its equivalent a day) during the acute inflammatory phase of the disorder (during the stage of extension of lesions) with tapering of the medication during the one- to three–week healing phase. If advanced tissue damage is already evident, secondary bacterial infections are a more prominent concern and steroid therapy is not advisable.[77]

TOXIC EPIDERMAL NECROLYSIS

Toxic epidermal necrolysis (TEN) is a severe exfoliative variant of erythema multiforme major characterized by the rapid onset of widespread erythema and epidermal necrolysis. Usually seen in adults 40 years of age or older and only rarely in children, the disorder is frequently, but not necessarily, related to a hypersensitivity to drugs: phenylbutazone, phenolphthalein, procaine, sulfonamides, penicillin or other antibiotics, barbiturates, tranquilizers, vaccines, salicylates, aminopyrine, allopurinol, and diphenylhydantoin (Dilantin). The reason for the decreased incidence of drug-induced toxic epidermal necrolysis in infants and young children may be related to the fact that infants and young children have less exposure to potentially sensitizing drugs and therefore have not had the opportunity to develop sensitization to those agents. Toxic epidermal necrolysis may also occur as a manifestation of a graft-versus-host reaction[71, 72] (Table 1–9). Originally described by Lyell in 1956[66] and by Lang and Walker in 1956 and 1957,[73, 74] the terms *toxic epidermal necrolysis* and *Lyell disease* should be reserved for the severe drug-induced disorder.[65, 67]

TABLE 1–9.—TOXIC EPIDERMAL NECROLYSIS
(LYELL'S DISEASE)

1. A hypersensitivity reaction (usually to drugs or as a
   manifestation of graft-vs.-host disease)
2. Universal erythema with subepidermal separation of the
   skin (between the dermis and epidermis)
   a. Nikolsky sign is positive
   b. With extensive involvement patients should be watched
      for evidence of shock, electrolyte imbalance, and
      secondary infection
3. High mortality (25%–50%)
4. Uncommon in young children

The pathogenesis of TEN involves a drug-induced necrosis of the basal cell layer of the epidermis with the production of subepidermal bullae rather than the superficial epidermal split seen in patients with staphylococcal scalded skin syndrome. This differentiating feature is important in the clinical differentiation of the two disorders.

CLINICAL MANIFESTATIONS.—In TEN, a widespread macular erythema and stomatitis may be common features with exfoliation of the skin occurring in limited areas or, in severe cases, along the entire body surface. As the erythema becomes universal, the skin begins to develop areas of separation between epidermis and dermis (these superficial blisters are usually first noticed on the face and upper trunk). During this stage of the disease, the upper layer of the epidermis may become wrinkled or may be removed (often peeling off like wet tissue paper) by light stroking, the characteristic Nikolsky sign. However, the Nikolsky sign is not specific for drug-induced toxic epidermal necrolysis; it may be seen in other bullous disorders (pemphigus, erythema multiforme major of the Stevens-Johnson type, epidermolysis bullosa, and the staphylococcal scalded skin syndrome). Shortly thereafter, the patient develops flaccid bullae and eventual exfoliation; death, when it occurs, is usually the result of sepsis and flud and electrolyte imbalance.

Drug-induced toxic erythema necrolysis carries a high mortality, varying between 25% and 50%, and the presence of mucosal lesions in patients with a great degree of cutaneous involvement present a particularly poor prognosis.[72]

DIAGNOSIS.—The diagnosis of TEN should be considered in the presence of generalized or focal erythema with exquisite tenderness, bullae, a positive Nikolsky sign, and large areas of exfoliation of the cutaneous surface. History of ingestion of a drug known to provoke toxic epidermal necrolysis in an older child or adult is further evidence suggesting a diagnosis of the drug-induced form of TEN. When the diagnosis is indeterminate, toxic epidermal necrolysis can be differentiated from staphylococcal scalded skin syndrome by a Tzanck test or histopathologic examination of a cutaneous punch biopsy. In the staphylococcal disorder, the disruption shows cleavage in the epidermis; in toxic epidermal necrolysis, separation is seen in the upper dermis below the basement membrane (similar to the cleavage plane seen in patients with bullous erythema multiforme). Histopathologic examination of a cutaneous punch biopsy also demonstrates eosinophilic necrosis of epidermal cells with a paucity of cellular infiltrate; these features, however, are not diagnostic of this disorder.

TREATMENT.—In patients with drug-induced toxic epidermal necrolysis, all drugs administered prior to onset of the eruption should be discontinued. If damage to the epidermis is extensive, treatment should be similar to that advocated for burn victims with special attention to fluid requirements, electrolyte balance, and avoidance of secondary infection. Although topical applications of silver sulfadiazine cream (Silvadene) are frequently beneficial, the risk of absorption and possible bone marrow suppression must be considered as a potential side effect.[78] In patients who recover, corneal scarring and blindness can complicate the picture. Ocular lesions, therefore, should be carefully monitored with ophthalmologic consultation, much as with patients with Stevens-Johnson syndrome, in an effort to avoid keratitis sicca, decreased visual acuity, corneal opacities and blindness.

Although systemic corticosteroids have been recommended for patients with toxic epidermal necrolysis, specific data confirming their efficacy is lacking. It is difficult to interpret their value in the management of this disorder. Recommendations regarding their use require further evaluation.

Hypereosinophilic Syndrome

The hypereosinophilic syndrome (HES) is a disorder characterized by persistent idiopathic eosinophilia of the blood and bone marrow associated with diffuse infiltration of various organs by eosinophils.[79, 80] Although virtually any organ system can be involved, affected patients generally demonstrate hepatosplenomegaly, cardiac, pulmonary, nervous system, or dermatologic involvement.[79–81] It is not clear whether the eosinophil itself is the primary cause of organ dysfunction or if the eosinophilia is secondary to whatever process is producing the tissue damage. Although the pathogenesis of HES remains unknown, it has been suggested that a hypersensitivity reaction to an unidentified antigen or antigens with abnormal immune reactivity may be involved in the production of eosinophilia and the mediation of organ damage seen in patients with this disorder.[81]

CLINICAL MANIFESTATIONS.—Seen primarily in males (90%), the hypereosinophilic syndrome occurs most frequently in middle-aged individuals (with the highest incidence in the 40- to 50–year age group), and is uncom-

TABLE 1–10.—THE HYPEREOSINOPHILIC SYNDROME

1. A group of disorders characterized by persistent eosinophilia and organ system involvement
   a. A hypersensitivity reaction?
   b. Male to female ratio 9:1
   c. Uncommon in children
2. Anorexia, weight loss, dyspnea, cough, fever, night sweats, chest pain, diarrhea, and arthralgia associated with hepatosplenomegaly, lymphadenopathy, cardiac disease and neurologic features
3. Cutaneous lesions:
   a. Pruritic erythematous or hyperpigmented macules, papules, nodules, or serpiginous lesions (often with secondary ulceration)
   b. Urticaria or angioedema (particularly on face and extremities)
   c. Erythematous papules over the trunk in a patchy sometimes perifollicular distribution

mon in children and adolescents[82] (Table 1–10). Presenting symptoms include anorexia, weight loss, dyspnea, cough, fever, night sweats, chest pain, diarrhea, and arthralgia. Clinical features include hepatosplenomegaly, lymphadenopathy, cardiac disease, and eosinophilia greater than 1500 eosinophils/mm^3 lasting for six months or longer. Except for the blood and bone marrow involvement, cardiovascular disease is the major cause of morbidity and mortality. Seen in 50% of affected patients, cardiac dysfunction is manifested by cardiomegaly, edema, dyspnea, mitral valve insufficiency, endocardial fibrosis, and myocardial inflammation, often with eosinophilic infiltration, mural thrombus formation, and congestive heart failure.[82–84]

Cutaneous lesions, seen in 25% to 50% of patients, may present as pruritic erythematous or hyperpigmented macules, papules, and serpiginous lesions with vesicles, or nodules, some of which may have an associated ulceration.[83] These lesions may appear anywhere on the body but are generally present over the trunk and extremities. Urticaria or angioedema may appear on the face and extremities and, in its most benign form, erythematous papules may be seen in a patchy and at times perifollicular distribution over the trunk.[83, 85, 86]

Pulmonary complications (seen in 40% of patients) include interstitial infiltrates, a persistent nonproductive cough, and pleural effusion. Neurologic findings include hemiparesis, dysesthesias or paresthesias, slurred speech, confusion, and, at times, coma. Hepatic dysfunction and diarrhea, with or without malabsorption, and renal involvement with persistent hematuria and hypouricemia have also been reported.[84]

Historically, the hypereosinophilic syndrome has been associated with a very poor prognosis with a mortality of 81% to 95% within one to three years of diagnosis. It now appears, however, that the course and eventual prognosis is variable and is dependent on the degree of systemic involvement, with some patients having no progression of the disease.[82, 87] Factors associated with a poor prognosis include evidence of heart failure, peripheral leukocytosis (90,000 or more), and the finding of myeloblasts in the peripheral blood with cases described as "eosinophilic leukemia" appearing at the severe end of the clinical spectrum.

DIAGNOSIS.—The diagnosis of the hypereosinophilic syndrome is dependent on its clinical features, an increased white blood count in the range of 10,000 to 250,000/mm^3, and an elevated eosinophilic count of 6,000 to 240,000 mm^3 when other causes of eosinophilia are ruled out. The histopathologic features of cutaneous lesions are characterized by a predominantly perivascular infiltrate of mature eosinophils, mononuclear cells, and, at times, polymorphonuclear cells.

TREATMENT.—Systemic corticosteroids are the treatment of choice for patients with progressive organ-system involvement. For patients unresponsive to steroids, the addition of chemotherapeutic agents such as hydroxyuria, vincristine, and cytarabine has been beneficial.[88, 89]

REFERENCES

1. Hurwitz S.: The skin and systemic disease, in Hurwitz S.: *Clinical Pediatric Dermatology.* W.B. Saunders Co., Philadelphia, 1981, pp. 384–434.
2. Braverman I.M.: Hypersensitivity syndromes, in Braverman I.M.: *Skin Signs of Systemic Disease,* ed. 2. W.B. Saunders Co., Philadelphia, 1981, pp. 453–515.
3. Champion R.H., Roberts, S.O.B., Carpenter, R.G., et al.: Urticaria and angioedema: a review of 554 patients. *Br. J. Dermatol.* 81:588–597, 1969.
4. Monroe E.W.: Urticaria, in Callen J.P.: *Cutaneous Aspects of Internal Disease.* Year Book Medical Publishers, Chicago, 1981, pp. 107–120.
5. Monroe E.W., Jones H.E.: Urticaria: An updated review. *Arch. Dermatol.* 113:80–90, 1977.
6. Warin R.P., Champion R.H.: *Major Problems in Dermatology, Vol. I.: Urticaria.* W.B. Saunders Co., Philadelphia, 1974.
7. Caputo R.V., Solomon L.M.: Vascular reactive diseases, in Solomon L.M., Esterly N.B., Loeffel E.D.: *Adolescent Dermatology.* W.B. Saunders Co., Philadelphia, 1978, pp. 404–432.
8. Hellgren L.: The prevalence of urticaria in the total population. *Acta Allerg.* 27:236–240, 1972.
9. O'Laughlin S., Schroeter A.L., Jordon R.E.: Chronic urticaria-like lesions in systemic lupus erythematosus. A review of 12 cases. *Arch. Dermatol.* 114:879–883, 1978.
10. Braverman I.M.: Urticaria as a sign of internal disease. *Postgraduate Med.* 41:450–454, 1967.
11. Dienstag J.L., Rhodes A.R., Bhan A., et al.: Urticaria associated with acute viral hepatitis type B. Studies of pathogenesis. *Ann. Intern. Med.* 89:34–40, 1978.

12. Greaves M., Marks R., Robertson I.: Receptors for histamine in human skin blood vessels. A review. *Br. J. Dermatol.* 97:225–228, 1977.
13. Beaven M.A.: Histamine. *N. Engl. J. Med.* 294:30–36, 320–325, 1976.
14. Christensen O.B., Maibach H.I.: Antihistamines in dermatology, in Rook A.J., Maibach H.I.: *Seminars in Dermatology* 2:270–280, 1983.
15. Wehrmeister J., Burkhart C.G.: Chronic urticaria: current modes of therapy. *Dermatology & Allergy* 6:21–24, 1983.
16. Kirby J.D., Matthews C.N.A., James J., et al.: The incidence and other aspects of factitious whealing (dermographism). *Brit. J. Dermatol.* 85:331–335, 1971.
17. Chalamidas S.L., Charles R.: Aquagenic urticaria. *Arch. Dermatol.* 104:541–564, 1971.
18. Shelley W.B., Rawnsley H.M.: Aquagenic urticaria. *J.A.M.A.* 189:895–898, 1964.
19. Harber L.C., Halloway R.M., Wheatley V.R., et al.: Immunologic and biophysical studies in solar urticaria. *J. Invest. Dermatol.* 41:439–443, 1963.
20. Ramsay C.A.: Solar urticaria treatment by inducing tolerance to artificial radiation and natural light. *Arch. Dermatol.* 113:1222–1225, 1977.
21. Bernhard J.D., Jaenicke K., Momtaz-T K., et al.: Ultraviolet A phototherapy in the prophylaxis of solar urticaria. *J. Am. Acad. Dermatol.* 10:29–33, 1984.
22. Ramsay C.A.: Solar urticaria. *Int. J. Dermatol.* 19:233–236, 1980.
23. Juhlin L., Shelley W.B.: Role of mast cell and basophil in cold urticaria with associated systemic reactions. *J.A.M.A.* 177:371–377, 1961.
24. Tindall J.P.: Cold urticaria. *Postgrad. Med.* 50:133–137, 1971.
25. Sarkany I., Gaylarde P.M.: Negative reactions to ice in cold urticaria. *Br. J. Dermatol.* 85:46–48, 1971.
26. Wanderer A.F., St. Pierre J., Ellis E.: Primary acquired cold urticaria. *Arch. Dermatol.* 113:1375–1377, 1977.
27. Parker C.W.: Serum sickness, in Demis D.J., Dobson R.L., McGuire J.: *Clinical Dermatology*, ed. 9. Harper and Row, Philadelphia, 1981. 13:1, pp. 22–23.
28. Stiehm E.R., Fulginiti V.A.: *Immunologic Disorders in Infants and Children.* W.B. Saunders Co., Philadelphia, 1973.
29. Schapira M., Silver L.D., Scott C.F., et al.: Prekallikrein activation and high-molecular-weight kininogen consumption in hereditary angioedema. *N. Engl. J. Med.* 308:1050–1054, 1983.
30. Frank M.M., Gelfand J.A., Atkinson J.A.: Hereditary angioedema: the clinical syndrome and its management. *Ann. Intern. Med.* 84:580–593, 1976.
31. Johnson A.M., Alper C.A., Rosen F.S., et al.: Evidence for decreased hepatic synthesis in hereditary angioneurotic edema. *Science* 173:553–554, 1971.
32. Klemperer M.R., Rosen F.S., and Donaldson V.H.: A polypeptide derived from the second component of human complement (C_2) which increases vascular permeability. *J. Clin. Invest.* 48:44a–44b, 1969.
33. Donaldson V.H.: Mechanisms of activation of C_1 esterase in hereditary angioneurotic edema plasma in vitro: the role of Hageman factor, a clot promoting agent. *J. Exp. Med.* 127:411–429, 1968.
34. Donaldson V.H., Rosen F.S.: Hereditary angioneurotic edema: a clinical survey. *Pediatrics* 37:1017–1027, 1966.
35. Soter N.A., Wasserman S.I.: Urticaria, angioedema (Review). *Int. J. Dermatol.* 18:517–532, 1979.
36. Austen K.F., Scheffer A.L.: Detection of hereditary angioneurotic edema by

demonstration of a reduction in the second component of human complement. *N. Engl. J. Med.* 272:649–656, 1965.

37. Gigli I., Rudd S., Austen K.G.: The stiochiometric measurement of the serum inhibitor of the first component of complement by the inhibition of immune hemolysis. *J. Immunol.* 100:1154–1169, 1968.

38. Berman B.A., Ross R.N.: Conversations in allergy and immunology. Hereditary angioedema. *Cutis* 31:124–168, 1983.

39. Maize J.C.: Hereditary angioneurotic edema, in Demis D.J., Dobson R.L., McGuire J.: *Clinical Dermatology,* ed. 9. Harper and Row, Philadelphia, 1982, 7–11:1–5.

40. Champion R.H., Lachman P.J.: Hereditary angioedema treated with E-aminocaproic acid. *Br. J. Dermatol.* 81:763–765, 1969.

41. Gelfand J.A., Sherrin R.J., Alling D.W., et al.: Treatment of hereditary angioedema with danazol. *N. Engl. J. Med.* 295:1444–1448, 1976.

42. Keil H.: The rheumatic erythema: a clinical survey. *Ann. Int. Med.* 11:2223–2272, 1938.

43. Perry C.B.: Erythema marginatum (rheumaticum). *Arch. Dis. Child.* 12:233–238, 1937.

44. McDonald E.C., Weisman M.H.: Articular manifestations of rheumatic fever in adults. *Ann. Int. Med.* 89:917–920, 1978.

45. Troyer C., Grossman M.E., Silvers D.: Erythema marginatum in rheumatic fever: early diagnosis by skin biopsy. *J. Am. Acad. Dermatol.* 8:724–728, 1983.

46. Canizares O.: Cutaneous lesions of rheumatic fever. *Arch. Dermatol.* 76:702–707, 1957.

47. Barnert A.L., Terry E.E., Persellin R.H.: Acute rheumatic fever in adults. *J.A.M.A.* 232:925–928, 1975.

48. Scrimenti R.J.: Erythema chronicum migrans. *Arch. Dermatol.* 102:104–105, 1970.

49. Mast W.E., Burrows W.M., Jr.: Erythema chronicum migrans in the United States. *J.A.M.A.* 236:859–860, 1976.

50. Steere A.C., Malawista S.E.: Cases of Lyme disease in the United States: location correlated with a distribution of *Ixodes dammini. Ann. Int. Med.* 91:730–733, 1979.

51. Steere A.C., Grodzicki R.L., Kornblatt A.N., et al.: The spirochetal etiology of Lyme disease. *N. Engl. J. Med.* 308:733–740, 1983.

52. Hardin J.E., Steere A.C., Malawista S.E.: Immune complexes and the evolution of Lyme arthritis. *N. Engl. J. Med.* 301:1358–1363, 1979.

53. Steere A.C., Malawista S.E., Hardin J.A., et al.: Erythema chronicum migrans and Lyme arthritis. The enlarging clinical spectrum. *Ann. Int. Med.* 86:685–698, 1977.

54. Steere A.C., Malawista S.E., Newman J.H., et al.: Antibiotic therapy in Lyme disease. *Ann. Int. Med.* 93:1–80, 1980.

55. Steere A.C., Hutchinson G.J., Rahn D.W., et al.: Treatment of early manifestations of Lyme disease. *Ann. Int. Med.* 99:22–26, 1983.

56. Hammer H., Ronnerfalt L.: Annular erythema in infants associated with autoimmune disorders in their mothers. *Dermatologica* 154:115–127, 1977.

57. Jillson O.F.: Erythema annulare centrifugum, in Demis D.J., Dobson R.L., McGuire J.: *Clinical Dermatology,* ed. 9. Harper and Row, Philadelphia, 1982, 7–5:1–3.

58. Martinez-Roiq A., Llorens-Terol J., Torres J.M.: Erythema nodosum and kerion of the scalp. *Am. J. Dis. Child.* 136:440–442, 1982.

59. Baden H.P., Holcomb F.D.: Erythema nodosum and oral contraceptives. *Arch. Dermatol.* 98:634–635, 1968.
60. Aetiology of erythema nodosum in children. A study by a group of pediatricians. *Lancet* 2:14–16, 1961.
61. Kibel M.A.: Erythema nodosum in children. *S. Afr. Med. J. Sci.* 44:873–876, 1970.
62. Winkelmann R.K., Förström L.: New observations in histopathology of erythema nodosum. *J. Invest. Dermatol.* 65:441–446, 1975.
63. Bean S.F., Quezada R.K.: Recurrent oral erythema multiforme. Clinical experience with 11 patients. *J.A.M.A.* 249:2810–2812, 1983.
64. Shelley W.B.: Herpes simplex virus, a cause of erythema multiforme. *J.A.M.A.* 201:153–165, 1967.
65. Huff J.C., Weston W.L., Tonnesen M.G.: Erythema multiforme: a critical review of characteristics, diagnostic criteria, and causes. *J. Am. Acad. Dermatol.* 8:763–775, 1983.
66. Lyell A.: Toxic epidermal necrolysis: an eruption resembling scalding of the skin. *Br. J. Dermatol.* 68:355–361, 1956.
67. Lyell A.: Toxic epidermal necrolysis (the scalded skin syndrome): A reappraisal. *Br. J. Dermatol.* 100:69–86, 1979.
68. Stevens A.M., Johnson F.C.: A new eruptive fever associated with stomatitis and ophthalmia: report of two cases in children. *Am. J. Dis. Child.* 24:526–533, 1922.
69. Bedi T.R., Pinkus H.: Histopathologic spectrum of erythema multiforme. *Br. J. Dermatol.* 95:243–250, 1976.
70. Kazmierowski J.A., Wuepper K.D.: Erythema multiforme: immune complex vasculitis of the superficial cutaneous microvasculature. *J. Invest. Dermatol.* 71:366–369, 1978.
71. Peck, G.L., Herzig G.P., Elias P.M.: Toxic epidermal necrolysis in a patient with graft-vs.-host reaction. *Arch. Dermatol.* 105:561–569, 1972.
72. McCarty J.R., Raimer S.S., Jarratt M.: Toxic epidermal necrolysis from graft-vs.-host disease. Occurrence in a patient with thymic hypoplasia. *Am. J. Dis. Child.* 132:282–284, 1978.
73. Lang R., Walker J.: An unusual bullous eruption. *S. Afr. Med. J.* 30:97–98, 1956.
74. Lang R., Walker J.: Toxic epidermal necrolysis: a report of four cases. *S. Afr. Med. J.* 31:713–716, 1957.
75. Snyder R.A., Elias P.M.: Toxic epidermal necrolysis and staphylococcal scalded skin syndrome, in Jegosathy B.V., Lazarus G.S.: *Symposium on Blistering Diseases. Dermatologic Clinics.* W.B. Saunders Co., Philadelphia, April 1983, Vol. 1, No. 2, pp. 235–248.
76. Rasmussen J.E.: Erythema multiforme in children—response to treatment with systemic corticosteroids. *Br. J. Dermatol.* 95:181–185, 1976.
77. Edmond B.J., Huff J.C., Weston W.L.: Erythema multiforme, in Rasmussen J.E. (Editor): *Symposium on Pediatric Dermatology II.* W.B. Saunders Co., Philadelphia, 1983, Vol. 30, No. 4. pp. 631–640.
78. Jarrett F., Ellerbe S., Demling R.: Acute leukopenia during topical burn therapy with silver sulfadiazine. *Am. J. Surg.* 135:818–819, 1978.
79. Chusid M.F., Dale V.C., West B.C., et al.: The hypereosinophilic syndrome: analysis of fourteen cases with a review of the literature. *Medicine* 54:1–25, 1975.
80. Faucy A.S., Harley J.B., Roberts W.C., et al.: The idiopathic hypereosino-

philic syndrome: clinical, pathophysiologic, and therapeutic considerations. *Ann. Intern. Med.* 97:78–92, 1982.

81. Parrillo J.E., Lawley T.J., Frank M.M., et al.: Immunologic reactivity in the hypereosinophilic syndrome. *J. Allergy Clin. Immunol.* 64:113–121, 1979.

82. Fisher M., Trusky D.E.: Fever and rash: update, in Moschella S. (Editor-in-Chief): *Dermatology Update.* Review for physicians. 1982 edition, Elsevier, New York, 1983, pp. 71–90.

83. Kazmierowski J.A., Chusid M.J., Parillo J.E., et al.: Dermatologic manifestations of the hypereosinophilic syndrome. *Arch. Dermatol.* 114:531–535, 1978.

84. Lugassey G., Michaeli J.: Hypouricemia in the hypereosinophilic syndrome. Response to treatment. *J.A.M.A.* 250:937–938, 1983.

85. Hardy W.R., Anderson R.E.: The hypereosinophilic syndrome. *Ann. Int. Med.* 68:1220–1229, 1968.

86. Rickles F.R., Miller D.R.: Eosinophilic leukemoid reaction. *J. Pediatr.* 80:418–428, 1972.

87. Sánches J.L., Padilla M.A.: Hypereosinophilic syndrome. *Cutis* 29:490–494, 1982.

88. Parillo J.E., Fauci A.S., Wolff S.M., et al.: Therapy of the hypereosinophilic syndrome. *Ann. Int. Med.* 89:167–172, 1978.

89. Van Slyck E.J., Adamson T.C.: Acute hypereosinophilic syndrome. *J.A.M.A.* 242:175–176, 1979.

2 / Vasculitic Syndromes

THE VASCULITIC DISORDERS are a group of conditions characterized by clinical evidence of vascular damage and histologic features of blood vessel necrosis, deposition of fibrinoid material in blood vessel walls, and the presence of scattered nuclear fragments, referred to as nuclear dust, resulting from disintegration of neutrophilic nuclei (leukocytosis) within the necrotic areas of the vessel wall and surrounding tissues.[1] The classification of cutaneous vasculitis is difficult and confusing since it is based on gross and morphologic features and encompasses a wide spectrum of vascular reactions to a variety of noxious stimuli and associated systemic disease. The vasculitic syndromes with systemic manifestations discussed in this chapter include leukocytoclastic vasculitis (Henoch-Schönlein purpura), acute febrile neutrophilic dermatosis (Sweet's syndrome), the vasculitic granulomatoses, Kawasaki disease, infantile and adult-types of periarteritis (polyarteritis) nodosa, and Behcet's syndrome.

Henoch-Schönlein (Anaphylactoid) Purpura

Henoch-Schönlein purpura (HSP) is a systemic disorder occurring primarily in children and young adults, and more often in boys than girls. It represents a diffuse leukocytoclastic angiitis caused by hypersensitivity to a variety of etiologic factors, and produces a vasculitis of the capillaries and pre- and postcapillary vessels in the upper dermis, gastrointestinal tract, synovial membranes, renal glomeruli, and lungs.[2, 3] Although the nature of the immunologic reaction is not completely clear, a history of frequent antecedent upper respiratory infections preceding the onset of symptoms and immunologic studies[4-7] suggests a hypersensitivity phenomenon precipitated by a number of provocative stimuli, resulting in localized or widespread vascular damage in an immunogenetically susceptible host[8] (Table 2–1). Bacterial or viral infections appear to be the most frequently implicated precipitating causes; drugs, food, insect bites, and chemical toxins have also been suggested as possible etiologic factors.[9, 10] Gairdner, in 1947, was the first to suggest a role for streptococcal infection in the etiology of this disorder.[2] More recent studies, however, fail to confirm a dominant etiologic role for the streptococcus.[11]

CLINICAL MANIFESTATIONS.—The clinical picture of Henoch-Schönlein vasculitis is distinctive. Mainly a disease of children and young adults (particularly those between three and ten years of age), the disorder is charac-

TABLE 2–1.—Henoch-Schönlein
(Anaphylactoid) Purpura

---

1. A disease of young children and young adults (highest incidence between 3 and 10 years of age)
2. A diffuse vasculitis (caused by hypersensitivity to a variety of etiologic factors)
3. Cutaneous lesions
   a. Small hemorrhagic macules, papules, and/or urticarial lesions
   b. A symmetrical distribution over buttocks and extensor surfaces of the arms and legs
   c. *Palpable purpura* (a hallmark of leukocytoclastic angiitis)
4. Systemic features (in two-thirds of patients)
   a. Gastrointestinal (colicky abdominal pain, vomiting, intussusception, hemorrhage)
   b. Arthritis (warm, tender, painful swollen joints, with or without overlying purpura)
   c. Renal involvement (the most frequent and serious complication) in 25% of children under 2 and 50% of those over 2 years of age

---

terized by a distinctive rash (erythematous papules followed by purpura), abdominal pain, and joint symptoms. Renal disease occurs frequently, but other organ involvement is less common. Generally the disease subsides within a few weeks, with frequent recurrences often related to an upper respiratory infection or reexposure to the offending agent.[2]

The skin lesions consist of small hemorrhagic macules, papules, and/or urticarial lesions, which appear in a symmetrical distribution over the buttocks and the extensor surfaces of the extremities (particularly the elbows and knees)[10] (Fig 2–1). In some instances, skin lesions may develop in patterns at pressure sites and, in more severe cases, hemorrhagic purpuric or necrotic lesions may be prominent. The disease usually consists of a single episode, which may last for several days to several weeks. In some cases, however, recurrent attacks may occur at intervals for weeks or months.

Individual lesions occur in crops, tend to fade after about five days, and are eventually replaced by areas of brownish pigmentation, purpura, or ecchymoses. New crops of lesions frequently occur over the fading lesions of a previous episode, giving a polymorphous appearance to the disorder. Although the lesions may be misinterpreted as drug reactions, erythema multiforme, or urticaria, the presence of *palpable purpura* (the hallmark of leukocytoclastic angiitis) will usually clarify the true nature of the disorder (Fig 2–2). This characteristic finding, created by edema and extravasation of erythrocytes, gives individual lesions their diagnostic palpable and purpuric appearance.

Rarely, the face, mucous membranes of the mouth and nose, and the

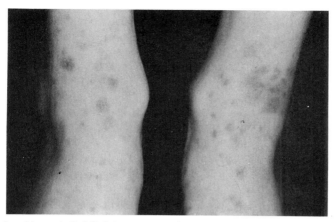

Fig 2–1.—Henoch-Schönlein purpura (anaphylactoid purpura). Hemorrhagic macules, papules, and urticarial lesions in a symmetrical distribution on the lower extremities of a 6-year-old girl.

anogenital regions may show petechial involvement. Children under 3 years of age often have an associated edema of the scalp, hands, feet, scrotum, and periorbital tissues. This edema occurs in the absence of renal or cardiac disease and appears to reflect an increased capillary permeability due to the underlying vasculitis.

SYSTEMIC MANIFESTATIONS.—Systemic involvement is seen in up to

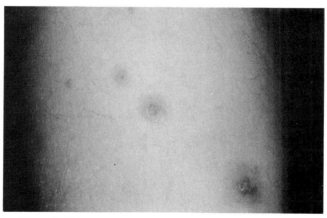

Fig 2–2.—Henoch-Schönlein purpura. Small hemorrhagic papules on the leg of a young child. Edema and extravasation of erythrocytes give individual lesions their diagnostic palpable and purpuric appearance ("palpable purpura").

two-thirds of children with severe forms of Henoch-Schönlein purpura. Since proper diagnosis depends on the characteristic cutaneous eruption, a significant diagnostic challenge occurs when systemic manifestations appear alone or precede the appearance of skin lesions.[12] The degree of systemic involvement may vary, with arthritic or gastrointestinal symptoms reportedly seen in as many as two-thirds of affected children. Gastrointestinal symptoms resulting from edema of the bowel wall and hemorrhage as a result of vasculitis are common. They usually include colicky abdominal pain and in severe cases, may consist of vomiting, intussusception, hemorrhage, or shock.[3] Intussusception, seen in up to 2% of patients, is more frequently seen in males, particularly those about 6 years of age. Since intussusception not associated with Henoch-Schönlein purpura generally occurs in young children under 2 years of age, when seen in older children. Henoch-Schönlein purpura must be strongly considered as a diagnostic possibility.[13] Intramural hematomas also may occur in the small or large bowel and on rare occasions eschemic necrosis and spontaneous intestinal perforation have been noted.[14] Although bowel involvement is the major cause of abdominal signs and symptoms in HSP, other abdominal organs (pancreatitis and cholecystitis) may also be affected, thus contributing to the abdominal pain and vomiting seen in patients with this disorder.[8]

Arthritis, when present, is characterized by warm, tender, painful swelling of joints, with or without overlying purpura. Although the ankles and knees are most frequently affected, arthropathy of the elbows, hands, and feet may also be seen in association with this disorder. Arthritic symptoms, when present, generally persist for several days and are frequently recurrent.

Renal involvement is probably the most frequent and serious complication of anaphylactoid purpura. It occurs in 25% of children under two and in 50% of those above 2 years of age.[15, 16] Nephritis may be demonstrated by gross or microscopic hematuria, with or without casts and proteinuria. Although often self-limited, if hematuria persists, it may progress to advanced glomerular disease and a poor prognosis, with death resulting from acute or chronic renal failure.[15–19]

Other systemic manifestations include hepatosplenomegaly and encephalopathy. Central nervous system involvement may result in headache and diplopia, and rarely subarachnoid hemorrhage may occur, with coma, seizures, and/or paresis.[20] Respiratory involvement, also uncommon, may range from an asymptomatic pulmonary infiltrate to recurrent episodes of pulmonary hemorrhage. Testicular and scrotal hemorrhage may occur in up to 20% of boys with this disorder. This may cause intense pain and scrotal swelling.[21] In one instance, torsion of the testicle requiring surgical intervention has occurred.

The prognosis for most patients with Henoch-Schönlein vasculitis is excellent, with full recovery without residue in most instances. In younger children, the disease is generally milder, of shorter duration, with fewer renal and gastrointestinal manifestations, and fewer recurrences.[3] In approximately 5% of patients with nephritis, the disorder progresses to end-stage renal disease. Serious gastrointestinal lesions and extensive kidney disease account for a mortality rate of up to 1% to 3%.

DIAGNOSIS.—The diagnosis of Henoch-Schönlein purpura is seldom difficult when all the components of the syndrome are present or when the typical eruption with palpable purpura is present. When the diagnosis remains in doubt, histopathologic examination of a cutaneous biopsy generally helps clarify the nature of the eruption. Histopathologic changes of Henoch-Schönlein purpura are characterized by leukocytoclastic vasculitis, with fibrinoid degeneration of vessel walls and a perivascular infiltrate consisting of neutrophils, some eosinophils, and only a few lymphocytes. Extravasation of erythrocytes is present in purpuric lesions, with deposits of hemosiderin in lesions of long duration. A highly characteristic feature is the presence of scattered nuclear fragments (nuclear dust), which result from the disintegration of the neutrophils.

TREATMENT.—There is no specific therapy for Henoch-Schönlein purpura. Bed rest and general supportive care are helpful. Throat cultures and appropriate antibiotics are indicated if a specific respiratory illness is identified. Since many cases of chronic glomerulonephritis in adults may be related to anaphylactoid purpura during childhood, serial urinalysis are indicated. The efficacy of corticosteroids is debatable. Although there is little evidence that corticosteroids influence the prognosis of Henoch-Schönlein purpura, they suppress the acute manifestations and may be justified for short periods in severe cases, particularly those with significant gastrointestinal complications or chronic glomerulonephritis. Corticosteroids alone or in combination with cytotoxic agents and anticoagulants have also been used in the treatment of HSP nephritis. Despite anecdotal reports of remarkable results, none of these agents has been proven effective in carefully controlled clinical trials.[22]

Acute Febrile Neutrophilic Dermatosis (Sweet's Syndrome)

Acute febrile neutrophilic dermatosis (Sweet's syndrome) is a rare disorder characterized by raised painful plaques on the limbs, face, and neck, accompanied by fever and leukocytosis[23] (Table 2–2). Although the etiology of this disorder is unknown, it appears to represent a hypersensitivity reaction to a bacterial or viral infection, or an immunologic response to a leukemic or preleukemic state.[24] The disorder has been described in an

TABLE 2–2.—Acute Febrile Neutrophilic
Dermatitis (Sweet's Syndrome)

1. High persistent fever
2. Irregular, somewhat nodular red tender nodules or plaques on face, neck and limbs
3. An immunologic response to infection, leukemia or a preleukemic state?
4. Histologic features
   a. Edema, polymorphonuclear leukocytes and nuclear dust in dermis
   b. Older lesions less characteristic (less infiltrate, and lymphocytes replace polymorphonuclear leukocytes)
5. Rapid response to systemic corticosteroids

infant as young as three months of age,[25] but is rare in children[26, 27] and most frequently seen in women between 35 and 66 years of age.[28, 29]

Although the etiology of Sweet's syndrome remains unknown, the presence of upper respiratory tract infection, high antistreptolysin titers, positive intracutaneous tests with bacterial antigens, and occasional kidney and joint involvement in affected patients suggests an allergic Arthus-like response to an infectious agent as the cause in many individuals.[30] In adults the disorder may also be associated with malignancy, presumably as a hypersensitivity reaction to tumor antigen. The eruption can frequently serve as a cutaneous sign of malignancy in adults. Although Sweet's syndrome appears to represent a hypersensitivity reaction with deposition of antigen-antibody complexes in dermal vessel walls and "nuclear dust", histopathologic examination of cutaneous lesions lack the characteristically vascular damage seen in typical lesions of leukocytoclastic angiitis.

Clinical manifestations.—Patients with acute febrile neutrophilic dermatosis usually have a spiking fever associated with raised brightly erythematous painful plaques and nodules on the face, neck and limbs (particularly the upper arms), with sparing of the areas between the upper chest and thighs. Although the lesions develop almost exclusively in sun-exposed regions, there is no evidence (clinical or experimental) to implicate a role for photosensitivity.[31] Elevated plaques measure one to several cm in diameter, are distributed in an asymmetric pattern, and tend to develop partial clearing, resulting in an arcuate pattern as the border of the lesion advances. They are indurated red to plum-colored in appearance and heal without scarring, often leaving a residual reddish-brown color which develops as a result of hemosiderin deposition. Larger plaques frequently have a mammillated surface simulating vesicles, and the borders of the plaques may develop vesicles or sterile pustules (Fig 2–3).

Leukocytosis ranging from 15,000 to 20,000 (with 80% to 90% polymorphonuclear leukocytes) is common in patients with Sweet's syndrome.

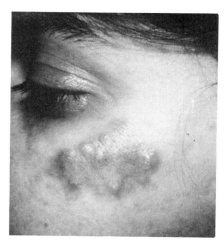

Fig 2–3.—Sweet's syndrome. A raised erythematous plaque with a mamillated vesiculopustular surface. (Courtesy of Dr. Louis Fragola, Providence, Rhode Island.)

Myalgia, polyarthralgia, and polyarthritis of large joints have been reported in 15% to 25% of patients afflicted with this disorder.[32] In at least 50% of patients, there is a history of a preceding febrile illness. Conjunctivitis and episcleritis may be present, and leukemia and carcinoma have been reported in adult patients with Sweet's syndrome.[23, 24, 33]

DIAGNOSIS.—Acute febrile neutrophilic dermatosis generally presents a characteristic clinical picture that can be confirmed by cutaneous biopsy. The histologic features of cutaneous lesions consist of edema and polymorphonuclear leukocytosis in the dermis. Initially seen as a dense perivascular infiltrate, as the disorder becomes more pronounced, the infiltrate frequently extends throughout the dermis and nuclear dust and, at times, polymorphonuclear involvement (described as an "exploding hand grenade") becomes apparent.[35] Older lesions present a less characteristic appearance with lessening of the infiltrate and lymphocytes replacing the polymorphonuclear leukocytes.

TREATMENT.—If untreated, lesions of Sweet's syndrome may increase in size and can persist for periods of 1 to 12 months and eventually resolve spontaneously without residual scarring.[31] Patients generally respond to systemic corticosteroids (2 mg/kg/day, up to a dosage of 30 to 60 mg per day of prednisone or its equivalent for a period of ten days). Once the patient responds, the systemic steroids should be tapered gradually over a period of one to two months in an effort to prevent recurrences. Potassium iodide has also been recommended for the treatment of Sweet's syndrome. Although the reason for the response to iodides is not clear, it appears to be related to an inhibitory effect on hypersensitivity in patients with this disorder.[34]

Allergic Granulomatoses

There are three systemic diseases in which necrotizing vasculitis is seen in association with necrotizing granuloma: Wegener's granulomatosis, allergic granulomatosis (Churg-Strauss syndrome), and lymphomatoid granulomatosis (Table 2–3). Primarily seen as adult disorders, cases of Churg-Strauss syndrome have recently been described in an adolescent boy,[35] and pediatric cases have been reported in retrospective studies of individuals with this disorder.[36] The mean age of the onset of Wegener's disease is 40 years with only a few cases reported in children. Except for a lower incidence of neurologic complications, Wegener's granulomatosis in pediatric patients is very similar to the disease in adults.[37]

Wegener's Granulomatosis

Wegener's granulomatosis (giant cell granulomatosis, WG) is a rare systemic disease characterized by necrotizing granulomatous vasculitis of the small vessels of the upper and lower respiratory tract (the nose, nasal sinuses, nasopharynx, glottis, trachea, bronchi and lungs) and focal necrotizing glomerulitis of the kidneys. Although the etiology is unknown, the presence of granulomatous inflammation with vasculitis and circulating immune complexes suggests a hypersensitive or immunologic basis to this disorder.[38, 39]

Presenting features are usually related to the upper respiratory tract and include rhinorrhea, paranasal sinus drainage and pain, nasal mucosal ulcerations and, at times, otitis media, cough, hemoptysis and pleurisy.[37] Cutaneous lesions are present in the early stage of the disease in about one-fourth and at the height of the disease in about one-half of patients with with disorder.[35] Mucocutaneous involvement appears as crusting, bleeding, nonhealing sores on the nostrils or nasal septum. Ophthalmologic findings (occurring in more than 50% of patients) include conjunctivitis, episcleritis, corneoscleral ulceration, retinal artery thrombosis, uveitis, proptosis, and pseudotumor of the orbits. Cutaneous lesions consist of petechiae, purpura, or ecchymoses (sometimes in association with ulcerations or blisters on the face, upper limbs and trunk); and erythematous papulonodular lesions measuring 1 to 5 cm in diameter, subcutaneous nodules, vesicles, pustules and ulcerations on the extremities, neck, upper chest and trunk caused by necrotizing vasculitis with thrombosis and necrosis.[37]

The diagnosis of Wegener's granulomatosis is suggested by cutaneous lesions; involvement of the respiratory tract, kidneys and other organs; and necrotizing granulomas with vasculitis on histopathologic examination of bi-

TABLE 2–3.—ALLERGIC GRANULOMATOSES

1. Wegener's granulomatosis
   a. A necrotizing granulomatous vasculitis of small vessels of upper and lower respiratory tracts with necrotizing glomerulitis of kidneys
   b. Cutaneous lesions in 25% to 50%
      (1) Crusting, bleeding, nonhealing sores on nostrils or nasal septum
      (2) Petechiae, purpura, or ecchymoses (at times, with ulcerations or blisters) on face, upper limbs and trunk
      (3) Papulonodular lesions, subcutaneous nodules, vesicles, pustules, and ulcerations on neck, upper chest, trunk and extremities
2. Churg-Strauss syndrome (allergic granulomatosis)
   a. Asthma, pneumonitis, peripheral eosinophilia, and vasculitis of skin, g.i. tract, and nervous system (generally sparing renal glomeruli)
   b. Cutaneous lesions in ⅔ of patients
      (1) Erythema-multiforme-like and hemorrhagic lesions (occasionally with necrotic ulcers); cutaneous and subcutaneous nodules
      (2) Nodular lesions reveal histologic picture of allergic granulomatosis
3. Lymphomatoid granulomatosis
   a. A serious systemic disease primarily affecting the lungs (also affects the skin, kidneys, liver, and nervous system)
   b. Skin lesions in 40% to 45%
      (1) Often the first clinical sign of disease
      (2) Symmetrical erythematous macules, papules, plaques, and dermal or subcutaneous nodules that tend to ulcerate

opsy specimens. Although Henoch-Schönlein purpura has a clinical picture similar to that of Wegener's granulomatosis (including palpable purpura), it lacks the characteristic necrotizing vasculitis of the upper and lower respiratory tract.

Prior to the advent of cytotoxic agents, WG was considered to be fatal with a mean survival of five months.[39] Untreated patients with Wegener's granulomatosis have a 50% survival at five months and a 90% mortality rate at two years.[40] Systemic corticosteroids are not very helpful, but immunosuppressive drugs, particularly cyclophosphamide, offer a better prognosis.[41] The usual starting dose of cyclophosphamide is 1 to 2 mg/kg body weight/day, increasing by 25 mg every 10 to 14 days (unless serious hematologic toxicity intervenes), until a favorable clinical response occurs. When a favorable clinical response is evident, the dose should be gradually reduced in an effort to prevent severe leukopenia.[37]

The Churg-Strauss Syndrome

Allergic granulomatosis (the Churg-Strauss syndrome), originally believed to be a form of polyarteritis nodosa, is a systemic disorder that can be differentiated from periarteritis nodosa by the presence of respiratory symptoms (usually asthma and pneumonitis); pronounced eosinophilia in the circulating blood and individual lesions; widespread vasculitis which may involve the skin, gastrointestinal tract and nervous system, and palisading granulomas in the connective tissue with involvement of small arteries and veins rather than small and medium-sized arteries. Although renal manifestations have been reported, the disorder tends to spare the renal glomeruli.[36] The etiology of Churg-Strauss syndrome remains unknown, but the respiratory tract appears to be the primary target. Its frequent association with a history of allergy in the patient and patient's family suggests the possibility of an inhaled antigen or pathogen in the pathogenesis of the disorder.

Respiratory symptoms usually precede the onset of allergic granulomatosis and cutaneous lesions, seen in about two-thirds of patients, consist of erythema, multiforme-like lesions, hemorrhagic lesions (varying from petechiae and palpable purpura to extensive ecchymoses) sometimes accompanied by necrotic ulcers and cutaneous and subcutaneous nodules.[36] The presence of granulomas in the dermis and in the subcutaneous nodules is of diagnostic value and the nodular lesions show the typical histopathologic picture of Churg-Strauss granuloma.

Patients with allergic granulomatosis of Churg-Strauss have a high incidence of abdominal pain, bloody diarrhea, hypertension, mild hematuria and albuminuria. Although spontaneous resolution of the disorder has been reported, untreated cases usually have a poor prognosis, the most frequent cause of death being congestive heart failure secondary to myocardial damage from the arteritis.[31] Systemic corticosteroids appear to be the treatment of choice (with reports of survival rates of 67% over a period of five years;[42] for those patients unresponsive to corticosteroid therapy, the addition of cytotoxic agents may prove to be beneficial.[43]

Lymphomatoid Granulomatosis

Lymphomatoid granulomatosis is a serious systemic disease primarily affecting the lungs, but also involving the skin, kidney, liver, and nervous system. First described in 1972, the disorder has been seen in children as young as 8½ years of age, but primarily affects adults (up to age 70) with an average onset between 30 and 60 years of age.[44] Lymphomatoid granulomatosis differs from Wegener's granulomatosis by the absence of glomerulitis and lesions in the upper respiratory tract and by the presence of a dense polymorphous cellular infiltrate which, especially in advanced lesions, contains lymphoid cells with larger hyperchromatic nuclei that are most pronounced in the deep layers of the dermis around the cutaneous appendages.[35]

The skin is involved in 40% to 45% of patients with the first clinical sign of the disease frequently consisting of symmetrical erythematous macules, papules, plaques, and dermal or subcutaneous nodules which often tend to ulcerate. Cutaneous lesions are often extensive and may resemble the cutaneous features of Wegener's granulomatosis (but without the purpura seen in the latter disorder). Other features include pulmonary symptoms (cough, shortness of breath, chest pain), fever, malaise, weight loss, myalgias, arthralgias, cranial nerve palsies, peripheral neuritis, ataxia, and diplopia.[45-47]

Although not considered a true malignant lymphoma, the prognosis of lymphomatoid granulomatosis is poor with a mortality rate of 40% in one year and 65% in four years.[31] Contrasting with previous reports of the mortality as high as 90%, a recent prospective study of 15 patients followed over a period of ten years has demonstrated good results in patients where prednisone and cyclophosphamide were included in the management of the disorder.[48]

Kawasaki Disease (Mucocutaneous Lymph Node Syndrome)

Kawasaki disease (mucocutaneous lymph node syndrome, MCLS, MCNS) is an acute febrile disorder of unknown etiology affecting infants and young children in Japan since around 1950. First reported by Dr. Tomisaku Kawasaki in 1967,[49] the Center for Disease Control in Atlanta, Georgia prefers the name "Kawasaki Disease" (KD) in honor of the Tokyo physician who contributed so much to our recognition of the syndrome. The first cases in the United States were reported from Hawaii in 1974[50] and patients with this multisystem disease have now been described worldwide.

Despite the vast number of well-documented case histories, the etiology of Kawasaki disease remains unknown. It currently represents an immunologic disorder triggered by an infectious, or perhaps toxic agent, with a possible relationship to a collagen vascular disorder.[51] The presence of generalized vasculitis, circulating immune complexes and occasional hypocomplementemia suggest an immunologic reaction and an association with collagen vascular disease; the acute onset, fever, and association with aseptic meningitis suggest an infectious agent. An epidemic of 26 cases following the use of a rug shampoo[52] suggests a possible relationship to a toxic agent.

Because this disease is most prevalent in Japan and its incidence is much higher in Japanese than in Caucasians or Blacks, and because Chinese,

Polynesian and Filipino children have an intermediate incidence, a unique genetic susceptibility has been hypothesized for this disorder.[51, 53] This genetic susceptibility appears to be further supported by an increased frequency of antigens that have a higher incidence in Japanese than in other races (i.e., HLA-BW22 and HLA-BW22J2 antigens) in patients with Kawasaki disease.[54] From a pathologic viewpoint, Kawasaki disease is an arteritis involving the small and medium-sized arteries, with a predilection for involvement of the main coronary vessels.

Kawasaki disease resembles the infantile form of periarteritis nodosa in many respects. Although it has been suggested that the small number of reported cases and the high rate of mortality in infantile periarteritis nodosa distinguishes this disorder from mucocutaneous lymph node syndrome, children with infantile periarteritis nodosa may represent the more severe fatal end of the Kawasaki disease spectrum.[55] However, infantile periarteritis nodosa should not be confused with the adult form of periarteritis nodosa. These two conditions differ in their clinical presentations, pathologic manifestations, and laboratory findings (see the adult form of periarteritis nodosa discussed later in this chapter).

CLINICAL MANIFESTATIONS.—Although occasional cases of Kawasaki disease have been reported in adults and children over 10 years of age, most patients (85%) are under 5, and 50% are under 2½ years of age.[49] Few cases of Kawasaki disease are actually seen in individuals beyond the age of 10 years, and most reports of Kawasaki syndrome in adults probably represent cases of toxic shock syndrome.[51, 55]

The clinical course of Kawasaki disease may be described as triphasic (Table 2–4) with phase I, *the acute febrile period,* lasting for approximately 12 days.[56] It begins abruptly with the onset of fever and is followed (usually

TABLE 2–4.—CLINICAL PHASES OF KAWASAKI DISEASE

Phase I	Acute febrile period
	a. Lasts approximately 12 days
	b. Begins abruptly with onset of fever
	c. Followed by other principal features (usually within 1 to 3 days)
Phase II	Subacute phase
	a. Lasts approximately until day 30 of illness
	b. Resolution of fever, thrombocytosis, desquamation, and (when present) arthritis, arthralgia, and carditis
	c. Highest risk for sudden death during this period
Phase III	Convalescent period
	a. Usually begins between 8 to 10 weeks after onset of illness
	b. Begins when all signs of illness have disappeared and ends when ESR returns to normal
	c. A small number of deaths occur during this period

within one to three days) by most of the other principal diagnostic criteria: conjunctival injection, changes on the lips and in the mouth, an erythematous rash, and lymphadenopathy. Associated features seen during this period include diarrhea, hepatic dysfunction, and aseptic meningitis.

Phase II, *the subacute phase*, lasts until approximately day 30 of the illness. It encompasses the period characterized by resolution of fever, desquamation, and thrombocytosis. Arthritis, arthralgia, and carditis, when present, usually appear in this period. This stage has the highest risk for sudden death due to coronary thrombosis.

Phase III, *the convalescent period*, begins when all signs of illness have disappeared, and lasts until the sedimentation rate returns to normal, usually eight to ten weeks after the onset of illness.[49] A small proportion of reported patients died suddenly during the convalescent phase (at a time when they were thought to be recovering from their illness).

PRINCIPAL CRITERIA.—The diagnosis of Kawasaki disease is based on strict adherence to clinical criteria, together with the exclusion of other clinically similar diseases. To make a diagnosis, the patient must meet five of six criteria (Table 2–5). These include fever lasting more than five days, with no other reasonable explanation for the illness, and four of the following five features: (1) bilateral conjunctival injection; (2) dry, red, and fissured lips, strawberry tongue, and redness of the oropharynx; (3) erythematous rash; (4) indurative edema of the hands and feet followed by desquamation of the fingertips; and (5) nonpurulent cervical adenopathy. In practice, most patients have all of the first five criteria while the sixth, lymphadenopathy, is seen in approximately 70% of patients in Japan and in 50% to 86% of patients seen in the United States.[51, 57]

Fever.—Fever, the first sign and principal symptom of Kawasaki disease, begins abruptly without prodromal signs. Seen in most patients (95%), it has a remittent pattern with several spikes in temperature up to 104° C each day, does not respond to antibiotics or intermittent doses of antipyretics, and lasts more than five days (5 to 23 days) with an average duration of eleven days.

Conjunctival injection.—Discrete bilateral injection of the bulbar con-

TABLE 2–5.—DIAGNOSTIC
CRITERIA OF KAWASAKI DISEASE

1. Fever lasting more than five days
2. Four of the five remaining criteria:
   a. Conjunctival injection
   b. Oral cavity changes
   c. Exanthem
   d. Changes in the extremities
   e. Lymphadenopathy

junctivae (seen in 88% of patients) generally appears within two days of the onset of fever and persists for three to five weeks (throughout the febrile course of the illness) (Fig 2–4). This is not a true conjunctivitis and consists chiefly of discrete dilatation of the bulbar conjunctival vessels without evidence of exudative discharge or corneal ulceration.

Oral cavity changes.—Changes in the mouth consist of erythema, fissuring, and, at times, bleeding and severe crusting of the lips (Fig 2–5). The lip changes (seen in 90% of the patients) may last for one to three weeks. Erythema and protuberance of the papillae of the tongue (seen in 77% of patients) produces a "strawberry tongue" appearance. When present, strawberry tongue and erythema of the oropharynx appear within one to three days after the onset of fever.

Exanthem.—On the third to fifth day of illness, a macular erythematous skin eruption appears (in 92% of patients) (Fig 2–6). Usually occurring simultaneously with or soon after the onset of fever, it generally begins with pronounced reddening of the palms and soles and gradually spreads to involve the entire trunk and extremities within two days. The rash is polymorphous in nature and usually begins on the extremities as erythematous macules measuring 5 mm or more in diameter. Individual lesions become larger and often coalescent. Although frequently pruritic, the eruption is

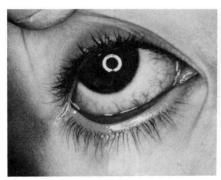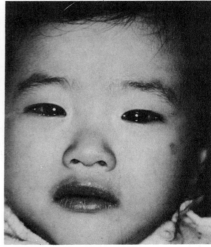

Fig 2–4 (left).—Congestion of bulbar conjunctivae in a patient with Kawasaki disease (mucocutaneous lymph node syndrome). (Courtesy of Dr. Tomisaku Kawasaki, Tokyo, Japan.)

Fig 2–5 (right).—Erythematous rash, bulbar conjunctival congestion and crusted fissured lips in a child with Kawasaki disease. (Courtesy of Dr. Tomisaku Kawasaki, Tokyo, Japan.)

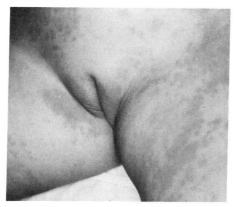

Fig 2–6.—Maculopapular urticarial rash in a patient with Kawasaki disease. (Courtesy of Dr. Tomisaku Kawasaki, Tokyo, Japan.)

not accompanied by vesicles, bullae, or crusts.[51] Deeply erythematous, symmetrical, and widespread, the rash may be maculopapular or morbilliform, urticarial, scarlatiniform, or erythema multiforme-like,[58] and generally persists for the duration of the fever. Symmetrical pruritic urticaria-like plaques are the most common exanthem seen in this disorder, maculopapular morbilliform lesions are the second most common, and less than 5% of eruptions are scarlatinal or erythema-multiforme-like. The eruption is not purpuric (it blanches with pressure) and is most severe and coalescent in the perineal area. The cutaneous exanthem generally persists for the duration of the fever and, in some patients, scattered areas of desquamation may appear sometime between the tenth and fifteenth days of the illness.

The histopathologic features of the cutaneous eruption are variable and generally nonspecific. Dilatation of the capillary loops of the dermal papillae, variable perivascular infiltration in arteries and arterioles of the dermis and mild dermal edema are described. Histopathologic findings reveal an arteritis involving small and medium-sized vessels, marked edema of the dermal connective tissue, swelling of the endothelial cells in postcapillary venules, dilatation of small blood vessels and lymphocytic and monocytic perivascular infiltrates of the microvessels.[49]

Changes in the extremities.—Changes in the hands and feet constitute the most distinctive clinical features of the syndrome.[49] Reddening of the palms and soles (seen in 90% of the patients) and a firm indurative edema of the hands and feet develop (in 75% of patients). The edema is characterized by deeply erythematous to violaceous brawny swelling of the palms and soles, fusiform swelling of the digits, and tightly stretched skin on the dorsal aspect of the hands and feet (Figs 2–7, 2–8).

Generally 14 to 20 days after the onset of fever, a highly characteristic pattern of desquamation begins. Seen in 94% of patients it lasts approximately one week. The desquamation generally begins on the tips of the fingers and toes at the junction of the nails and skin (just beneath the tips of the nails) and, over a period of ten days, gradually progresses to include the fingers, toes, and areas of the palms and soles (Fig 2–9).

As with many other severe illnesses, Beau's lines (transverse furrows on the nail surface) may develop one or two months after the onset of the illness. This horizontal groove, although seen in almost all patients with Kawasaki disease, is not diagnostic of this disorder since they develop as a nonspecific reaction to any stress that temporarily interrupts nail growth and become visible on the surface of the nail several weeks later.

Lymphadenopathy.—Cervical lymphadenopathy (the least reliable clinical feature of this disorder) is said to occur in 70% of patients with Kawasaki disease in Japan and in 50% to 86% of patients seen in the United States.[57] When present, it is unilateral and is generally seen as a single

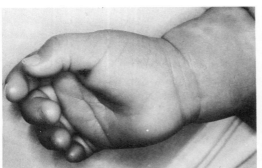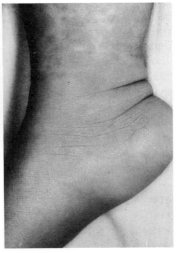

Fig 2–7 (left).—Kawasaki disease. Erythematous brawny swelling of the hands with fusiform swelling of the fingers. (Courtesy of Dr. Tomisaku Kawasaki, Tokyo, Japan.)

Fig 2–8 (right).—Erythematous firm brawny edema of the feet in Kawasaki disease (mucocutaneous lymph node syndrome). (Courtesy of Dr. Tomisaku Kawasaki, Tokyo, Japan.)

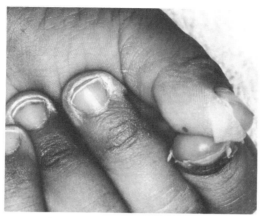

Fig 2–9.—Desquamation at the tips of the fingers at the junction of the nails in a patient with mucocutaneous lymph node syndrome (Kawasaki disease). (Courtesy of Dr. Tomisaku Kawasaki, from Hurwitz S.: *Clinical Pediatric Dermatology.* W.B. Saunders Co., Philadelphia, 1981. Used by permission.)

enlarged lymph node in the cervical region. Measuring more than 1.5 cm in diameter, the enlarged node is usually not warm, red, tender, or fluctuant, and in most cases, the lymphadenopathy disappears as the fever subsides. Histopathologic examinations of lymph nodes from patients with Kawasaki disease are nonspecific and reveal hypertrophy of germinal centers, medullary edema, and an inflammatory infiltrate consisting of lymphocytes and large atypical mononuclear cells.

Other clinical features.—Other clinical features of Kawasaki disease include cardiac manifestations, central nervous system involvement, extreme irritability, lethargy, aseptic meningitis, pyuria, uveitis, rheumatic complications (arthritis and arthralgia), and gastrointestinal manifestations. The prognosis of mucocutaneous lymph node syndrome is good in most cases, with improvement usually beginning about the 14th day of illness. ECG abnormalities (prolongation of the PR and QT intervals, and ST segments and T-wave changes), however, have been found in 70% to 90% of children with this disorder; 27% of patients demonstrate abnormalities in coronary angiography one to six months after the onset of the disease.

Cardiac effects.—Clinical cardiac disease occurs in at least 20% of patients with Kawasaki syndrome. During the acute febrile phase of the disease, severe tachycardia and gallop rhythm are the most common manifestations. Toward the end of the febrile phase (at a mean time of 11 days) more serious cardiac abnormalities appear, including congestive heart failure, pericardial effusion, mitral insufficiency, and cardiac arrhythmias manifesting as first and second degree A-V block, premature ventricular contractions or paroxysmal atrial tachycardia.

Sudden death due to coronary occlusion has been reported in 1% to 2% of patients, generally young infants with Kawasaki disease. Recent studies, however, indicate that such deaths in Japan have decreased to 0.4%.[59] Male infants are at special risk (since 80% of fatalities have been in boys). Although death due to coronary occlusion has been noted a short time after apparent recovery from the illness, most deaths (90%) occur suddenly between three and seven weeks after the onset of the disease, and several deaths have been reported two to four years after apparent recovery.[60–62] Children at high risk of sudden death or carditis are boys less than one year of age, particularly those who have prolonged or recurrent fever and rash, extreme elevation of the erythrocyte sedimentation rate, and cardiac signs such as gallop rhythm, arrhythmia, cardiomegaly, and ECG abnormality.[51] These factors are only a guide and not always reliable in predicting the prognosis for patients with Kawasaki disease.

Pathologic examination of the hearts of patients who died of Kawasaki disease reveal acute perivasculitis of the arterioles, capillaries, and venules of the small arteries, acute perivasculitis and endarteritis of the major coronary arteries, myocarditis, coagulation necrosis, lesions of the conduction system, pericarditis, and endocarditis with vasculitis. The causes of sudden death in such individuals are myocarditis, inflammation of the A-V conduction systems, ischemic heart disease, and rupture of aneurysms.[59]

Arthritis and arthralgia.—Arthritis and arthralgia (seen in 20% to 40% of patients respectively) occur late in the febrile stage of the illness, or shortly thereafter. Large joints such as the knees, hips, and elbows are the most commonly affected. Although ultimately self-limiting, arthritis and effusion may last for two to four weeks.

Central nervous system effects.—Central nervous system effects are seen in nearly all patients with Kawasaki disease. They consist of negativistic behavior, sleep disturbances, severe irritability, and frequent episodes of crying and whining. Approximately one-third of patients have severe lethargy, semicoma, or coma during the acute febrile stage. One-fourth of patients are found to have an associated aseptic meningitis with mononuclear pleocytosis (25 to 100 WBC/cu mm) with normal glucose and normal to slightly elevated protein values.[51]

Gastrointestinal manifestations.—Gastrointestinal manifestations (diarrhea and abdominal pain) are seen in approximately one-fourth of affected patients. Hepatitis, with modest to moderate bilirubin elevation and moderate elevations of serum SGOT and SGPT, is seen in about 10% of patients in the acute febrile stage of the illness. Diarrhea, consisting of frequent watery stools, generally without blood, pus, or mucous, and acute hydrops of the gall bladder have also been reported. Appearing late in the acute febrile phase of the illness or early in convalescence, the hydrops is frequently self-limiting, may disappear spontaneously in two or three weeks, and can be monitored by repeated ultrasound evaluations.[63]

Pyuria.—Pyuria, seen in 70% of patients, occurs in the acute stage of the disease. It appears to be urethral in origin, and although a small portion of patients may have a transient hematuria, proteinuria is not a feature of the disease.

Laboratory studies.—Laboratory tests show leukocytosis, polycythemia, a mild anemia, normal flora in the throat and stools and sterile cultures of the blood and cerebrospinal fluid. Thrombocytosis, a universal laboratory finding in Kawasaki disease, appears to coincide with the period of highest risk of coronary thrombosis. Generally beginning after the tenth day of illness, it reaches a peak of 600,000 to 1,800,000 between the 15th and 25th days, and then falls to normal values by the 30th day of the disorder.[51] Other laboratory findings may include an increased erythrocyte sedimentation rate, positive C-reactive protein, increased serum alpha$_2$ proteins, elevated IgM and IgE levels, and reduced serum protein levels with reversal of the A/G ratio.

DIAGNOSIS.—The diagnosis of Kawasaki disease is dependent on strict adherence to the previously described clinical criteria (Table 2–5) and the exclusion of other disorders considered in its differential diagnosis. These include scarlet fever, viral exanthems, erythema multiforme and Stevens-Johnson syndrome, rickettsial disease, atypical measles, juvenile rheumatoid arthritis, systemic lupus erythematosus, toxic epidermal necrolysis, herpetic stomatitis, drug reactions, acrodynia (mercury poisoning, pink disease) and toxic shock syndrome.

MANAGEMENT.—To date there is no definitive treatment for this disease or its catastrophic sequelae. Once the diagnosis has been established, the most important step in management is the ability to detect and prevent coronary aneurysm and myocardial infarction. Coronary angiography and, at times, bypass surgery have been recommended for children who develop myocardial infarction,[62] and biplaner echocardiography is suggested as an effective noninvasive technique for the detection of aneurysms, mitral valve dysfunction, myocardiopathy, and pericardial effusion.[64, 65] Present treatment requires a careful program of repeated clinical and laboratory evaluations to detect and manage potentially serious cardiac and vascular complications (Table 2–6).[51] Hospitalization during the acute febrile stage is helpful and facilitates diagnostic testing. Blood, urine and throat cultures, viral and Leptospira diagnostic tests should be done to rule out other diseases. Chest x-ray, EKG and liver function tests should be performed

TABLE 2–6.—OUTLINE FOR MANAGEMENT OF PATIENTS WITH
KAWASAKI DISEASE

1. Hospitalization during acute stage facilitates diagnosis
2. Chest x-ray, EKG, and liver function studies
3. Aspirin
   a. 80–100 mg/kg/24 hrs. initially (aim for salicylate level between 18 and 28 mg/dl)
   b. 10 mg/kg/24 hrs. after fever, rash, acute symptoms, and ESR subside
4. Monitor for arthritic and cardiac abnormalities (twice weekly during second and fourth weeks, then weekly until ESR and PE normal)
5. EKG, CBC, sed rate, platelet and salicylate levels weekly
6. Two-mode echocardiography (between 7th to 12th days and 28th to 35th days), followed by angiography if evidence of aneurysm, ischemia or severe cardiac disease

and, once the diagnosis has been established, if there is no evidence of cardiomegaly, cardiac failure, or mitral insufficiency, the patient may be discharged and observed at home with supportive treatment and repeated clinical laboratory evaluations to detect and manage systemic toxicity, arthritis, and serious cardiovascular abnormalities.

The patient should be checked twice a week through the second and fourth week, then weekly until the sedimentation rate has dropped and physical examination is normal. Weekly monitoring of the blood count, platelet count, erythrocyte sedimentation rate, salicylate levels, and EKG should be performed. Two-mode echocardiography should be done between the seventh and 12th days and again between the 28th and 35th days of the illness.[64, 65] Angiography is recommended if there is evidence of aneurysm, ischemia, or severe cardiac disease.

Aspirin, in dosages of 80 to 100 mg/kg/day, appears to shorten the duration of the fever. Salicylate levels should be monitored 48 hours after the initiation of aspirin therapy, aiming for a level between 18 and 28 mg/dl, with adjustment upward or downward as indicated by the clinical picture.[56] Approximately two-thirds of patients become afebrile within two days of treatment, and in the remaining one-third of cases the temperature remains elevated for several days. Once the patient has become afebrile, if there is no evidence of arthritis or arthralgia, the dosage of aspirin may be reduced to 10 mg/kg/day and, in patients without complications, aspirin should be continued until the sedimentation rate has become normal (this usually occurs approximately six to ten weeks after the onset of illness). Although systemic corticosteroids have been suggested for treatment of Kawasaki disease, recent studies suggest that corticosteroids are contraindicated since there appears to be a higher incidence of coronary aneurysms and/or thrombosis in patients so treated.[66]

Careful, long-term follow-up of all patients with Kawasaki syndrome is necessary. At present, the disease appears to be nonrecurrent and self-limiting, and the short-term outlook for most children is hopeful. Delayed deaths, however, have been reported up to ten years after onset of the illness,[67, 68] and the ultimate outcome of this multisystem vasculitis remains unknown.[51]

Periarteritis Nodosa

Periarteritis nodosa, also known as polyarteritis nodosa, is a relatively uncommon systemic disorder characterized by a severe necrotizing inflammation of small and medium-sized arteries. Classified as "adult" or "infantile" types, periarteritis nodosa has two disease spectra in childhood. The adult form affects older children and adults; the infantile disorder characteristically affects children in the first two years of life[69] (Table 2–7). Although the cause of periarteritis nodosa is unknown, it is presumed to represent a hypersensitivity-type immune-complex vasculitis with deposits of IgM, C_3 or both in affected vessel walls.[69]

Infantile Periarteritis Nodosa

Infantile periarteritis nodosa (IPN, infantile polyarteritis), a disorder characteristically affecting children in the first two years of life, usually manifests as an overwhelming acute illness diagnosed at autopsy by evidence of coronary artery occlusion and vasculitis. It frequently begins as a febrile illness (suggesting a viral infection) and affects both sexes equally. As the disorder progresses, cardiac arteritis leads to aneurysms, infarction, cardiomegaly, congestive heart failure, and renal peripheral artery and ner-

TABLE 2–7.—PERIARTERITIS NODOSA

1. Infantile form (usually in first 2 years of life)
   a. An overwhelming acute illness (usually begins with fever)
   b. Bears pathologic similarity to Kawasaki disease
   c. The severe fatal end of the KD spectrum?
2. Adult form (older children and adults)
   a. A necrotizing arteritis of small and medium-sized muscular-type arteries (gastrointestinal tract, pancreas, kidney, heart, muscles, and skin)
   b. Death, when it occurs, usually associated with renal failure, cardiac involvement or intracranial or intra-abdominal hemorrhage
   c. Cutaneous features in 25% to 50% of patients (livedo reticularis, purpura, bullae, necrotic vesicles or pustules, urticaria, and tender subcutaneous nodules or ulcerations along course of medium-sized arteries)

vous system involvement, resulting in hypertension, abnormal urinary findings, peripheral ischemia, neuritis, paralysis, and seizures. Prognosis is poor and death is usually related to cardiac decompensation. Although it has been suggested that the small number of reported cases and the high rate of mortality of infants with infantile periarteritis nodosa distinguish this disorder from Kawasaki disease, IPN appears to represent a fatal form of Kawasaki disease.[68]

Adult-Type Periarteritis Nodosa

Adult-type periarteritis (polyarteritis) nodosa, a disorder of older children and adults, is characterized by crops of subcutaneous nodules along the course of the superficial arteries of the trunk and extremities with fever, calf pain, arthritis, abdominal pain, Raynaud's phenomenon, hypertension, peripheral neuropathy, and myocardial infarction.[70–72]

Cutaneous lesions, seen in about half the cases, are usually limited to the lower extremities and range from livedo reticularis, purpura, urticaria and bullae to maculopapular eruptions, necrotic vesicles, pustules, and, at times, tender subcutaneous nodules or ulcerations that follow the course of medium-sized arteries of the trunk and extremities (Fig 2–10). The nodules vary in size from 0.5 to 1.0 cm, are tender to palpation, and usually are red to purple in color. They may persist for days or months, often disappear spontaneously, or, as a result of acute infarction (depending on the degree of necrosis), may go on to develop ulceration and scar formation. Other cutaneous manifestations include ecchymoses and peripheral gangrene of fingers and toes.

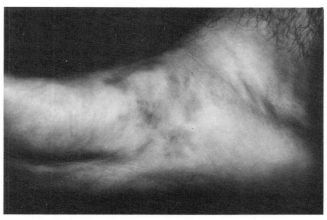

Fig 2–10.—Adult-type periarteritis nodosa. Livedo reticularis, purpura, and subcutaneous nodules on the foot of a 20-year-old male.

Benign cutaneous periarteritis nodosa is a clinical variant in which cutaneous lesions predominate and there is no visceral involvement. In some instances, however, fever, peripheral neuropathy, myalgia, or arthralgia may be present.[35, 73, 74] After many years' duration, the disorder gradually subsides. The term *nodosa* is based on the fact that the arteritis is focal and thus causes nodose swellings in the affected blood vessels.[35] Since subcutaneous nodules are present in the benign cutaneous form and are rarely encountered in the systemic disorder, they generally suggest a good prognosis.[72]

In the systemic disease, coronary arteritis may lead to aneurysms and infarction, thus producing cardiomegaly, congestive heart failure, and (in 70% to 80% of patients) kidney disease.[75] Peripheral artery and nervous system involvement may result in hypertension, abnormal urinary sediment, peripheral ischemia, paralysis, and convulsions. Death, when it occurs, is usually associated with renal failure, intracranial or intra-abdominal hemorrhage, hypertensive heart failure, and myocardial involvement.

DIAGNOSIS.—The diagnosis of periarteritis nodosa is suggested by the presence of multiple organ involvement with dilatation of medium-sized arteries demonstrable by angiography.[75] Histopathologic examination of cutaneous lesions reveals a necrotizing vasculitis (a panarteritis) in medium-sized and small muscular arteries with fibrinoid necrosis of the media, endothelial proliferation, and predominantly polymorphonuclear leukocytic infiltration of affected vessel walls.

TREATMENT.—The adult-type of periarteritis nodosa follows an intermittent course and used to be uniformly fatal within a few months to a few years. With present-day therapy, however, the prognosis is not as grim as previously thought (half of these patients currently survive).[76–78] Management of the adult-type of periarteritis nodosa consists of general supportive therapy and corticosteroids (1–2 mgm/kg per day of prednisone or its equivalent). In patients in whom the disease persists or worsens despite the use of systemic corticosteroids, immunosuppressive agents (azathioprine or cyclophosphamide) may be utilized, with cyclophosphamide appearing to be the more effective modality. Since systemic corticosteroids appear to be contraindicated for patients with Kawasaki disease,[66] nonsteroidal, anti-inflammatory agents such as aspirin currently are a more logical choice for the treatment of the infantile form of periarteritis nodosa.[70]

The Behcet Syndrome

The Behcet syndrome is a chronic multisystem disease of unknown etiology characterized by a triad of recurrent oral aphthous stomatitis, recurrent aphthous ulcers on the external genitalia, and inflammatory disease of the eye (uveitis, iritis, or iridocyclitis). Originally described in 1937, the spectrum of the disease has been broadened with the recognition of multiple organ system involvement: dermal vasculitis, synovitis, arthritis, central nervous system involvement (meningoencephalitis), myocarditis, colitis, phlebitis, and focal necrotizing glomerulonephritis[79, 80] (Table 2–8). Although onset in early childhood has been reported, this rare syndrome usually begins in patients between 10 and 45 years of age and has a marked predilection (between 2:1 and 5:1) for males.

A precise etiology has not been delineated, but aberrations in humoral and cellular immunity play a role in aphthosis and Behcet's syndrome. Phenomena of lymphocyte transformation and lymphocyte cytotoxity suggest a cellular immunogenesis. In favor of a humoral mechanism are the presence of circulating antibodies directed against oral and other mucosal epithelial cells, the finding of elevated levels of immune complexes, and the demonstration of immunoglobulins and complement within and around blood vessel walls and/or in the subepithelial zone.[81–83]

CLINICAL MANIFESTATIONS.—Cutaneous and oral lesions are the most common clinical features of Behcet's disease. Oral lesions are an almost constant feature and are the initial manifestation in about 60% of cases. The ulcerations begin as vesicles or pustules, may occur anywhere on the oral mucosa, and present as superficial erosions (indistinguishable from aphthous stomatitis) or as deeply punched-out necrotic ulcers. They tend to appear in crops and are characterized by superficial grayish erosions that vary in size from a few millimeters to a centimeter in diameter.[85] The ulcer base is covered with a yellowish-gray exudate and the margin is surrounded by a red halo. The aphthous lesions, whether in the mouth or genitalia, generally persist for periods of 7 to 14 days and usually heal without scar-

TABLE 2–8.—BEHCET'S SYNDROME

1. Etiology: an aberration of humoral and cellular immunity?
2. Cutaneous lesions
   a. Widely scattered papules, pustules, furuncles, vesicles, ulcerations, or acneform lesions
   b. Painful nodose lesions resembling erythema nodosum in severe chronic forms
3. Oral ulcerations frequently the first manifestation
4. Ocular lesions (in up to 80%)
   a. Intense periorbital pain and photophobia
   b. Conjunctivitis, iritis, uveitis, vitreous opacification, and hypopyon
5. Genital ulcers (in 10%)
6. Other clinical findings
   a. Fever, thrombophlebitis, arthralgia, gastrointestinal ulceration
   b. Pericarditis, myocarditis, and focal glomerulonephritis
   c. CNS involvement in 20%–50% (the most severe prognostic feature)

ring. Deep crateriform necrotic ulcerations with raised margins, called periadenitis mucosa necrotica recurrence (Sutton's disease), are distinctive, usually very painful, and frequently heal with scarring. Whether Sutton's disease is a separate entity or a form of Behcet's disease is still uncertain.

Cutaneous lesions present a varied picture. Seen in approximately 70% of patients, they consist of vesicles, pustules, pyoderma, acneform lesions, furuncles, ulcerations, and angiitic lesions on the legs, suggesting a diagnosis of erythema nodosum.[84]

Genital ulcerations, since they define the disease, are seen in virtually 100% of patients with Behcet's syndrome. Generally less painful than oral lesions, they are found on the scrotum or penis in males and the vulva and vagina of females, are similar in appearance to the oral ulcerations, and are occasionally overlooked by the patient, his or her parents, and, unless carefully sought for, the physician.[85]

Ocular lesions, seen in two-thirds to 80% of patients, generally begin with intense periorbital pain and photophobia. Conjunctivitis may be an early ocular finding, followed by iritis, optic neuritis, arteritis of retinal vessels or uveitis, often with loss of vision from vitreous opacification and, eventually, hypopyon.

Fever and constitutional symptoms are variable. Other findings include recurrent thrombophlebitis of the superficial veins of the legs (in about 45% of paients), arthralgia (in 35% to 50%), gastrointestinal ulceration, pericarditis, orchitis, and epididymitis. In patients with arthritic manifestations, the episodes of arthritis are often accompanied by fever and erythema nodosum.

Gastrointestinal complaints in Behcet's disease range from vague abdominal pain and anorexia to diarrhea and may be due to an ulcerating, hemorrhagic colitis. The esophagus, stomach, small intestine, colon, and anal mucosa may all be involved, and radiological findings are often consistent with those seen in patients with regional enteritis.[85]

Vascular involvement including arteritis with aneurysm formation and thrombophlebitis may also be seen in patients with Behcet's disease, with the phlebitis involving superficial veins at the site of venipuncture, the deep veins, or the vena cavae.[85]

Central nervous system involvement, often the most severe prognostic feature of this disorder, is seen in 20% to 50% of patients (generally an average of two to five years after the disease has begun).[80] Neurological manifestations may be divided into four patterns: (1) a brain stem syndrome with extraocular muscle palsies, nystagmus, ataxia, and hyperreflexia; (2) a meningitic syndrome with headaches and nuchal rigidity; (3) a state of progressive confusion eventually leading to dementia; and (4) a pseudotumor cerebri-like syndrome with increased intracranial pressure, headache, vomiting, and papilledema.[85]

Renal involvement is an uncommon complication of Behcet's disease. It may be seen as acute glomerulonephritis, proteinuria with hematuria, and amyloidosis, with a spectrum ranging from asymptomatic abnormalities detected on urinalysis to a rapidly progressive glomerulonephritis. Although the incidence of renal involvement is unknown, Behcet's syndrome should be included in the differential diagnosis of patients with rapidly progressive glomerulonephritis.[84]

DIAGNOSIS.—The diagnosis of Behcet's syndrome in a patient with the full triad of features is not difficult. In those without the classic triad, two or more major criteria (oral, genital, ocular, or cutaneous involvement) or a combination of major and minor criteria (vascular, neurologic, skeletal, or intestinal) may constitute a diagnosis.[86]

TREATMENT. —There is no entirely satisfactory treatment of the Behcet syndrome. Treatment of the aphthous ulcers with a tetracycline suspension (250 mg swished around in the mouth for two minutes and then swallowed) four times a day for a period of five to ten days may be beneficial. Intralesional steroid injection (triamcinolone acetonide, 0.2 to 0.3 ml, in concentrations of 10 mg per ml) may give rapid relief and resolution of large ulcerations. Milder cases may be treated with topical application of silver nitrate ($AgNO_3$) or oral rinses with Elixir of Benadryl (diphenhydramine) or Viscous Xylocaine (lidocaine). Application of a steroid such as Kenalog (triamcinolone) in Orabase to the lesions four times daily may also give symptomatic relief. Although favorable results are inconsistent, indomethacin (Indocin; Merck Sharp & Dohme)[83] and, in severe cases, systemic corticosteroids may suppress many of the inflammatory features of this disorder, particularly for those individuals with central nervous system involvement. Colchicine, perhaps due to its inhibition of leukocyte chemotaxis, has also been found to be effective for the treatment of Behcet's syndrome (especially its cutaneous manifestations) and may have a corticosteroid-sparing effect.[87–89]

The overall mortality rate of Behcet's disease is 3% to 4%. When death occurs, it usually is attributed to intestinal perforation, a ruptured aneurysm, CNS involvement, or a complication of therapy for central nervous system disease.[84, 85] Although the incidence in childhood is uncommon, the younger the patient at the onset of illness, the worse the prognosis.

REFERENCES

1. Sams W.M., Jr., Thorne E.G., Small P., et al.: Leukocytoclastic vasculitis (Review). *Arch. Dermatol.* 112:219–226, 1976.
2. Gairdner D.: The Schönlein-Henoch syndrome (anaphylactoid purpura). *Q. J. Med.* 17:95–122, 1948.
3. Allen D.M., Diamond L.K., Howell D.A.: Anaphylactoid purpura in children (Schönlein-Henoch syndrome). *Am. J. Dis. Child.* 99:833–854, 1960.

4. Sams W.M., Jr., Claman H.N., Kohler P.F., et al.: Human necrotizing vasculitis: immunoglobulins and complement in vessel walls of cutaneous lesions and normal skin. *J. Invest. Dermatol.* 64:441–445, 1975.
5. Giangiacoma J., Tsai C.C.: Dermal and glomerular deposition of IgA in anaphylactoid purpura. *Am. J. Dis. Child.* 131:981–983, 1977.
6. Levinsky R.J., Barratt M.: IgA immune complexes in Henoch-Schönlein purpura. *Lancet* 2:1100–1103, 1979.
7. Kuno-Sakai H., Sakai H., Nomoto Y., et al.: Increase of IgA-bearing peripheral blood lymphocytes in children with Henoch-Schönlein purpura. *Pediatr.* 64:918–922, 1979.
8. Saulsbury F.T.: Henoch-Schönlein purpura. *Pediatric Dermatology*, Vol. 1. No. 3, pp. 195–201, 1984.
9. Vernier R.L., Worthen H.C., Peterson R.D., et al.: Anaphylactoid purpura, 1. Pathology of the skin and kidney and frequency of streptococcal infection. *Pediatrics* 27:181–193, 1961.
10. Michaelsson G., Pettersson L., Juhlin L.: Purpura caused by food and drug additives. *Arch. Dermatol.* 109:49–52, 1974.
11. Ayoub E.M., Hoyer J.: Anaphylactoid purpura: streptococcal antibody titers and B1$_C$-globulin levels. *J. Pediatr.* 75:193–201, 1969.
12. Byrn J.R., Fitzgerald J.F., Northway J.D., et al.: Unusual manifestations of Henoch-Schönlein syndrome. *Am. J. Dis. Child.* 130:1335–1337, 1976.
13. Wolfsohn H.: Purpura and intussusception. *Arch. Dis. Child.* 22:242–247, 1947.
14. Smith H.J., Krupski W.C.: Spontaneous intestinal perforation in Schönlein-Henoch purpura. *South. Med. J.* 73:603–606, 1980.
15. Wedgewood R.J.P., Klaus M.H.: Anaphylactoid purpura (Schönlein-Henoch syndrome)—a long-term follow-up study with special reference to renal involvement. *Pediatrics* 16:196–206, 1955.
16. Ansell B.M.: Henoch-Schönlein purpura with particular reference to the prognosis of the renal lesion. *Br. J. Dermatol.* 82:211–215, 1970.
17. Counahan R., Winterborn M.H., White R.H.R., et al.: Prognosis of Henoch-Schönlein nephritis in children. *Br. Med. J.* 2:11–14, 1977.
18. West C.D., McAdams A.J.: The chronic glomerulonephritides of childhood. Part I. *J. Pediatr.* 93:1–12, 1978.
19. Meadow R.: Schönlein-Henoch syndrome. *Arch. Dis. Child.* 54:822–824, 1979.
20. Lewis I.C., Philpott, M.G.: Neurologic complications in the Schönlein-Henoch syndrome. *Arch. Dis. Child.* 31:369–371, 1956.
21. Naiman J.J., Harcke T., Sebastianelli J., et al.: Scrotal imaging in the Henoch-Schönlein syndrome. *J. Pediatr.* 92:1021–1022, 1978.
22. Meadow S.R.: The prognosis of Henoch-Schönlein nephritis. *Clin. Nephrol.* 9:87–90, 1978.
23. Sweet R.D.: An acute febrile neutrophilic dermatosis. *Br. J. Dermatol.* 76:349–361, 1964.
24. Spector J.I., Zimbler H., Levine R., et al.: Sweet's syndrome. Association with acute leukemia. *J.A.M.A.* 244:1131–1132, 1980.
25. Itami S., Nishioka K.: Sweet's syndrome in infancy. *Br. J. Dermatol.* 103:449–451, 1980.
26. Levin D., Esterly N.D., Herman J.J., et al.: The Sweet syndrome in children. *J. Pediatr.* 99:73–78, 1981.

27. Hazen P.G., Kark E.C., Davis B.R., et al.: Acute febrile neutrophilic dermatosis in children. *Arch. Dermatol.* 119:998–1002, 1983.
28. Sweet R.D.: Further observations on acute febrile neutrophilic dermatosis. *Br. J. Dermatol.* 80:800–805, 1968.
29. Chmel H., Armstrong D.: Acute febrile neutrophilic dermatosis: Sweet's syndrome. *South. Med. J.* 71:1350–1352, 1978.
30. Hofmann C., Braun-Falco O., Petzoldt D.: Acute febrile neutrophilic dermatosis (Sweet's syndrome). *Dtsch. Med. Wochensher* 101:1120–1128, 1976.
31. Braverman I.M.: Neutrophilic dermatoses; the angiitides, in Braverman I.M.: *Skin Signs of Systemic Diseases.* W.B. Saunders Co., Philadelphia, 1981, pp. 378–452, 740–760.
32. Trentham D.E., Masi A.T., Bale G.F.: Arthritis with inflammatory dermatosis resembling Sweet's syndrome. *Am. J. Med.* 61:424–432, 1976.
33. Raimer S.S., Duncan W.C.: Febrile neutrophilic dermatosis in acute myelogenous leukemia. *Arch. Dermatol.* 114:413–414, 1978.
34. Horio T., Imamura S., Danno K., et al.: Treatment of acute febrile neutrophilic dermatosis (Sweet's syndrome) with potassium iodide. *Dermatologica* 160:341–347, 1980.
35. Lever W.P., Schaumburg-Lever G.: Vascular diseases, in Lever W.P., Schaumburg-Lever G.: *Histopathology of the Skin.* ed. 6. 1983, J.B. Lippincott Co., Philadelphia, pp. 164–189.
36. Wishnick M.M., Valensi Q., Doyle E.F., et al.: Churg-Strauss syndrome: development of cardiomyopathy during corticosteroid treatment. *Am. J. Dis. Child.* 136:339–344, 1982.
37. Chyu J.Y.H., Hagstrom W.J., Soltani K., et al.: Wegener's granulomatosis in childhood: cutaneous manifestations as the presenting signs. *J. Am. Acad. Dermatol.* 10:341–346, 1984.
38. Donald K.J., Edwards R.L., McEvoy J.D.S.: An ultrastructural study of the pathogenesis of tissue in limited Wegener's granulomatosis. *Pathology* 8:161–169, 1976.
39. Fauci A.S., Wolff S.M.: Wegener's granulomatosis: studies in eighteen patients and a review of the literature. *Medicine* 52:535–561, 1973.
40. Walton E.W.: Giant cell granuloma of the respiratory tract (Wegener's granulomatosis). *Br. Med. J.* 2:265–270, 1958.
41. Reza M.J., Dornfeld L., Goldberg L.S., et al.: Wegener's granulomatosis: long-term follow-up of patients treated with cyclophosphamid. *Arthritis Rheum.* 18:501–506, 1975.
42. Chumbley L.C., Harrison E.G., Jr., De Remee R.A.: Allergic granulomatosis and angiitis (Churg-Strauss syndrome): report and analysis of 30 cases. *Mayo Clin. Proc.* 52:477–484, 1977.
43. Cooper B.J., Bacal E., Patterson R.: Allergic angiitis and granulomatosis: prolonged remission induced by combined prednisone-azathioprine therapy. *Arch. Int. Med.* 138:367–371, 1978.
44. Liebow A.A., Carrington C.R.B., Friedman P.J.: Lymphomatoid granulomatosis. *Hum. Pathol.* 3:457–558, 1972.
45. Minars N., Kay S., Escobar M.R.: Lymphomatoid granulomatosis of the skin. *Arch. Dermatol.* 111:493–496, 1975.
46. Rosen T., Chernoski M.E.: Lymphomatoid granulomatosis. *Int. J. Dermatol.* 18:497–498, 1979.
47. James W.D., Odom R.B., Katzenstein A.A.: Cutaneous manifestations of lym-

phomatoid granulomatosis: report of 44 cases and review of the literature. *Arch. Dermatol.* 117:196–202, 1981.

48. Fauci A.S., Haynes B.F., Costa J., et al.: Lymphomatoid granulomatosis: prospective clinical and therapeutic experience over 10 years. *N. Engl. J. Med.* 306:68–74, 1982.
49. Kawasaki T., Kosaki F., Okawa S., et al.: A new infantile acute febrile mucocutaneous lymph node syndrome (MLNS) prevailing in Japan. *Pediatrics* 54:271–276, 1974.
50. Melish M.E., Hicks R.M., Larson E.: Mucocutaneous lymph node syndrome (MLNS) in the United States (abstr.). *Pediatr. Res.* 8:427, 1974.
51. Melish M.E.: Kawasaki syndrome (mucocutaneous lymph node syndrome). *Pediatrics in Review* 2:107–114, 1980.
52. Patriarca P.A., Rogers M.F., Morens D., et al.: Kawasaki's syndrome: association with the application of a rug shampoo. *Lancet* 2:578–580, 1982.
53. Morens D.M., Anderson L.J., Hurwitz E.S.: National surveillance of Kawasaki disease. *Pediatr.* 65:21–25, 1980.
54. Kato S., Kimura M., Tsuji K., et al.: HLA antigens in Kawasaki disease. *Pediatrics* 61:252–255, 1978.
55. Raimer S.S., Tschen E.H., Walker M.K.: Toxic shock syndrome: possible confusion with Kawasaki disease. *Cutis* 28:33–36, 1981.
56. Melish M.E.: Kawasaki syndrome (mucocutaneous lymph node syndrome), in Gellis S.S., Kagan B.M.: *Current Pediatric Therapy 11.* W.B. Saunders Co., Philadelphia, 1984, pp. 449–450.
57. Melish M.E., Hicks R.M., Larson E.J.: Mucocutaneous lymph node syndrome in the United States. *Am. J. Dis. Child.* 130:599–607, 1976.
58. Bitter J.J., Friedman S.A., Peltzik R.L., et al.: Kawasaki disease appearing as erythema multiforme. *Arch. Dermatol.* 115:71–73, 1979.
59. Fujiwara H., Hamashima Y.: Pathology of the heart in Kawasaki disease. *Pediatrics* 61:100–107, 1978.
60. Shigematsu I., Shibata S., Tamashico H., et al.: Kawasaki disease continues to increase in Japan. *Pediatrics* 64:386, 1979.
61. Yanigasawa M., Kobayashi N., Matsuya S.: Myocardial infarction due to coronary thromboarteritis following acute febrile mucocutaneous lymph node syndrome (MLNS) in an infant. *Pediatrics* 54:277–281, 1974.
62. Kitamura S., Kawashima Y., Fujita T., et al.: Aortocoronary bypass grafting in a child with coronary artery obstruction due to mucocutaneous lymph node syndrome. *Circulation* 53:1035–1040, 1976.
63. Magilavy D.B., Speert D.P., Silver T.M., et al.: Mucocutaneous lymph node syndrome: report of 2 cases complicated by gallbladder hydrops and diagnosed by ultrasound. *Pediatrics* 61:699–702, 1978.
64. Neches W.H., Young L.W.: Mucocutaneous lymph node syndrome. Coronary artery disease and cross-sectional echocardiography. *Am. J. Dis. Child.* 113:1233–1235, 1979.
65. Yoshida H., Funabashi T., Nakaya S., et al.: Mucocutaneous lymph node syndrome: a cross-sectional echocardiographic diagnosis of coronary aneurysms. *Am. J. Dis. Child.* 133:1244–1247, 1979.
66. Kato H., Koike S., Yokoyama T.: Kawasaki disease. Effect of treatment of coronary artery involvement. *Pediatrics* 63:175–179, 1979.
67. Kegel S.M., Dorsey T.J., Rowen M., et al.: Mitral insufficiency secondary to mucocutaneous lymph node syndrome. *Am. J. Cardiol.* 40:282–286, 1977.

68. Tanaka N.: Kawasaki disease (acute febrile mucocutaneous lymph node syndrome) in Japan: Relationship with infantile periarteritis nodosa. *Pathol. Microbiol.* (Basel) 43:204–218, 1975.

69. Roberts F.B., Fetterman G.H.: Polyarteritis nodosa in infancy. *J. Pediatr.* 63:519–529, 1963.

70. Hollister J.R.: Collagen vascular disease: polyarteritis nodosum, in Gellis S.S., Kagan B.M.: *Current Pediatric Therapy 10.* W.B. Saunders Co., Philadelphia, 1981, p. 346.

71. Blau E.B., Morris R.F., Yunis E.J.: Polyarteritis in older children. *Pediatrics* 60:227–234, 1977.

72. Magilavy D.B., Petty R.E., Cassidy J.T., et al.: A syndrome of childhood polyarteritis. *J. Pediatr.* 91:25–30, 1977.

73. Borrie P.: Cutaneous polyarteritis nodosa. *Br. J. Dermatol.* 87:87–95, 1972.

74. Diaz-Perez J.L., Schroeter A.L., Winkelmann R.K.: Cutaneous periarteritis nodosa. *Arch. Dermatol.* 116:56–58, 1980.

75. Travers R.L., Allison D.J., and Brettle R.P., et al.: Polyarteritis nodosa: a clinical and angiographic analysis of 17 cases. *Semin. Arthritis Rheum.* 8:184–199, 1979.

76. Cohen R.D., Conn D.L., Ilstrup D.M.: Clinical features, prognosis and response to treatment in polyarteritis. *Mayo Clin. Proc.* 55:146–155, 1980.

77. Fauci A.S., Doppman J.L., and Wolff S.M.: Cyclophosphamide-induced remissions in advanced polyarteritis nodosa. *Am. J. Med.* 64:890–894, 1978.

78. Leib E.S., Restivo C., Paulus H.E.: Immunosuppressive and corticosteroid therapy for polyarteritis nodosa. *Am. J. Med.* 67:941–947, 1979.

79. Kansu E., Deglin S., Cantor R.I., et al.: The expanding spectrum of Behcet syndrome—a case with renal involvement. *J.A.M.A.* 237:1855–1856, 1977.

80. Gorlin R.J., Pindborg J.J., Cohen M.M., Jr.: Behcet's syndrome, in *Syndromes of the Head and Neck,* ed. 2. McGraw-Hill, Inc., New York, 1976. pp. 48–51.

81. Lehner T.: Stimulation of lymphocyte transformation by tissue homogenates in recurrent oral ulceration. *Immunology* 13:159–166, 1967.

82. Levinsky R.J., Lehner T.: Circulating immune complexes in recurrent oral ulceration and Behcet's syndrome. *Clin. Exp. Immunol.* 32:193–198, 1978.

83. Macijewski W., Bandmann H.J.: Immune complex vasculitis in a patient with Behcet's syndrome. *Arch. Dermatol. Res.* 264:253–256, 1979.

84. Tokoro Y., Seto T., Abe Y., et al.: Skin lesions in Behcet's disease. *Int. J. Dermatol.* 16:227–244, 1977.

85. Mundy T.M., Miller J.J. III: Behcet's disease presenting as chronic aphthous stomatitis in a child. *Pediatrics* 62:205–208, 1978.

86. Wray D.: Behcet's syndrome, in Maddin S.: *Current Dermatologic Therapy.* W.B. Saunders Co., Philadelphia, 1982, pp. 51–53.

87. Raynor A., Askari A.D.: Behcet's disease and treatment with colchicine. *J. Am. Acad. Dermatol.* 2:396–400, 1980.

88. Scarlett J.A., Kistner M.L., Yang L.C.: Behcet's syndrome: report of a case associated with pericardial effusion and cryoglobulinemia treated with indomethacin. *Am. J. Med.* 66:146–148, 1979.

89. Jorizzo J.L., Hudson D., Schmalstieg F.C., et al.: Behcet's syndrome: immune regulation, circulating immune complexes, neutrophil migration, and colchicine therapy. *J. Am. Acad. Dermatol.* 10:205–214, 1984.

3 / Infectious Diseases With Systemic Manifestations

THERE ARE MANY INFECTIOUS DISEASES in infants and children that have systemic manifestations. Unfortunately, because of limitations of space, all of them cannot be included in this review. This chapter deals with some of the more significant infections encountered in the practice of pediatric dermatology with emphasis on their cutaneous and systemic involvement and their relationship to the diagnosis and management of these disorders.

Staphylococcal Scalded Skin Syndrome

The staphylococcal scalded skin syndrome (SSSS), first described by Ritter von Rittershain more than 100 years ago[1] and previously known as Ritter's disease or pemphigus neonatorum, is a distinctive dermatosis caused by an exfoliative toxin termed "exfoliation" (or epidermolytic toxin). It is generally elaborated by coagulase-positive Group II staphylococci, usually but not necessarily phage-type 55 or 71, and occasionally Group I, type 52.[2-3] Originally classified as a form of toxic epidermal necrolysis, staphylococcal scalded skin syndrome comprises a distinct disorder associated with staphylococcal infection that occurs primarily in children. When seen in adults, it generally occurs in individuals with immunosuppression, renal impairment, or both.[4] Staphylococcal scalded skin syndrome has now been differentiated from and should not be classified as or confused with toxic epidermal necrolysis (Lyell's disease), a disorder of cutaneous exfoliation induced by sensitivity to drugs or as a manifestation of graft-vs.-host reaction.[5]

Bullous impetigo is considered a localized form of staphylococcal scalded skin syndrome[6] (Fig 3–1). The reason for the increased incidence of staphylococcal scalded skin syndrome (SSSS) in infants and young children as opposed to adults appears to be related to the fact that adults and 85% of children over 10 years of age have specific staphylococcal antibody, metabolic differences, or greater ability to localize the infection, thus allowing the development of localized staphylococcal bullous impetigo but limiting widespread bloodstream dissemination of the toxin.[4]

CLINICAL MANIFESTATIONS.—Staphylococcal scalded skin syndrome usually begins in children, particularly under five years of age, with fever,

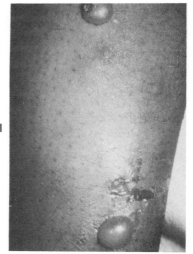

Fig 3–1.—Bullous impetigo. Characteristic of a localized group II staphylococcal infection.

a generalized macular erythema (the erythematous phase) and a fine stippled sandpaper or nutmeg-like appearance which quickly progresses to a tender scarlatiniform phase over a period of one or two days (Table 3–1). From the intertriginous and periorificial areas and trunk, the erythema and tenderness spread over the entire body, usually sparing the hairy parts. Affected children are extremely irritable, uncomfortable, and difficult to hold because of the extreme tenderness of the skin.

Within two or three days, frequently over a period of a few hours, the upper layer of the epidermis may become wrinkled or may be removed by

TABLE 3–1.—STAPHYLOCOCCAL SCALDED SKIN
SYNDROME

1. Generally in children under 5 years of age
2. Caused by an exfoliative toxin ("exfoliatin")
    a. Usually Gp II staph (phage-type 55 or 71)
    b. Occasionally Gp I type 52
3. Clinical features
    a. Fever, tender erythematous skin
    b. Exfoliation with exudation and crusting around mouth, eyes, and paranasal areas
    c. Positive Nikolsky sign
4. Diagnosis:
    a. Tzanck test—cleavage in the epidermis
    b. Bacterial cultures positive for staphylococci (from skin, conjunctivae, ala nasi, nasopharynx, stools, or blood— *not* from blisters)

light stroking (often peeling off like a wet tissue paper), the characteristic Nikolsky sign. The exfoliative phase is heralded by exudation and crusting around the mouth and sometimes the orbits (Fig 3-2). Large fragments of crust become separated, leaving radial fissures surrounding the mouth, which give this disorder its characteristic and diagnostic appearance. Shortly thereafter, the patient develops flaccid bullae and eventual exfoliation of the skin (the desquamative phase). Unless further infection of other skin irritation supervenes, the entire skin heals without scarring within 14 days of the onset of the process.[4, 7–9]

DIAGNOSIS.—Diagnosis of staphylococcal scalded skin syndrome can be verified by isolation of coagulase-positive *Staphylococcus aureus*. In patients with this disorder, the exfoliative (epidermolytic) toxin is disseminated from a primary infection site, usually in the nose or around the eyes. The organism may be recovered from pyogenic foci on the skin, conjunctivae, ala nasi, nasopharynx, stools, and occasionally the blood. The organism is usually not recovered from blisters or areas of exfoliation.

When the diagnosis is indeterminate, differentiation of the staphylococcal disease from drug-induced toxic epidermal necrolysis and other bullous diseases can be made by a Tzanck test, the examination of frozen sections

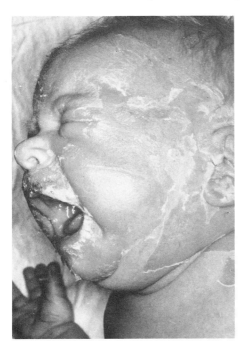

Fig 3–2.—Staphylococcal scalded skin syndrome. Generalized erythema with a fine sandpaper appearance; tenderness of the skin, crusting around the eyes, nose, and mouth; and exfoliation.

of desquamating skin, or a cutaneous biopsy.[10] In staphylococcal scalded skin syndrome (SSSS), cleavage occurs in the epidermis, usually at the level of the granular cell layer. In toxic epidermal necrolysis (TEN), conversely, the split occurs in the upper dermis (below the dermal-epidermal junction).[11]

TREATMENT.—Although controversy exists over the importance of antibiotic therapy in the treatment of staphylococcal scalded skin syndrome, SSSS has an appreciable mortality, slightly less than 4% of cases in children,[12] with most fatalities occurring in neonates with generalized involvement. In adults, however, the mortality rate exceeds 50%, death usually being associated with coexistent disease or immunosuppressive therapy.[13]

The treatment of SSSS should be directed at the eradication of staphylococci from the focus of infection, thus terminating the production of toxin. One of the penicillinase-resistant antistaphylococcal agents (e.g., dicloxacillin) is preferred, since most of the organisms are resistant to penicillin and some are resistant to erythromycin. While oral therapy is generally sufficient for limited bullous impetigo and those without evidence of sepsis or systemic involvement, parenteral antibiotics should be given to those with extensive skin disease and to those who are severely ill.[4] Fluid and electrolyte imbalance should be treated with careful measurements of body weight, input and output, electrolytes, and renal function. Corticosteroids, however, are contraindicated, as they have a detrimental effect and enhance susceptibility of the host to infection.[4] In the late desquamatous phase, the skin may be lubricated with bland ointments or lubricating lotion. Topical antibiotics, however, are unnecessary once systemic antibiotics are initiated.

Toxic Shock Syndrome

Toxic shock syndrome (TSS), an acute febrile disorder with mucocutaneous manifestations and multisystem involvement, is a severe illness characterized by the sudden onset of high fever with vomiting, diarrhea, myalgia, hypotension, and, in severe cases, shock. Originally described by Todd and his associates in 1978,[14] similar cases may have been reported as staphylococcal scarlet fever as far back as 1927.[15] This disorder, generally seen in adolescent females and young women, is caused by a phage-group-I *Staphylococcus aureus*, with a toxin or group of toxins having features of an enterotoxin and a pyrogenic exotoxin.[16–19] The exotoxin appears to be responsible for the fever, rash, and desquamation of the skin. The endotoxin (enterotoxin E) produces the nausea and vomiting, much like that seen in patients with staphylococcal food poisoning. The term "migma toxin" (from the Greek word "migma" meaning "mixture") has been coined for this unique combination.[17]

Patients of both sexes and all age and racial groups have been affected by toxic shock syndrome. Most cases, however, are women during the reproductive years of life. Having an incidence of 6.2 per 100,000 menstruating women, 95% of afflicted individuals are women who contract the disorder at the time of their menses.[20, 21] Although the youngest patient reported to date was a 15-month-old male, there is one report of suspected TSS in a newborn delivered by a mother who had toxic shock syndrome at the time of her delivery.[22] It is still uncertain, however, as to what role tampons (including highly absorbent brands) play in the pathogenesis of the disorder. In spite of much national publicity over the association of TSS with the use of specific tampons, data regarding this linkage are poor and recommendations for a change in the choice or use of tampons remain unproven.[23–25]

Approximately 15% of cases reported to the Centers for Disease Control in Atlanta are not related to menstruation and tampon use. They include cases associated with surgical wound infections; infection following submucous resection and rhinoplasty;[26] deep or superficial abscesses; infected burns, abrasions, insect bites and herpes zoster; cellulitis; adenitis; bursitis; empyema; fasciitis; septic abortion; osteomyelitis; and women during their postpartum period (caused by mastitis as well as vaginal infection), after cesarean section as well as after vaginal delivery.[27]

CLINICAL FEATURES.—Toxic shock syndrome was first reported in seven patients, ages 8 to 17 years, who developed high fever, headache, confusion, conjunctival hyperemia (Fig 3–3), a scarlatiniform rash, subcutaneous edema, vomiting, watery diarrhea, oliguria, a propensity to acute renal failure, hepatic abnormalities, disseminated intravascular coagulation, severe prolonged shock, redness and swelling of the palms (Fig 3–4) and soles, fine desquamation of affected skin, and peeling of the palms and soles during convalescence.[14] Criteria for the diagnosis of toxic shock syndrome, although still disputed,[24] have been defined by the Centers for Disease Control[28] (Table 3–2).

Typically, fever, hypotension, gastrointestinal symptoms, myalgias, and diffuse erythroderma appear on the first day of the illness, but mucous membrane changes are frequently not manifested until the third to fifth days of the illness (at which time the erythroderma frequently has disappeared). Petechiae may be noted late in the first week of the disorder. Desquamation (generally seen on the palms, soles, and tips of the fingers and toes) often does not become apparent until one or two weeks later. Gastrointestinal involvement (typically present at the onset of the illness) is characterized by vomiting and diarrhea with elevation of bilirubin levels and, in some cases, clinical or subclinical jaundice. The nails may be shed and telogen effluvium may occur approximately two months later.[29–32]

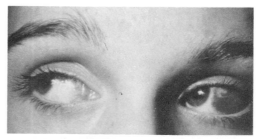

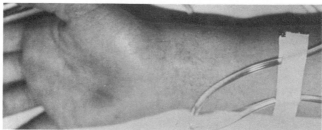

Fig 3–3 (left).—Bulbar erythema and hemorrhage in a 13-year-old girl with toxic shock syndrome. (Courtesy of Dr. Andrew Margileth, Bethesda, Md.)

Fig 3–4 (right).—Toxic shock syndrome. Redness and swelling of the palms in a 13-year-old girl with TSS. (Courtesy of Dr. Andrew Margileth, Bethesda, Md.)

Diagnosis.—The patient with toxic shock syndrome is typically but not necessarily a young healthy menstruating woman with high fever; vomiting; diarrhea; headache; muscular or abdominal pain and diffuse erythroderma followed by prostration; postural hypotension; hyperemia of pharyngeal, conjunctival and vaginal mucous membranes; mental disorientation; cardiac malfunction; severe pulmonary congestion; palmar edema; extensive mucous membrane ulceration and desquamation; a fine generalized desquamation, and extensive desquamation localized to the palms, soles, and digits that occurs seven to 14 days after onset of the disease.[31, 33, 34] Although petechiae are uncommon, most patients have thrombocytopenia. The creatine phosphokinase level is often elevated (occasionally to extremely high levels) and some patients have myoglobinuria. When tampons are found in place and removed by medical personnel, they frequently emit a foul odor. Diffuse myalgia is almost always present, and many patients complain of exquisite skin or muscle tenderness when they are touched or moved.

The pathology of skin biopsies and postmortem material suggests that patients with toxic shock syndrome present a diffuse vasculitis and/or a perivascular infiltration in the dermis.[24] Flaccid bullae with subepidermal blister formation have also been seen in some infants with TSS.

For the present we should adhere to strict criteria for the diagnosis of toxic shock syndrome (Table 3–2). When the diagnosis is suspected, a thorough search for a possible site of infection should be made and cultures should be obtained from a variety of sites (vagina, throat, nares, conjunctiva, blood, or stool) and any cutaneous or subcutaneous lesions, no matter how benign they appear.[27]

TREATMENT.—Because of the high morbidity and mortality rate, the treatment of patients with toxic shock syndrome should be aggressive with early initiation of beta-lactimase resistant antistaphylococcal antibiotics. Although the reported case fatality is still significant, with appropriate treatment the mortality has fallen from 15% to approximately 3%.[24] In severe cases, aggressive fluid replacement is essential and vasopressors to maintain normal blood pressure and other supportive measures such as respiratory assistance or dialysis should be utilized when necessary. If a tampon is present, it should be removed and vaginal irrigation with sterile water, saline, or provadine iodine (Betadine) should be performed in an effort to remove organisms, toxin, and possible related pieces of tampon.

If menstruating women wish to reduce the risk of TSS they probably should avoid or minimize the use of tampons, or restrict tampon use to only part of the menstrual period or only part of the day or night.[21] Because of high risk for recurrence (30%), women with a history of toxic shock syndrome should avoid the use of tampons. Those who continue the use of tampons should have two negative anterior nares and vaginal cultures before they resume this practice.[35]

TABLE 3–2.—TOXIC SHOCK SYNDROME

1. Fever—temperature equal to or greater than 38.9°C (102°F)
2. Rash (diffuse macular erythroderma)
3. Desquamation, particularly palms and soles (1–2 weeks after onset of illness)
4. Hypotension or orthostatic syncope
5. Involvement of three or more of following organ systems:
   a. Gastrointestinal (vomiting and diarrhea)
   b. Muscular (severe myalgia or elevated CPK)
   c. Hyperemia of mucous membranes (vaginal, conjunctival, or oropharyngeal)
   d. Renal
   e. Hepatic
   f. Hematologic (thrombocytopenia)
   g. CNS (disorientation or alterations in consciousness)
6. Negative results of following studies (if obtained):
   a. Cultures of blood, throat, or CSF
   b. Serologic tests for RMSF, leptospirosis, or measles

Lyme Disease

Lyme disease, first recognized in southeastern Connecticut and named for the town where the first cases were recognized in 1975,[36] is an acute febrile syndrome which begins in 95% of cases with lesions of erythema chronicum migrans (Fig 3–5) (see Chapter 1). It is followed after several weeks or months by attacks of arthritis in 50% to 59% and by neurologic or cardiac involvement in 18% of patients.[37]

Until 1982 the mechanism of formation of lesions of erythema chronicum migrans and the cause of Lyme disease were unknown, but studies suggested an association with an antibiotic-sensitive microbial agent transmitted by an arthropod vector (*Ixodes dammini* or related ticks) and mediated by an immunological agent.[38–41] It was subsequently found that antibiotics (penicillin, tetracycline or erythromycin), if given early in the course of the illness, could shorten the duration of erythema chronicum migrans and either attenuate or prevent subsequent sequelae such as arthritis[41–44] (Table 3–3). This suggested that a bacterium, possibly a spirochete, could be the causative agent of erythema chronicum migrans and Lyme disease. This hypothesis was subsequently confirmed by the isolation of spirochetes from the blood, skin and cerebrospinal fluid of patients and ticks found in areas endemic for Lyme disease, and the finding of elevated antibody titers to the spirochete in the skin, blood and cerebrospinal fluid of patients with erythema chronicum migrans and Lyme disease.[45–47] This spirochete has now been determined to be a Borrelia and has been termed *Borrelia burgdorferi*.

CLINICAL FEATURES.—The acute illness of Lyme disease has its onset 3

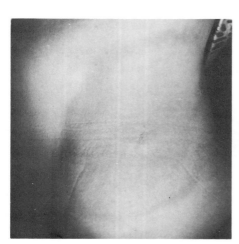

Fig 3–5.—A lesion of erythema chronicum migrans of three weeks duration with central tick bite papule. (Courtesy of Burrows W.M., Jr.[39]).

TABLE 3–3.—LYME DISEASE

1. A spirochetal infection transmitted by a tick of the *Ixodes* variety
2. Erythema chronicum migrans
   a. Expanding ringed lesions 4 to 20 days after a tick bite
   b. May be single or multiple (with clearing in a period of three days to two months)
   c. Tetracycline, penicillin or erythromycin for treatment of ECM may prevent arthritis and perhaps other sequelae
3. Arthritis, cardiac, or neurologic complications

to 21 days following the bite of the *Ixodes* tick. Since the tick bite is painless, it generally goes unnoticed, and 90% of patients with erythema chronicum migrans and Lyme disease do not recall being bitten.[38] There is no age predilection and patients range in age from toddlers to 70–year–old adults. The major correlation is that of summer activity or travel in endemic areas.[40, 48]

The acute illness is characterized by malaise and easy fatigability (90% of cases), fever and chilly sensation (80%), and cutaneous lesions of erythema chronicum migrans (90%).[37] The skin lesions of erythema chronicum migrans are the initial clue to the diagnosis of Lyme disease (formerly known as Lyme arthritis). The typical lesion begins as a small erythematous macule or papule that occurs 4 to 20 days after a tick bite and expands rapidly with central clearing to form a ring which may attain a size of 20 to 30 cm or more, and then clears spontaneously (in a period of three days to two months) (see Fig 3–5). Lesions are generally flat; may be single or multiple; may be asymptomatic or may itch, sting, or burn; and frequently are accompanied by fever, headache, vomiting, fatigue, and regional adenopathy (see Chapter 1).

The systemic features of Lyme disease are characterized by the sudden onset (in the summer or fall) of a swollen joint (usually one, occasionally several), most often in the knee (70%); fatigue; lymphadenopathy; and, in some individuals, Bell's palsy. Weeks or months later, certain patients have meningoencephalitis, cranial or peripheral neuropathies, myocarditis or atrioventricular-node block, or migratory musculoskeletal pain. Still later, frank arthritis may develop with attacks of arthritis generally recurring for several years. The initial attack of Lyme disease generally lasts a week to a month, but the duration varies and recurrences are common. Other features of Lyme disease include an elevated erythrocyte sedimentation rate, decreased levels of C_3 in the serum and, in many cases, increased IgM and IgG cryoprecipitates in the sera of patients during acute attacks.[38, 48]

Although Lyme disease was initially described in Connecticut, ticks of the *Ixodes* complex have been found along the eastern coast of the United States, from Massachusetts to Florida, and as far west as Texas, Utah and the west coast.[40, 41] Of further importance is the fact that this disorder has been recognized in a child from Florida who spent summer vacations in southern Connecticut,[49] in three campers who were bitten by ticks in northeastern Wisconsin[50] and central Minnesota.[51] Such cases emphasize the fact that Lyme disease is not merely a disorder restricted to Connecticut and its adjoining states, but one that has national and (with our highly mobile society) worldwide significance, with cases reported in at least 24 states, France, Switzerland, Canada and Australia.[52, 53]

Patients with arthritis as a manifestation of Lyme disease generally present with an acutely swollen joint with pain on movement or weight bearing, but without associated erythema or tenderness. The arthritis may develop while the acute symptoms of erythema chronicum migrans are still present or up to a period of two years after the onset of the disorder. It usually appears one week to six months (the average being one month) after the acute illness.[38] Seen in up to 48% of patients with Lyme disease, the arthritis may be monoarticular or oligoarticular. In order of prevalence, the knee, shoulder, elbow, temporomandibular joint, ankle, hip, wrist, and small joints of the fingers are most frequently involved.[39] Chronic arthritis occurs in 10% of patients, and severe disability requiring synovectomy has been a significant feature in a small number of patients.

Patients with erythema chronicum migrans who have cryoglobulin containing IgM associated with high serum IgG levels appear to be at risk for developing arthritis.[48] Although the mechanism by which erythema chronicum migrans and Lyme disease occur is not completely understood, a prevalence of B cell alloantigen DRw2 in affected individuals suggests an immunologic susceptibility or a disordered or inappropriate immune response to the infectious agent.[54]

Cardiac abnormalities, when present, appear four days to three months after the onset of the acute illness with electrocardiographic abnormalities including fluctuating a-v block (in 90% of patients with carditis), complete a-v block (in 40%), nonspecific T-wave flattening or inversion and diffuse ST segment depression.[38, 55] Two-thirds of patients with associated cardiac abnormality also have concomitant arthritis, and one-third have signs and symptoms of neurologic involvement.

Neurologic signs and symptoms (seen in 15% of patients with Lyme disease), with the interval following onset of the acute illness being similar to that seen in patients with cardiac abnormality, is generally manifested as a meningoencephalitis with superimposed cranial or peripheral neuropathy (Bell's palsy and sensory or motor radiculoneuritis of the trunk or extremities).[56] Meningeal symptoms are characterized by recurrent attacks of headache, stiff neck, nausea, vomiting, and photophobia; encephalitic symptoms include somnolence, emotional lability, changes in behavior, depression, and poor memory and concentration. These symptoms generally run a fluctuating course which, with remissions and exacerbations, last from one to nine months.

DIAGNOSIS.—Although the diagnosis of Lyme disease is frequently difficult in nonepidemic settings, a history of erythema chronicum migrans followed within weeks to months by recurrent arthritis and/or neurologic and cardiac abnormalities is highly suggestive. Cultures of the *I. dammini* spirochete from patients, although a low-yield procedure, may allow a more definitive diagnosis. Antibody response may be aborted by antibiotic therapy, but 90% of patients have an elevated IgM antibody titer of 1:128 or greater between the time that cutaneous lesions appear and the convalescent phase. Although patients with other treponemal infections may have false positive reactions, an optical density ratio of 0.2 by the Elisa test or an indirect immunofluorescence assay (IFA) which measures IgG class antibodies against the spirochete isolated from *Ixodes dammini* ticks in a titer of 1:256 is considered diagnostic. Since serologic response may be aborted by early antibiotic therapy, and may be absent in patients with erythema chronicum migrans (ECM) alone, a negative result does not exclude the diagnosis of Lyme disease. This test alone is not specific since cross reactivity with other treponomes may result in false positive reactions.

TREATMENT.—Antibiotics such as penicillin, erythromycin, and tetracycline (the last of which should not be administered to children under the age of 12 years) given for a period of ten days early in the illness shortens the duration of erythema chronicum migrans and appears to prevent or attenuate subsequent arthritis and major complications (meningoencephalitis, myocarditis, or recurrent attacks of arthritis). Of these, tetracycline appears to be the most effective followed closely by penicillin and then erythromycin.[44] High-dose intravenous penicillin are currently under investigation for patients with cardiac and/or neurologic complications. It is reasonable to treat all patients who did not receive a previous course of antibiotic therapy, regardless of the duration of their disease.[39, 43]

Gianotti-Crosti Syndrome (Papular Acrodermatitis of Childhood)

Gianotti-Crosti syndrome (papular acrodermatitis of childhood) is a distinctive, self-limiting dermatosis of childhood characterized by the abrupt onset of nonpruritic erythematous lichenoid papules on the face, buttocks, and extremities lasting about three weeks (occasionally longer), with mild constitutional symptoms, lymphadenopathy and acute, usually anicteric, hepatitis[57] (Table 3–4). First recognized in Milan in 1953 and described by

TABLE 3–4.—Features of Gianotti-
Crosti Syndrome

1. Children 3 months to 15 years (particularly between 1 and 6 years of age)
2. Lichenoid papules (face, buttocks, extremities, palms, soles)
3. Anicteric hepatitis
4. Lymphadenopathy, hepatosplenomegaly, fever, leukopenia
5. Hepatitis-B surface antigen and other viruses implicated in some cases

Gianotti in 1955 and later by Crosti and Gianotti in 1956, the term "infantile papular acrodermatitis" was designated in 1957.[58, 59]

Infection with hepatitis B virus subtype ayw has frequently been associated with the Gianotti-Crosti syndrome.[59, 60] Further confirmation of this infectious agent's role as the cause of Gianotti-Crosti syndrome is the report of a child with Gianotti-Crosti syndrome and the subsequent development of acute icteric hepatitis B in the child's mother ten weeks later.[61] Recent reports of other hepatitis subtypes (adw)[62] and other infectious agents (Coxsackievirus A-16,[63] cytomegalovirus, Epstein-Barr virus and parainfluenza virus[64, 65]), however, suggest that the disorder may represent a self-limited cutaneous response to a number of infectious agents.

Clinical manifestations.—Since its original description, it now appears that the Gianotti-Crosti syndrome, although frequently unrecognized, is probably worldwide in distribution.[58, 59, 66, 67] Since the disorder is frequently related to subtype ayw of the hepatitis B virus, a subtype common in the Mediterranean countries, it is not surprising that Gianotti-Crosti disease was first recognized in Italy.[57] The condition begins abruptly and the eruption is often preceded by an upper respiratory infection, generalized lymphadenopathy, hepatomegaly and occasionally splenomegaly, and mild constitutional symptoms. Although adults have occasionally been affected by this disorder, children between 3 months and 15 years of age appear to be most susceptible. The peak incidence in children is between 1 and 6 years of age.[68]

The clinical features of Gianotti-Crosti syndrome are quite distinctive (Table 3–4). The eruption consists of a monomorphous, nonpruritic, generally but not necessarily symmetrical, flat-topped 1 to 10 mm flesh-colored, pale pink or coppery red papules that appear in crops and involve the face (Fig 3–6), buttocks, extremities, palms, soles, and occasionally the upper aspect of the back.[57, 69] Although the trunk is generally spared, a transient eruption may be seen in this region during the early phase of the disorder. In infancy the lesions are generally large (5 to 10 mm in diameter) and in older children the eruption is often micropapular (one to two mm

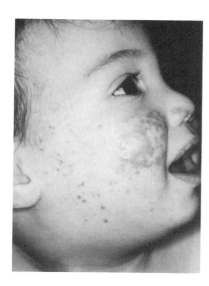

Fig 3–6.—Flat-topped erythematous papules on the face of a 1-year-old child with Gianotti-Crosti syndrome.

in diameter). At times the lesions may have a purpuric appearance and, on occasion, a coarse infiltrated tumor-like appearance has been noted. As the rash progresses, lesions frequently become confluent and, particularly on areas subject to trauma, may merge to form plaques of flat-topped lichenoid papules.

Constitutional symptoms and systemic manifestations include malaise, low-grade fever, mild generalized lymphadenopathy, hepatomegaly, splenomegaly, and, at times, diarrhea. Hepatitis, when present, begins at the same time or a week or two after the onset of the cutaneous eruption, lasts at least two months, and only rarely progresses to chronic liver disease.[57] The rash resolves spontaneously after a variable period of two to eight weeks (usually 15 to 20 days). The lymphadenitis (mainly inguinal and axillary) generally lasts two to three months, and hepatomegaly, when present, generally persists for a three-month period.

Leukopenia with a relative increase in monocytes (up to 20%) and mild hypochromic anemia have been reported. Abnormal liver function with elevation of SGOT, SGPT, LDH, alkaline phosphatase, and bromsulphalein retention without abnormal bilirubin levels have been noted. Australian antigen, when present, is generally detectable ten days or more after the onset of the skin eruption and persists for periods of two months to several years. Liver biopsies done during the dermatitis phase of the disorder in patients with evidence of hepatitis antigen reveal a histologic picture indistinguishable from that of acute viral hepatitis.[58]

Papulovesicular acrolocalized syndrome.—Gianotti also described a similar disorder that generally affects children of a more limited age group (2 to 6 years) not associated with hepatomegaly or hepatitis virus B surface antigenemia.[70] This disorder has been termed "papulovesicular acrolocalized syndrome" (PAS) and consists of small 1 to 5 mm alabaster to rosepink or purple spherical or hemispherical vesicular papules that are often covered with a hemorrhagic crust. The eruption is symmetrically located on the cheeks, ears, buttocks, and extremities. Pruritus is common, splenomegaly is absent, liver function studies are normal, and hepatitis virus B surface antigenemia (HBS Ag) is absent. Whether this disorder warrants separate classification is still uncertain.

DIAGNOSIS.—The diagnosis of Gianotti-Crosti syndrome is dependent upon the characteristic clinical findings and histopathologic examination of cutaneous lesions. Microscopic features of the cutaneous eruption, although nonspecific, are frequently helpful in the diagnosis of this disorder. Histologic features include acanthosis, hyperkeratosis, focal spongiosis with extensive exocytosis of mononuclear cells, liquefactive degeneration of the basal layer, a dense perivascular lymphomonocytic and histiocytic dermal infiltrate, swelling of the vascular endothelium, and dilatation of dermal capillaries.

TREATMENT.—Since the Gianotti-Crosti syndrome is benign and self-limiting (with a low incidence of familial involvement), treatment with other than symptomatic measures is unnecessary. In view of its apparent association with hepatitis B virus in some patients, however, children with this disorder should be observed for possible hepatitis and associated liver involvement. Topical shake lotions such as calamine lotion and oral antihistamines are helpful if pruritus is troublesome. Steroid creams have been reported to have an adverse effect on the cutaneous eruption.[66]

Infectious Mononucleosis

Infectious mononucleosis is an acute, self-limiting, infectious disease caused by the Epstein-Barr virus. Most frequently seen in adolescents and young adults, it is manifested by fever and lymphadenopathy accompanied by pharyngitis, hepatosplenomegaly, atypical lymphocytes in the peripheral blood, and, in 10% to 15% of cases, a cutaneous eruption. Although infection with EB virus is quite common in young children, infectious mononucleosis in this age group is rare, inapparent, or so mild and atypical that a diagnosis frequently is recognized. In contrast, the incidence is high in adolescents and young adults between the ages of 15 and 25 years. The higher incidence of infectious mononucleosis parallels the age-related increase in social activities accompanied by close interpersonal contacts in this age group.

CLINICAL MANIFESTATIONS.—Transmitted by direct contact with a low degree of contagiousness, the incubation period is said to be between 33 and 49 days. The disorder begins insidiously with headache and malaise, and the early course is frequently marked by fevers of 101° to 104°F. Fever usually lasts 4 to 14 days, rarely up to three or four weeks. A sore throat commonly develops a few days after the onset of the illness, and an extensive membranous tonsillitis is characteristic. Lymphadenopathy begins early, is often generalized, and the cervical glands are usually the most conspicuously affected. The spleen is moderately enlarged in one-half to two-thirds of cases, hepatomegaly is common, and icteric hepatitis is reported in 5% to 10% of affected individuals (Table 3–5).

An exanthem occurs in 10% to 15% of cases, usually between the fourth and sixth days, and appears as a macular or maculopapular morbilliform eruption of the trunk (Fig 3–7) or upper arms, and occasionally the face, forearm, thighs, and legs. The eruption may last only a few days and be followed by an urticarial or erythema-multiforme-like eruption. The face is often puffy, the conjunctivae suffused, and in up to 50% of patients, upper eyelid edema may occur, frequently with narrowing of the eyelid aperture. An enanthem also appears on the palate in 25% of cases between the fifth and 17th days of the illness. Manifested by discrete bright red petechiae 0.5 to 1.0 mm in diameter, these lesions, seen at the junction of the hard and soft palates, fade to a brownish hue in two days and are considered to be highly characteristic of the disorder.

In most cases, spontaneous recovery occurs in 10 to 20 days, and virtually all patients return to their normal state of health and activity within four to six weeks after the onset of the illness. Deaths are extremely rare and, when reported, are generally associated with splenic rupture.

DIAGNOSIS.—The diagnosis of infectious mononucleosis is established on the basis of the clinical picture, a white blood count of 10,000 to 40,000, with lymphocytosis, and abnormally large basophilic-staining lymphocytes containing foamy cytoplasm. Heterophile antibody studies (agglutination of

TABLE 3–5.—CLINICAL FEATURES OF INFECTIOUS MONONUCLEOSIS

1. Headache, malaise, fever, sore throat, lymphadenopathy, hepatosplenomegaly
2. Exanthem (in 10% to 15% of patients)
   a. Macular, maculopapular, or morbilliform (may be followed by urticaria or EM-like rash)
   b. Facial puffiness with eyelid edema may be present
3. Enanthem (in 25%)—petechiae at junction of hard and soft palate
4. Ampicillin gives a rash (in 70% to 90%)

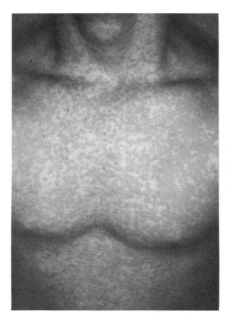

Fig 3–7.—Infectious mononucleosis. Erythematous maculopapular eruption (see in 10% to 15% of patients with this disorder).

sheep erythrocytes by the Paul-Bunnell test) resulting in titers of 1:112 or higher are diagnostic, and the Mono-spot test, a slide test utilizing formalized horse cells (available from Wampole Laboratories), is a valuable presumptive test for rapid diagnosis. Because of its enhanced sensitivity, the Mono-spot test may yield positive results for months after resolution of infectious mononucleosis. It is useful to confirm the Mono-spot test with the classic, more short-lived sheep cell agglutination test.

TREATMENT.—The treatment of infectious mononucleosis is symptomatic. During the acute phase, rest is the most important aspect of treatment. In severe forms of the disorder, corticosteroids reduce the duration and severity of the illness and are effective in the relief of symptomatic cervical adenopathy and tonsillar hyperplasia, frequently with relief of associated discomfort and respiratory problems within 24 to 48 hours. Twenty percent to 25% of patients with infectious mononucleosis may have a concurrent secondary pharyngeal infection with beta-hemolytic streptococci. Penicillin and erythromycin are beneficial in such instances, but ampicillin should be avoided because of a high incidence of sensitivity causing a cutaneous eruption in patients with infectious mononucleosis. [72, 73]

Ampicillin rashes in infectious mononucleosis.—As stated previously, the frequency of cutaneous eruptions in patients with infectious mononucleosis is between 10% and 15%. However, if penicillin is administered, this incidence increases to 44%. If ampicillin is administered, the incidence of sensitivity to this drug, characterized by copper-colored maculopapular lesions that occur five to eight days after the initiation of therapy, increases to 80% to 90%.[71–74] Viral infections, especially Epstein-Barr virus and cytomegalovirus, create an altered immunologic state with abnormal lymphocytes. The increased incidence of sensitivity reaction to ampicillin appears to be related to a transient serologic abnormality involving a number of antigens during infection with these disorders. This concept is supported by the fact that patients with infectious mononucleosis who receive ampicillin demonstrate high levels of ampicillin-specific IgM and IgG which persist for 15 to 17 months following the disease. Since this association is not permanent, it is reassuring to know that on reexposure to ampicillin 1 to 17 months after the acute illness, only 5% of patients continue to display this cutaneous reaction.[72–74]

Rickettsial Diseases

The rickettsial diseases are arthropod-borne disorders caused by a family of microorganisms that have characteristics common to both bacteria and viruses. Spread by blood-sucking insects such as body lice, fleas, ticks and mites, the rickettsial disorders seen in the United States include epidemic louse-borne typhus fever, endemic or murine typhus, rickettsialpox, Q fever and Rocky Mountain spotted fever.

Epidemic (louse-borne) typhus fever.—Epidemic louse-borne typhus fever is an acute, potentially fatal infectious disease transmitted to humans by the body louse, *Pediculosis humanus.* Caused by *Rickettsia prowazekii,* the disorder is characterized clinically by high fever, headaches, general aches and pains, and a centripetal maculopapular eruption that begins on the fourth to seventh day of the illness as a pink macular eruption (that, in severe cases, becomes hemorrhagic) on the trunk and in the axillae and spreads to the rest of the body, usually sparing the face, palms and soles.

Diagnosis of epidemic typhus fever can be established by the clinical picture, isolation of *R. prowazekii* from the blood, and a positive Weil-Felix agglutination reaction with *Proteus* OX-19. Epidemic during periods of war, famine, and social upheaval, the disorder only occurs sporadically in the United States with several cases attributed to contact with infected flying squirrels.[75] The mortality of epidemic typhus is uncommon in children but reaches 10% in young adults and may run as high as 60% to 70% in individuals over 50 years of age. Central nervous system and cardiac manifestations occur when the disease is severe and treatment with tetracycline (except in children under 9 years of age) or chloramphenicol is required.

Endemic (murine, flea-borne) typhus fever.—Endemic typhus fever (flea-borne or murine typhus) is an acute, relatively mild infection caused by *Rickettsia mooseri* and characterized chiefly by headaches, fever, malaise, and a centripetal maculopapular eruption. Essentially a modified version of epidemic typhus, it is spread to man by the rat flea *Xenopsylla cheopis* and is diagnosed on the basis of the clinical picture, isolation of the organism by inoculation of the patient's blood into guinea pigs and adult white mice, and a positive Weil-Felix agglutination reaction with *Proteus* OX-19.

The incubation period of murine typhus ranges from 6 to 14 days. Signs and symptoms are similar to those of epidemic louse-borne typhus, the principal differences being that the course of murine typhus is milder and shorter. The temperature tends to be remittent, terminates after 9 to 13 days, and generally does not rise much above 39°C (102°F). The headache is less severe and the maculopapular rash is less extensive and of shorter duration than that seen in patients with epidemic typhus. Complications are uncommon, and the mortality is 1% or less. Since murine typhus is a mild disease and the rash may be evanescent, it is frequently confused with other illnesses. The disorder seldom lasts longer than two weeks, is usually not complicated by visceral involvement, and, as in other rickettsial disorders, tetracyclines or chloramphenicol are the antibiotics of choice.

Rickettsialpox.—Rickettsialpox is an acute infectious disease caused by *Rickettsia akuri,* an organism antigenically related to the spotted fever group. Spread by the rodent mite *Allodermanyssus sanguineus* and ectoparasites of the mouse, *Mus musculus* (the reservoir of the infection), the disorder is characterized by an initial papule at the site of the bite, a grippe-like syndrome, and a papulovesicular eruption (papules surmounted by vesicles) with an irregular distribution. Most cases of rickettsialpox in the United States have been reported from New York City and other cities in the northeastern United States.[76] Diagnosis can be made on the basis of the clinical picture, isolation of the causative agent from the blood during the acute stage of the disease, negative Weil-Felix agglutinations, a complement fixation test that shows a fourfold or greater rise in antibody titer in paired sera obtained early and late in the disease, or immunofluorescent tests using either RMSF or rickettsialpox antigens. The tetracyclines are helpful (but should not be used for children less than 12 years of age) and shorten the course of this illness.

Q fever.—Q fever, an acute infection of worldwide occurrence, is caused by a rickettsia *(Coxiella burnetti).* Characterized by fever, headache, acute pneumonitis and hepatitis, it is unique in that it is primarily a disease of animals transmitted to humans by inhalation of the agent rather than an arthropod bite, and is not characterized by a cutaneous eruption. Diagnosis is confirmed by complement-fixation or immunofluorescent tests. Death from uncomplicated Q fever is rare and the disease responds promptly to tetracycline or chloramphenicol therapy.

Rocky Mountain spotted fever.—Rocky Mountain spotted fever is an acute febrile exanthematous illness caused by *Rickettsia rickettsii* and transmitted by the bite of a wood or dog tick. Although for years a disorder primarily confined to the Rocky Mountain states, the condition is also endemic in the South Atlantic states and cases are now reported from all parts of the United States.[77] In the western United States, *Dermacentor andersonii* (the wood tick) is the most important vector, and the disease usually occurs in men who acquire the tick bite in wooded areas. In the eastern United States, a dog tick *(Dermacentor variabilis)* is the usual vector, and most patients are women and children.[78] For a decade after the discovery of the broad-spectrum antibiotics (in the early 1950s), the incidence of Rocky Mountain spotted fever began to decline. However, in the 1960s its incidence began to soar in the eastern United States and today it has become the most prevalent rickettsial disease in this country. With this predominance in the eastern coastal and southeastern states, where it is carried by the dog tick, it is not surprising that nearly two-thirds of patients are under the age of 15 years.[79]

CLINICAL MANIFESTATIONS.—The incubation period is usually five to seven days. Most often the rash begins on the third or fourth day of illness as a maculopapular eruption on the extremities (the flexors of the wrists and ankles), spreads centrally to involve the back, chest, and abdomen, and within two days becomes generalized. At first the macules are erythematous, later become purpuric (Fig 3–8), and the palms and soles usually are involved. Occasionally the face is also affected. The lesions are at first discrete, macular, and maculopapular, blanching on pressure. Within one or two days, however, the rash becomes hemorrhagic, with the severity and extent of the eruption directly proportional to the severity of the disease (Table 3–6).

DIAGNOSIS.—The history of a tick exposure in a child with fever, headache, a peripherally distributed hemorrhagic eruption, conjunctivitis, peripheral and periorbital edema, low serum sodium concentration, and thrombocytopenia suggests the possibility of Rocky Mountain spotted fever.[78, 79] Diagnosis can usually be confirmed by Weil-Felix agglutinations positive with OX-19 and OX-2 strains by the second or third week of the infection and by complement fixation tests. Since the pathogenic organism cannot routinely be cultured and the Weil-Felix or complement fixation tests may be negative during the early stages of the disorder, a high index of suspicion and careful epidemiologic history are important. Rapid diagnosis can be obtained as early as the fourth or fifth day after onset of the illness by direct immunofluorescent staining of a cutaneous punch biopsy.[80]

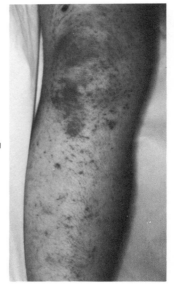

Fig 3–8.—Maculopapular purpuric eruption on the leg of a 4-year-old girl with Rocky Mountain spotted fever.

When complement fixation or immunofluorescent tests are used for diagnosis, antigenic crossovers between typhus and spotted fever are common. In such instances, clinical, geographic, and epidemiological features will aid in the differentiation of these disorders.

TREATMENT.—Rocky Mountain spotted fever (RMSF) is a potentially fatal disease (particularly in children and young adults) with an overall mortality of 13% to 40% (usually 20% to 25%) without treatment.[81] With early diagnosis and rapid therapy, however, this mortality can be lowered to a level of 5% to 7%. Patients treated during the first week of illness almost invariably improve promptly. On the other hand, if the disease is untreated into the second week, therapy is less effective.[81, 82]

Tetracyclines and chloramphenicol have replaced para-aminobenzoic acid in the treatment of Rocky Mountain spotted fever. The preferred

TABLE 3–6.—ROCKY MOUNTAIN SPOTTED FEVER

1. Eruption begins on third to fourth day of illness
2. Erythematous and maculopapular, later purpuric (especially on palms and soles)
3. Diagnosis:
   a. Weil-Felix agglutination OX-19 and OX-2
   b. Direct immunofluorescence of skin biopsy for early diagnosis
4. Rx: tetracycline or chloramphenicol

drug, tetracycline, may be administered orally (to children over 9 years of age) in a dosage of 40 mg/kg per day, in four equally divided doses, with a maximum of 2 gm daily for seven to ten days. When administered intravenously, the dosage of tetracycline is 20 mg/kg/per day. In the more severely ill, intravenous chloramphenicol (50 to 100 mg/kg/per day, with a maximum of 2 to 4 grams per day) may be utilized. When chloramphenicol is administered, however, patients and their families should be advised of the potential toxicity of this preparation. Complete blood counts should be done every two days (or daily if the white blood count is below 7000/cu/mm), and chloramphenicol should be replaced with tetracycline if the white blood count decreases to below 5000/cu/mm or the polymorphonuclear cell count becomes less than 30%.

All patients with Rocky Mountain spotted fever have vasculitis to a varying degree. The more severely ill patients may have edema involving the periorbital area, face, and extremities, disseminated intravascular coagulopathy (purpura fulminans), myocarditis, and, at times, heart failure. Though rarely necessary, the platelet deficit may be lessened temporarily by platelet or whole blood transfusion and intravenous heparin (50 to 100 units/kg intravenously every four to six hours appears to decrease or stop the progression of the coagulopathy). Central nervous system vasculitis, when present, is manifested by delirium, confusion, stupor, and seizures.[83] Phenobarbital sodium, intravenously, in a dose of 4 mg/kg will usually control the seizures. Widespread capillary permeability and hyponatremia may be prominent abnormalities in patients with Rocky Mountain spotted fever. Intravenous therapy with plasma, whole blood transfusions, and appropriate fluid and electrolyte replacement is frequently necessary for those severely affected by this disorder.[84]

Systemic Candidiasis

Candidiasis (moniliasis), an acute or chronic fungus infection, although usually limited to the skin and mucous membranes, is also capable of producing serious systemic disease. Superficial cutaneous and mucosal infections are common. Serious *Candidal* infections, however, are encountered much less frequently. In recent years, the problem of systemic candidiasis has become greater because of increasing use of systemic antibiotics and the opportunistic nature of candidal organisms in immunologically depressed individuals. Although the digestive tract is the principal reservoir, candida is harbored in the vagina in up to 35% of asymptomatic women. Its incidence is increased by pregnancy, menstrual changes, diabetes, and the administration of systemic antibiotics or anovulatory drugs, with many infants being infected at birth from the mother's vaginal tract.[85]

Systemic candidiasis presents a major challenge to the clinician since neither diagnostic nor therapeutic measures are entirely satisfactory. The disorder may affect the lungs, bronchial tree, meninges, kidneys, bladder, joints and, less commonly, the liver, myocardium, endocardium, and eyes. Drug addiction, in-dwelling intravenous catheters and direct trauma during intracardiac surgery have also been implicated in this disorder.[86]

DIAGNOSIS.—Although almost indistinguishable from corresponding bacterial, viral, or other fungal diseases, systemic candidiasis should be suspected in patients with intermittent, spiking, therapy-resistant fever, in those with cutaneous or unusual candidal lesions, cellulitis at the site of an intravenous catheter, on corticosteroid therapy, following open heart surgery, on peritoneal dialysis, with in-dwelling urinary catheters and with drug addiction.[86] The diagnosis is confirmed by isolation of *Candida* from blood, abscesses, urine, or other body fluids; by demonstration of the organism in cutaneous biopsy or other surgical specimens; and by the presence of hypergammaglobulinemia and precipitating antibodies to cytoplasmic antigens of *C. albicans*.

TREATMENT.—Treatment is directed toward removal of iatrogenic factors, management of the underlying illness, and specific antifungal therapy. Nystatin, 1 to 1.5 million units per day in infants or 3 to 6 million units per day in older children, may be administered as an oral suspension (for infants) or in tablet form (for older individuals). Amphotericin may be administered in dosages of 0.25 mg/kg to 1 mg/kg intravenously daily, or 1.5 mg/kg every other day, but the toxicity of amphotericin B (anemia, thrombocytopenia, and nephrotoxicity) requires caution with the use of this preparation. In such instances, oral clotrimazole (60 to 150 mg/kg per day) in three divided doses, flucytosine (100 mg/kg/day) divided into four doses, or intravenous miconazole (30 to 60 mg/kg daily), given at eight-hour intervals, may be administered.[87-90] Side effects to clotrimazole include gastrointestinal intolerance, leukopenia, and elevated liver enzymes, all of which are reversible. Because the drug induces hepatic microsomal enzymes that affect its metabolism, the manufacturer (Delbay Pharmaceuticals) recommends that it be administered for courses of two weeks, followed by two-week rest periods. Although flucytosine may be given orally and is relatively safe, resistant strains of *Candida* often develop during therapy.[90]

Oral ketoconazole (Nizoral), a broad-spectrum antifungal agent, has been approved by the FDA for the treatment of the following fungal infections: candidiasis, chronic mucocutaneous candidiasis, oral thrush, candiduria, paracoccidiomycosis, chromomycosis, histoplasmosis, and coccidiomycosis.[91, 92] It also has been utilized for the treatment of dermatophytosis, tinea versicolor, and vaginal candidiasis. The dosage for older individuals varies from 100 mg to 400 mg/day. Although the dosage for young children has not been established, 4 to 10 mg/kg/day has been suggested,[93] and 3.3 mg/kg/day appears to be an appropriate dosage for children. Unlike other imidazole antifungals, ketoconazole acts on the cytoplasmic membrane of the sensitive fungi by selectively inhibiting the absorption of precursors of DNA, RNA, and mucopolysaccharide, thus creating defects in the cell membrane. The most frequent side effects seen in association with this medication include gastrointestinal upset, liver disturbance, and mental confusion.

It has recently been recognized that hepatic toxicity may occur in 1 of 12,000 patients treated systemically with ketoconazole. Accordingly, it has been suggested that ketoconazole should be reserved for severe systemic or incapacitating disorders such as recurrent dermatophytoses or chronic mucocutaneous candidiasis unresponsive to other agents. Oral ketoconazole, however has not been approved for the treatment of dermatophytosis. It has further been suggested that liver function studies be evaluated before the initiation of therapy and at semimonthly intervals during its use. Physicians and patients should watch for possible pruritus or jaundice and the medication should be discontinued if any of these symptoms occur.[92, 93]

Chronic mucocutaneous candidiasis.—Chronic mucocutaneous candidiasis is a progressive candidal infection that may be congenital or acquired and usually is associated with endocrinopathy (hypoadrenalism, hypothyroidism, diabetes, hypoparathyroidism), vitiligo, immunologic deficiency, and defects in the thymus-controlled lymphocyte defense system. Although the disorder may have its onset in the neonatal period, it usually manifests itself later in infancy or early childhood.

It may begin as an oral candidiasis (thrush), candidal diaper dermatitis, candidial intertrigo or paronychia that is persistent and resistant to the usual modes of therapy. The disorder persists and spreads to involve the scalp, eyelids, nose, hands, and feet, and may be characterized by intertrigo, pathognomonic satellite pustules, erythematous lesions covered with dry scaly patches, or thick macerated crusts. Coalescence of individual lesions often leads to the formation of crusted granulomatous areas with verrucous surfaces and horn-like projections. Dystrophy of the nails, scarring, and loss of hair are common sequellae. Although the disorder is frequently refractory to therapy, systemic involvement is uncommon.[94]

TREATMENT.—In the past, nystatin and amphotericin B have been the treatments of choice for chronic mucocutaneous candidiasis. Unfortunately, neither of these antifungal antibiotics is absorbed from the gastrointestinal tract sufficiently to be of value in the oral treatment of systemic infection. Although the intravenous or prolonged administration of amphotericin B may result in clearing of chronic mucocutaneous candidiasis, it invariably recurs when treatment is discontinued, and nephrotoxicity precludes its continued use.

In recent years, there have been reports of successful treatment of chronic mucocutaneous candidiasis with the newer antifungal agents, clotrimazole, intravenous miconazole, and ketoconazole,[95] but again the possibility of hepatotoxicity associated with the use of ketoconazole should be watched for and monitored with appropriate liver studies.

Chronic Granulomatous Disease of Childhood

Chronic granulomatous disease of childhood (CGD) is an X-linked disorder predominantly affecting young males during the first year of life and, prior to the availability of prophylactic antibiotics, generally resulted in death during childhood.[96, 97] Formerly termed fatal granulomatous disease of childhood, the disorder is characterized by severe recurrent chronic granulomatous reactions to a number of common bacteria that require phagocytic production of hydrogen peroxide for death. The organisms usually associated with this disease are *Staphylococcus aureus*, *Klebsiella*, *Enterobacter aerogenes*, *Salmonella*, and *Serratia*.

The primary abnormality in chronic granulomatous disease is a defect in the ability of peripheral leukocytes (both neutrophils and monocytes) to kill bacteria. This defect is not a failure of the cells to phagocytize organisms, but an abnormality in the intracellular killing process of the phagocytic cells. One mechanism by which granulocytes kill bacteria involves halogenation of bacterial cell walls by a process that involves hydrogen peroxide and peroxidase. In chronic granulomatous disease of childhood, there is an abnormality in peroxide and superperoxide production after phagocytosis caused either by a defect in pyridine nucleotide-dependent, superoxide-forming oxidase or an abnormality in the activation of oxidase in the phagocytic neutrophils of patients with this disorder.[98] A few families have also been described in which females were affected, probably as a result of an autosomal recessive type of inheritance.[94, 95] Deficient glutathione peroxidase activity of leukocytes has been described in these individuals.[99, 100] Male patients with chronic granulomatous disease outnumber females by a 7 to 1 ratio and are more severely affected (Table 3–7).

CLINICAL MANIFESTATIONS.—The earliest characteristic feature of chronic granulomatous disease is an eczematous eruption in infancy. Pa-

TABLE 3–7.—CHRONIC GRANULOMATOUS DISEASE
OF CHILDHOOD

1. X-linked, affects males during 1st year of life (male-female ratio 7 to 1)
2. A defect in intracellular killing of bacteria by phagocytic cells
3. NBT (nitro-blue tetrazolium test) diagnostic

tients often have infectious eczematoid dermatitis, purulent miliaria, frequent pustules, paronychia, small indolent papules about the margins of the eyelids and lips, and apple-jelly nodules about the face, particularly about the nares, the postauricular and periorbital areas, the scalp, the axillae, and the inguinal region.[101] Other clinical manifestations include pyoderma, stomatitis, conjunctivitis, osteomyelitis, chronic draining lymphadenitis (particularly in the cervical and inguinal regions), meningitis, pneumonia, peritonitis, septicemia, and abscesses or interstitial infiltrative granulomatous processes of the lungs, bone marrow, pericardium, and gastrointestinal tract.

DIAGNOSIS.—The diagnosis of chronic granulomatous disease is suggested in a child, particularly a male, who has impetiginized eczema, suppurative lymphadenopathy, incompletely clearing infections (especially those caused by *Staphylococcus aureus* or unusual organisms such as *Serratia marcescens*), or in children in a family where male siblings died from infection in infancy or have documented CGD. The leukocyte defect can be diagnosed by the nitro-blue tetrazolium (NBT) slide test. Whereas leukocytes from normal individuals reduce nitro-blue tetrazolium dye during phagocytosis, cells from patients with this disorder have an inability or marked decrease in the ability to reduce the dye from a colorless to a deep blue state during phagocytosis.

TREATMENT.—Treatment of children with chronic granulomatous disease has, in general, been frustrating. Genetic counseling, including carrier states in sisters of affected males, is recommended in all cases. Although the value of continuous courses of antibiotics remains questionable, treatment with a bactericidal antibiotic specific for the patient's infecting organism for long periods of time appears to prolong symptom-free intervals in patients affected with this disorder.

Job Syndrome

The Job syndrome appears to be an autosomal recessive variant of chronic granulomatous disease.[102] In this disorder, there is also a defect in polymorphonuclear function in which certain species of bacteria are ingested but not destroyed, but the granulomatous reactions seen in X-linked chronic granulomatous disease of childhood do not occur. Studies by Hill suggest that chemical mediators released by interaction of leukocytes, IgE, and specific antigen are responsible for the functional leukocyte dysfunction seen in this disorder (Table 3–8).[103]

CLINICAL MANIFESTATIONS.—The few patients described with this condition are young and fair-haired girls. Symptoms generally begin in the first year of life with a persistent seborrheic form of eczema of the scalp, ears, periorbital areas, and inguinal regions. Scalp folliculitis and staphylococcal

TABEL 3–8.—JOB SYNDROME

---

1. A defect in PMN function in young fair-haired girls
2. Persistent eczema of scalp, ears, periorbital areas and inguinal regions
3. Recurrent infections
   a. Scalp folliculitis and staphylococcal abscesses of skin, subcutaneous tissues, or lymph nodes
   b. Recurrent pneumonia, otitis media, and abscess of liver and lung
4. Elevated IgE levels and immunoglobulins with normal management of other bacterial and viral infections

---

abscesses of the skin, subcutaneous tissues or lymph nodes with little overt inflammation (suggestive of tuberculous "cold abscesses") are prominent features, and recurrent upper respiratory infection, otitis media, pneumonia, and abscesses of the lung and liver are commonly seen in this disease. Other features include extremely elevated IgE levels, elevated immunoglobulins, and a generally normal history of management of other bacterial and viral infections.

TREATMENT.—Treatment of patients with Job syndrome requires appropriate cultures and the administration of a semisynthetic penicillinase-resistant penicillin.

REFERENCES

1. Ritter von Rittershain G.: Die exfoliative Dermatitis jüngerer Säuglinge. *Centralzeitschrift für kinderheilkunde.* 2:3–23, 1978.
2. Lillibridge C.B., Melish M.E., Glasgow L.A.: Site of action of exfoliative toxin in the staphylococcal scalded-skin syndrome. *Pediatrics* 50:723–738, 1972.
3. Melish M.E., Glasgow L.A.: The staphylococcal scalded skin syndrome—development of an experimental model. *N. Eng. J. Med.* 282:1114–1119, 1970.
4. Melish M.E.: Staphylococcal infections, in Feigin R.D., Cherry J.D. (eds.): *Textbook of Pediatric Infectious Disease.* W.B. Saunders Co., Philadelphia, 1981, pp. 956–985.
5. Lyell A.: Toxic epidermal necrolysis (scalded skin syndrome): a reappraisal. *Br. J. Dermatol.* 100:69–86, 1979.
6. Elias P.M., Levy S.W.: Bullous impetigo: occurrence of localized scalded skin syndrome in an adult. *Arch. Dermatol.* 112:856–858, 1976.
7. Melish M.E., Glasgow L.A.: Staphylococcal scalded skin syndrome: the expanded clinical syndrome. *J. Pediatr.* 78:958–967, 1971.
8. Elias P.M., Fritsch P., Mittermeyer H.: Staphylococcal toxic epidermal necrolysis: species and tissue susceptibility and resistance. *J. Invest. Dermatol.* 66:80–89, 1976.
9. Koblenzer P.J.: Toxic epidermal necrolysis (TEN: Ritter's disease) and staphylococcal scalded-skin syndrome (SSSS). A description and review. *Clin. Pediatr.* 15:724–730, 1976.
10. Amon R.B., Diamond R.L.: Toxic epidermal necrolysis: rapid differentiation

between staphylococcal- and drug-induced disease. *Arch. Dermatol.* 111:1433–1437, 1975.

11. Manzella J.P., Hall C.B., Green J.C., et al.: Toxic epidermal necrolysis in childhood: differentiation from staphylococcal scalded skin syndrome. *Pediatrics* 66:291–294, 1980.

12. Elias P.M., Fritsch P., Epstein E.H., Jr.: Staphylococcal scalded skin syndrome (Review). *Arch. Dermatol.* 113:207–219, 1977.

13. Ridgway H.B., Lowe N.J.: Staphylococcal syndrome in an adult with Hodgkin's disease. *Arch. Dermatol.* 115:589–590, 1979.

14. Todd J., Fishaut N., Kapral F., et al.: Toxic-shock syndrome associated with phage-group-I staphylococci. *Lancet* 2:1116–1118, 1978.

15. Stevens F.A.: The occurrence of *Staphylococcus aureus* infection with a scarlatiniform rash. *J.A.M.A.* 88:1957–1958, 1927.

16. Altermeier W.A., Lewis S., Schlievert P.M., et al.: Studies on the staphylococcal causation of toxic-shock syndrome. *Surg. Gynecol. Obstet.* 153:481–485, 1981.

17. Schlievert P.M., Shands K.N., Dan B.B., et al.: Identification and characterization of an exotoxin from *Staphylococcus aureus* associated with toxic shock syndrome. *J. Infect. Dis.* 143:509–516, 1981.

18. Bergdoll M.S., Crass B.A., Reiser R.F., et al.: A new staphylococcal enterotoxin, enterotoxin F, associated with toxic-shock syndrome *Staphylococcal aureus* isolates. *Lancet* 1:1017–1021, 1981.

19. Schlievert P.M., Osterholm M.T., Kelly J.A., et al. Toxin and enzyme characterization of *Staphylococcus aureus* isolated from patients with and without toxic shock syndrome. *Ann. Int. Med.* 96(Part 2):937–940, 1982.

20. Whitfield J.W., Valenti W.M., Magnussen R.: Toxic shock syndrome in the puerperium. *J.A.M.A.* 246:1806–1807, 1981.

21. Shands K.N., Schmid G.P., Dan B.B., et al.: Toxic-shock syndrome in menstruating women. Association with tampon use and *Staphylococcal aureus* and clinical features in 52 cases. *N. Engl. J. Med.* 303:1436–1443, 1980.

22. Green S.L., LaPeter K.S.: Evidence for postpartum toxic-shock syndrome in a mother-infant pair. *Am. J. Med.* 72:169–172, 1982.

23. Reingold A.L., Hargrett N.T., Shands K.N.: Toxic shock syndrome surveillance in the United States, 1980–1981. *Ann. Int. Med.* 96:875–880, 1982.

24. Todd J.K.: Toxic shock syndrome—scientific uncertainty and the public media. *Pediatrics* 67:921–923, 1981.

25. Todd J.K.: Toxic shock syndrome: a perspective through the looking glass. *Ann. Intern. Med.* 96:839–842, 1982.

26. Thomas S.W., Baird I.M., Frazier G.D.: Toxic shock syndrome following submucous resection and rhinoplasty. *J.A.M.A.* 247:2402–2403, 1982.

27. Reingold A.C.: Nonmenstrual toxic shock syndrome: the growing picture. *J.A.M.A.* 249:932, 1983.

28. Center for Disease Control: Follow-up toxic shock syndrome—United States. *Morbidity Mortality Weekly Rep.* 29:297, 1980.

29. Weston W.L., Todd J.K.: Toxic-shock syndrome. *J. Am. Acad. Dermatol.* 4:478–488, 1981.

30. Tofte R.W., Williams D.N.: Toxic shock syndrome: evidence of a broad clinical spectrum. *Ann. Int. Med.* 96(Part 2) 843–847, 1982.

31. Chesney P.J., Davis J.E., Purdy W.K., et al.: Clinical manifestations of toxic shock syndrome. *J.A.M.A.* 264:741–748, 1981.

32. Hansen R.C.: Staphylococcal scalded skin syndrome, toxic shock syndrome, and Kawasaki disease, in Rasmussen, J.E. (guest editor): Symposium on Pediatric Dermatology (Part I), *Pediatric Clinics of North America*. W.B. Saunders Co., Philadelphia, 1983, pp. 533–544.

33. Chesney P.J., Jaucian R.M., McDonald R.A., et al.: Exfoliative dermatitis in an infant: association with enterotoxin F-producing staphylococci. *Am. J. Dis. Child.* 137:899–901, 1983.

34. Bach M.C.: Dermatologic signs in toxic shock syndrome—clues to diagnosis. *J. Am. Acad. Dermatol.* 8:343–347, 1983.

35. Davis J.P., Chesney P.J., Wand P.J., et al.: Toxic-shock syndrome: epidemiological features, recurrence, risk factors, and prevention. *N. Engl. J. Med.* 303:1429–1435, 1980.

36. Steere A.C., Malawista S.E., Syndman D.R., et al.: Lyme arthritis, an epidemic of oligoarticular arthritis in children and adults in three Connecticut communities. *Arthritis and Rheumatism* 20:7–17, 1977.

37. Hardin J.A., Steere A.C., Malawista S.E.: Immune complexes and the evolution of Lyme arthritis. *N. Engl. J. Med.* 301:1358–1363, 1979.

38. Steere A.C., Malawista S.E., Hardin J.A., et al.: Erythema chronicum migrans and Lyme arthritis. The enlarging clinical spectrum. *Ann. Int. Med.* 86:685–698, 1977.

39. Burrows W.M., Jr.: Erythema chronicum migrans and Lyme disease. *J. Assoc. Military Dermatologists*, VIII: 18–21, 1982.

40. Steere A.C., Malawista S.E.: Cases of Lyme disease in the United States: location correlated with distribution of *Ixodes dammini. Ann. Int. Med.* 91:730–733, 1979.

41. Wallis R.C., Brown S.E. Kloter K.O., et al.: Erythema chronicum migrans and Lyme arthritis: field study of ticks. *Am. J. Epidemiol.* 108:322–327, 1978.

42. Mast W.E., Burrows W.M.: Letters to the editor: Erythema chronicum migrans and "Lyme arthritis". *J.A.M.A.* 236:2392, 1976.

43. Steere A.C., Malawista S.E., Newman J.H., et al.: Antibiotic therapy in Lyme disease. *Ann. Int. Med.* 93:1–8, 1980.

44. Steere A.C., Hutchinson J., Rahn D.W., et al.: Treatment of early manifestations of Lyme Disease. *Ann. Int. Med.* 99:22–26, 1983.

45. Steere A.C., Grodzicki R.L., Kornblatt A.N., et al.: The spirochetal etiology of Lyme disease. *N. Engl. J. Med.* 308:733–740, 1983.

46. Burgdorfer W., Barbour A.G., Hayes S.F., et al.: Lyme disease—a tick-borne spirochetosis? *Science* 216:1317–1319, 1982.

47. Benach J.L., Bosler E.M., Hanrahan J.P., et al.: Spirochetes isolated from the blood of two patients with Lyme disease. *N. Engl. J. Med.* 308:740–742, 1983.

48. Steere A.C., Hardin J.A., Riddy S., et al.: Lyme arthritis: Correlation with serum and cryoglobulin IgM with activity, and serum IgG with remission. *Arth. Rheum.* 22:471–489, 1979.

49. Zakem J.M., Germain B.F.: Lyme arthritis in Florida. *J. Fla. Med. Assoc.* 66:281–283, 1979.

50. Dryer R.F., Goeliner P.G., Carney A.S.: Lyme arthritis in Wisconsin. *J.A.M.A.* 241:498–499, 1979.

51. Schrock C.G.: Lyme disease: additional evidence of widespread distribution: recognition of tick-borne dermatitis-encephalitis-arthritis syndrome in an area of known *Ixodes* tick distribution. *Am. J. Med.* 72:700–702, 1982.

52. Gerster J.C., Guggi J., Perroud H., et al.: Lyme arthritis appearing outside the United States: a case report from Switzerland. *Br. Med. J.* 283:951–952, 1981.
53. Stewart A., Glass J., Patel A., et al.: Lyme arthritis in the Hunter Valley. *Med. J. Australia* 1:139, 1982.
54. Steere A.C., Gibofsky A., Patarroyo M.E., et al.: Chronic Lyme arthritis: clinical and immunologic differentiation from rheumatoid arthritis. *Ann. Int. Med.* 90:896–901, 1979.
55. Steere A.C., Batsford W.P., Weinberg M., et al.: Lyme carditis: cardiac abnormalities of Lyme disease. *Ann. Intern. Med.* 93:8–16, 1980.
56. Reik L., Steere A.C., Bartenhagen N.H., et al.: Neurologic abnormalities of Lyme disease. *Medicine* 58:281–294, 1979.
57. Gianotti F.: Papular acrodermatitis of childhood and other papulovesicular acro-located syndromes. (Review) *Br. J. Dermatol.* 100:49–59, 1979.
58. Gianotti F.: Papular acrodermatitis of childhood: an Australian antigen disease. *Arch. Dis. Child.* 48:794–799, 1973.
59. Gianotti F.: Papular acrodermatitis of childhood: an Australian antigen disease. *Mod. Probl. Paediat.* 17:180–189, 1975.
60. Ishimaru Y., Ishimaru H., Toda G., et al.: An epidemic of infantile papular acrodermatitis (Gianotti's disease) in Japan associated with hepatitis-B surface antigen subtype ayw. *Lancet* 1:707–709, 1976.
61. San Joaquin V.H., Ward K.E., Marks M.I.: Gianotti disease in a child and acute hepatitis B in a mother. *J.A.M.A.* 246:2191–2192, 1981.
62. Schneider J., Poley J.R., Millunchick E.W., et al.: Papular acrodermatitis (Gianotti-Crosti syndrome) in a child with anicteric hepatitis B, virus sub-type adw. *J. Pediatr.* 101:219–221, 1982.
63. James W.D., Odom A.B., Hatch M.H.: Gianotti-Crosti-like eruption associated with Coxsackievirus A-16 infection. *J. Amer. Acad. Dermatol.* 6:862–866, 1982.
64. Spear K.L., Winkelmann R.K.: Gianotti-Crosti syndrome. A review of ten cases not associated with hepatitis B. *Arch. Dermatol.* 120:891–896, 1984.
65. Kanno M., Kikuta H., Ishiwaka N., et al.: A possible association between hepatitis-B antigen-negative infantile papular acrodermatitis and Epstein-Barr virus infection. *J. Pediatr.* 101:222–224, 1982.
66. Hjorth N., Kopp H., Osmundsen P.E.: Gianotti-Crosti syndrome—papular eruption of infancy. *Trans. St. John's Hosp. Derm. Soc.* 53:46–56, 1967.
67. Rubenstein D., Esterly N.B., Fretzin D.: The Gianotti-Crosti syndrome. *Pediatrics* 61:433–437, 1967.
68. Claudy A.L.: Adult papular acrodermatitis. *Ann. Derm. Venereol.* 104:190–194, 1977.
69. Eiloart M.: The Gianotti-Crosti syndrome. Report of forty-four cases. *Br. J. Dermatol.* 78:488–492, 1966.
70. Gianotti F.: Infantile papular acrodermatitis: acrodermatitis papulosa and infantile papulovesicular acrolocalized syndrome. *Hautarzt* 27:467–472, 1976.
71. Patel B.M.: Skin rash with infectious mononucleosis. *Pediatrics* 40:910–911, 1967.
72. Kraemer M.J., Smith A.L.: Rashes with ampicillin. *Pediatrics in Review* 1:197–201, 1980.
73. Levene G., Baker H.: Ampicillin and infectious mononucleosis. *Br. J. Dermatol.* 80:417–418, 1978.

74. Lund A., Bergan T.: Temporary skin reactions to penicillins during acute stage of infectious mononucleosis. *Scand. J. Dis.* 7:21–28, 1975.
75. Duma R.J., Sonenshine D.E., Bozeman M., et al.: Epidemic typhus in the United States associated with flying squirrels. *J.A.M.A.* 245:2318–2323, 1981.
76. Wong B., Singer C., Armstrong D., et al.: Rickettsialpox. Case report and epidemiologic review. *J.A.M.A.* 242:1998–1999, 1979.
77. Cawley E.P., Wheeler C.E.: Rocky Mountain spotted fever. *J.A.M.A.* 163:1003–1007, 1957.
78. Haynes R.E., Sanders D.Y., Cramblett H.G.: Rocky Mountain spotted fever in children. *J. Pediatr.* 76:685–693, 1970.
79. Bradford W.D., Hawkins H.K.: Rocky Mountain spotted fever in childhood. *Am. J. Dis. Child.* 131:1228–1232, 1977.
80. Woodward T.E., Peterson C.E., Jr., Oster C.N., et al.: Prompt confirmation of Rocky Mountain spotted fever. Identification of Rickettsia in skin tissues. *J. Infect. Dis.* 134:297–305, 1976.
81. Krugman W., Ward R., Katz S.L.: *Infectious Diseases of Children.* The C.V. Mosby Company, St. Louis, 1977.
82. Murray E.S.: Rickettsial diseases, in Feigin R.D., Cherry J.D. (eds.): *Textbook of Pediatric Infectious Diseases.* W.B. Saunders Co., Philadelphia, 1981, pp. 1437–1439.
83. Gorman R.J., Saxon S., Snead O.C. III: Neurologic sequelae of Rocky Mountain spotted fever. *Pediatrics* 67:354–357, 1981.
84. Hattwick M.A.W., Retalliau H., O'Brien R.J., et al.: Fatal Rocky Mountain spotted fever. *J.A.M.A.* 240:1499–1503, 1978.
85. Fitzpatrick R.E., Newcomer V.D.: Dermatophytosis and candidiasis, in Feigin R.D. and Cherry J.D. (eds.): *Textbook of Pediatric Infectious Diseases.* W.B. Saunders Co., Philadelphia, 1981, pp. 608–643.
86. Keller M.A., Sellers B.B., Jr., Melish M.E., et al.: Systemic candidiasis in infants. A case presentation and literature review. *Am. J. Dis. Child.* 131:1260–1263, 1977.
87. Rockoff A.S.: Chronic mucocutaneous candidiasis. Successful treatment with intermittent oral doses of clotrimazole. *Arch. Dermatol.* 115:322–323, 1979.
88. Fisher T.J., Klein R.B., Kershnar H.E., et al.: Miconazole in treatment of chronic mucocutaneous candidiasis: Preliminary report. *J. Pediatr.* 91:815–819, 1977.
89. Leikin S., Parrott R., Randolph J.: Clotrimazole treatment of chronic mucocutaneous candidiasis. *J. Pediatr.* 88:864–866, 1976.
90. Logan R.I., Goldberg M.J.: *C. albicans* resistance to 5-fluorocytosine. *Br. Med. J.* 3:531, 1972.
91. Hanifin J.M.: Ketoconazole—an oral antifungal with activity against superficial and deep mycoses. *J. Am. Acad. Dermatol.* 2:537–539, 1980.
92. Jones H.E., Simpson J.G., Artis W.M.: Oral ketoconazole, an effective and safe treatment for dermatophytosis. *Arch. Dermatol.* 117:129–133, 1981.
93. Hurwitz S., Kahn G.: Meeting report. IXth Postgraduate Seminar in Pediatric Dermatology, Miami, Florida, Feb. 25–28, 1982. *J. Am. Acad. Dermatol.* 271–278, 1983.
94. Higgs J.M., Wells R.S.: Chronic mucocutaneous candidiasis: new approaches to treatment. *Br. J. Dermatol.* 89:179–190, 1973.
95. Zachariae H., Laurberg G., Thestrup-Pedersen K.: Ketoconazole in a case of

chronic mucocutaneous candidiasis. *Acta Dermatovenereol* (Stockh.) 62:87–89, 1982.

96. Berendes H., Bridges R.A., Good R.A.: A fatal granulomatosis of childhood. *Minn. Med.* 40:309–312, 1957.
97. Bridges R.A., Berendes H., Good R.A.: A fatal granulomatous disease of childhood—the clinical, pathological, and laboratory features of a new syndrome. *AMA J. Dis. Child.* 97:387–408, 1959.
98. Curnutte J.T., Kipnes R.S., and Babior B.M.: Defect in pyridine nucleotide dependent superoxide producton by a particulate fraction from the granulocytes of patients with chronic granulomatous disease. *N. Engl. J. Med.* 293:628–632, 1975.
99. Quie P.G., Kaplan E.L., Page A.R., et al.: Defective polymorphonuclear-leukocyte function and chronic granulomatous disease in two female children. *N. Engl. J. Med.* 278:976–980, 1968.
100. Holmes B., Park B.H., Malawista S.E., et al.: Chronic granulomatous disease in females—a deficiency of leukocyte glutathione peroxidase. *N. Engl. J. Med.* 283:217–221, 1970.
101. Windhorst D.R., Good R.A.: Dermatologic manifestations of fatal granulomatous disease of childhood. *Arch. Dermatol.* 103:351–357, 1971.
102. Bannatyne R.M., Skoworn P.N., Weber J.L.: Job's syndrome: a variant of chronic granulomatous disease. *J. Pediatr.* 75:236–242, 1969.
103. Hill H.R., Quie P.G., Pabst H.F., et al.: Defect in neutrophil granulocyte chemotaxis in Job's syndrome of recurrent "cold" staphylococcal abscesses. *Lancet* 2:617–619, 1974.

4 / Disorders of Connective Tissues

THE CONNECTIVE TISSUE OF THE DERMIS consists of collagen, reticulum, and elastic fibers (elastin) embedded in an amorphous ground substance consisting of glycosaminoglycans or acid mucopolysaccharides. This chapter will cover the systemic disorders of childhood associated with collagen and elastic tissue.

Disorders of Collagen

Ehlers-Danlos Syndrome (cutis hyperelastica)

The Ehlers-Danlos syndrome (E-D, EDG, cutis hyperelastica) is a group of inherited disorders of collagen biosynthesis characterized by increased cutaneous elasticity, hyperextensibility of the joints, and fragility of the skin with impaired wound healing and the formation of pseudotumors and large atrophic or gaping scars. It has now been divided into nine or ten subgroups, each with a characteristic and clinical pattern or unique biochemical defect reflecting genetic abnormalities within the collagen component of the connective tissue.[1, 2] Approximately 50% of patients with stigmata of Ehlers-Danlos syndrome do not fit into one of the ten subtypes and are designated as EDS, type unspecified.[2] The collagenous defect appears to be the manner in which collagen bundles are joined to one another (a defective wickerwork arrangement), which results in increased mobility and rubber-like stretchability of the skin, joints, and many of the other features seen in individuals with this disorder.[3-5]

CLINICAL MANIFESTATIONS.—Many infants with Ehlers-Danlos syndrome are prone to premature birth because of early rupture of membranes (the placenta is determined entirely by the fetal genotype and its membranes have the same fragility as other structures in this disorder). The skin of affected individuals is velvety and soft in texture and on palpation has a peculiar, doughy consistency. It is hyperelastic, yet not lax, except in late stages. After being stretched, it returns to its normal position as soon as the skin is released (Fig 4–1).

In addition to this abnormal elasticity, the skin is extremely fragile, and minor trauma may produce gaping "fish-mouth" wounds. It has poor tensile strength and cannot hold sutures properly. This leads to frequent dehiscence, poor healing, and the formation of wide, papyraceous, wrinkled

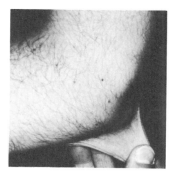

Fig 4–1.—Ehlers-Danlos syndrome. Hyperelasticity of skin overlying the elbow. Contrary to the lax skin seen in patients with cutis laxa, after being stretched it returns to its normal position as soon as released.

hernia-like scars, particularly over areas of trauma (such as the forehead, elbows, and knees) (Fig 4–2). Blood vessels are fragile, resulting in hematomas. The resolution of hematomas is accompanied by fibrosis, which produces soft subcutaneous pseudotumors.

Hyperextensible joints may result in "double-jointed" fingers or frequent subluxation of larger joints (Fig 4–3). This may occur spontaneously or following slight trauma. Muscle tone is often poor, and inguinal and diaphrag-

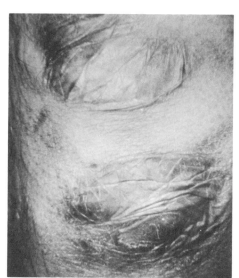

Fig 4–2.—Pseudotumors and papyraceous scars on the knee in Ehlers-Danlos syndrome.

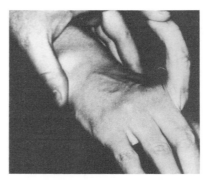

Fig 4–3.—Hyperextensibility of the fingers in Ehlers-Danlos syndrome.

matic hernias are common. Anomalies of the heart and dissecting aortic aneurysms have been described, and although life expectancy is generally normal, premature deaths have occurred from gastrointestinal bleeding, rare bowel perforation, and rupture of cardiovascular defects.[6]

Clinical Types of Ehlers-Danlos Syndrome

E-D types I, II, and III.—The most common forms of Ehlers-Danlos syndrome are inherited in an autosomal dominant pattern and are distinguished by the extent and severity of their clinical features. No biochemical defect has been detected as yet for this group of patients[7] (Table 4–1). Patients with *E-D type I* (the "gravis type") have soft, velvety skin characterized by marked hyperextensibility, fragility and bruising; generalized severe hypermobility of the joints; friability of tissues at surgery, thin "cigarette paper" or wide spreading atrophic, wrinkled, or hyperpigmented scars; frequent, venous varicosities and hernias; and prematurity caused by early rupture of fetal membranes. Life expectancy is normal.

E-D type II (the mitis form) is characterized by milder cutaneous and joint manifestations with soft skin, moderate skin hyperextensibility, and hypermobility of the joints which is generally limited to the hands and feet. Prematurity and friability of the tissues are not usually seen in patients with type II disease.

E-D type III (the benign familial hypermobile type) is manifested by marked generalized joint hypermobility with dislocations, soft but otherwise minimally affected skin, mild cutaneous hyperextensibility, and bleeding problems. The "floppy mitral valve syndrome" (a disorder characterized by redundant chordae tendinae and valve cusps) has been associated with this variant.

TABLE 4–1.—EHLERS-DANLOS SYNDROME

TYPE	NAME	INHERITANCE	CLINICAL FEATURES	TISSUE DEFECT
I	Gravis	Autosomal dominant	Premature birth, soft velvety fragile hyperextensible skin, marked bruising, cigarette paper and fish-mouth scars, marked hypermobility of joints	Unknown
II	Mitis	Autosomal dominant	Less severe, prematurity uncommon, moderately hypermobile joints, moderately hyperextensible skin, varicosities, hernias	Unknown
III	Benign hypermobile	Autosomal dominant	Minimal cutaneous manifestations, marked joint hypermobility, floppy mitral valve may occur	Unknown
IV	Ecchymotic, arterial, or Sack type	Autosomal dominant and recessive forms	Arterial and gastrointestinal rupture, thin skin, EPS common	Deficiency of type III collagen
V	X-linked	X-linked recessive	Similar to type II, skin highly extensible, floppy mitral valve may occur	Lysyl oxidase deficiency
VI	Ocular	Autosomal recessive	Intraocular bleeding, soft velvety skin, cigarette paper scars, severe scoliosis, hyperextensible skin and joints	Lysyl hydroxylase deficiency
VII	Arthrocalasis	Autosomal recessive	Markedly lax joints with multiple dislocations, microcornea, moderate skin fragility, short stature, scoliosis	Structural mutation of type I collagen
VIII	Periodontal	Autosomal dominant	Severe early periodontitis, moderate skin fragility with pretibial scarring, minimal joint hypermobility	Unknown
IX	Fibronectin type	Autosomal recessive	Striae, moderate extensibility of skin, hypermobility of joints, platelet aggregation defect	Dysfunction of plasma fibronectin
X	Maternal	?	Disorders of pregnancy, sinus of Valsalva aneurysms, myocardial infarction, emphysema, normal hemostasis and wound healing	Abnormal fibronectin and collagen (pregnancy seems to improve the abnormality)

E-D type IV (the ecchymotic, arterial, or Sack type), a severe but rare disorder with both autosomal dominant and autosomal recessive forms, is characterized by a deficiency of type III collagen, thin skin, ecchymoses, pinched facies, acrogeria (premature aging of the skin of the hands and feet), and a tendency toward rupture of the great vessels, gastrointestinal tract and uterus. Elastosis perforans serpiginosa, arteriovenous fistulae and varicose veins are also seen in patients with type IV E-D.[8]

E-D type V is an X-linked recessive disorder with clinical features similar to those of patients with E-D II. This variant, in one family at least, is caused by a deficiency of lysyl oxidase, suggesting an increased turnover of collagen and elastin because of a decrease in cross-links (lysyl oxidase is required for cross-linking in collagen and elastin)[9] and a lack of collagen

III.[10, 11] "Floppy mitral valve syndrome" is also associated with this variant.

E-D type VI (the ocular type) is characterized by an autosomal recessive inheritance, a deficiency of lysyl hydroxylase (in some patients), blue sclerae, epicanthal folds, myopia, microcornea with glaucoma, intraocular bleeding, soft, velvety skin, cigarette paper scars and severe scoliosis.[12]

E-D type VII (the arthrochalasis type) is an autosomal recessive disorder characterized by markedly lax joints which result in the development of multiple dislocations, short stature, microcornea, and scoliosis.[13]

E-D type VIII (the periodontal type) is inherited as an autosomal dominant disorder. Individuals with E-D VIII have severe periodontitis at an early age with loss of permanent teeth and moderate skin fragility with ecchymoses that resolve normally (except on the shins where the pretibial skin heals with tender hypopigmented telangiectatic scars). Patients have no evidence of skin hyperextensibility or visceral involvement, and joint hypermobility is minimal.[14]

E-D type IX (the fibronectin type) is an autosomal recessive disorder manifested by striae, moderate extensibility of the skin, joint hypermobility and a platelet aggregation defect caused by a dysfunction of plasma fibronectin.[15]

E-D type X (maternal Ehler-Danlos syndrome) was recently described in a patient with abnormal fibronectin, abnormal collagen fibrils, sinus of Valsalva aneurysms, myocardial infarction, panacinar emphysema, cerebral heterotopias, and disorders of pregnancy.[2, 16] In E-D type X, pregnancy appears to alter the function or level of fibronectin, and patients seem to have normal hemostasis and wound healing. As a result, normal pregnancy and childbearing are possible in patients with this disorder, and the presence of this variant does not seem to be a contraindication to conception (but a cautious approach to such patients is still warranted).[16]

DIAGNOSIS.—The diagnosis of Ehlers-Danlos syndrome is made on the characteristic clinical features of the disorder and its various subgroups. Except for skin that has been altered by trauma, histopathologic examination generally reveals no obvious alteration in thickness of the skin or in the appearance of collagen or elastic fibers. Occasionally, some patients may demonstrate thin collagen fibers that are not united to collagen bundles. In such cases, the skin may be reduced in thickness and a relative increase in elastic fibers may be noted.[17]

TREATMENT.—Management of patients with Ehlers-Danlos syndrome is mainly supportive in nature and should include genetic counseling. The possibility of premature birth should be discussed and cutaneous, skeletal, and ocular difficulties (possible retinal detachment and abnormalities of the lens) should be emphasized. Surgical procedures present problems because tissues are friable and difficult to suture. Edges of gaping wounds should be kept approximated with appropriate sutures and adhesive closure to facilitate healing. Precautions must be taken to minimize trauma to the skin and joints. Pressure bandages over hematomas may help prevent pseudotumor formation.

Ascorbic acid stimulates collagen synthesis in tissues by serving as a cofactor for prolyhydroxylase and lysylhydroxylase, enzymes that catalyze the formation of hydroxyproline and hydroxylysine. Large doses of ascorbic acid, in doses of 2 to 4 grams a day, have been utilized in some patients with type 6 Ehlers-Danlos syndrome with apparent clinical response.[18]

Lipoid Proteinosis (Hyalinosis Cutis et Mucosae)

Lipoid proteinosis (hyalinosis cutis et mucosae) is a rare, chronic, autosomal recessively inherited disorder of lipid metabolism characterized by hoarseness and hyaline deposition in the skin, mucous membranes, upper respiratory tract and occasionally the upper gastrointestinal tract and other visceral organs. The exact cause of lipoid proteinosis is unknown, but appears to be related to an abnormal deposition of hyaline material (believed to be a glycoprotein) elaborated by and associated with a enzyme deficit of fibrocytes.[19–21] Although termed *lipoid* proteinosis, the hyaline consists of type IV collagen and lipids do not appear to be an essential feature of this disorder.[22]

CLINICAL MANIFESTATIONS.—Hoarseness secondary to vocal cord involvement is a clinical feature in virtually every case of lipoid proteinosis. Persons with this disorder can be easily recognized because of their husky voice and thickened eyelids. The voice may be hoarse from birth or within the first few years of life and become progressively worse during early childhood. Further examination of such individuals commonly reveals hyperkeratotic plaques on elbows and knees, morphea-like plaques on the trunk, and yellowish papular and nodular infiltrates on the skin and mucous membranes[21] (Table 4–2).

In a typical case, the skin is yellow-white in color and resembles old ivory. Individual lesions consisting of discrete or confluent 2 to 3 mm yellowish-white to yellowish-brown papules are found most frequently on the face, eyelids, neck, and hands. In about 50% of individuals, a string of bead-like papules, often followed by a loss of cilia, appear on the free eyelid margins. Also characteristic are eversion of the lips (with their surfaces studded with tiny yellow nodules), hypertrophic or vegetative lesions at the corners of the mouth, and round papules just below the lip on the midline of the chin. Skin lesions, particularly in children, may also occur as vesicles, pustules, or bullae. Ulcerations; atrophic or varioliform scars; plaques simulating localized scleroderma; radiating fissures at the corners

TABLE 4–2.—Lipoid Proteinosis
(Hyalinosis cutis et mucosae)

1. Autosomal recessive with increase in type IV collagen
2. Clinical manifestations
   a. Husky voice with thick woody tongue, thickened eyelids with loss of cilia and bead-like papules on free eyelid margins
   b. Yellowish papular and nodular infiltrates in skin and mucous membranes
   c. Yellowish white skin, morphea-like plaques on trunk, and hyperkeratotic plaques on elbows and knees
   d. CNS involvement (attacks of rage, psychomotor or grand mal seizures)
3. Histology: hyperkeratotic epidermis and PAS-positive amorphous material in upper dermis with patchy distribution surrounding bvv, sweat gg and arrector pili muscles

of the mouth; alopecia of the scalp, eyebrows, eyelashes, or bearded area; impaired nail growth; and multiple confluent papules seen as verrucous plaques on the elbows, knees, hands, and feet help complete the picture.

The tongue becomes thick, firm and woody (because of hyaline deposition), and is bound to the floor of the mouth and difficult to extrude. Dysphagia caused by pharyngeal infiltration and respiratory obstruction as a result of severe laryngeal involvement can complicate the disorder. The abnormal glycoprotein has also been found in the stomach, intestine, trachea, lungs, eyes, pancreas, bladder, kidney, vagina, testes, lymph nodes, and striated muscle. A diabetic tendency has also been stated to be part of the syndrome (in 20% of family members and affected individuals). This finding, however, requires further investigation and documentation.

Central nervous system involvement has been associated with attacks of rage and psychomotor or grand mal epilepsy. Although intracranial calcification seen as bilateral bean-shaped opacities above the sella turcica on radiographic examination have been held responsible for convulsive seizures in patients with hyalinosis cutis et mucosae, the central nervous systemic involvement is restricted to asymptomatic calcification in 70% of patients above 10 years of age.

DIAGNOSIS.—Diagnosis is aided by a history of hoarseness from early childhood; thickening, stiffening, and difficulty in extrusion of the tongue; an impaired ability to swallow; characteristic involvement of the skin and mucous membranes; and histopathologic examination of involved tissue. Histologic features consist of a hyperkeratotic and occasionally papillomatous epidermis and thick homogeneous bands of eosinophilic, PAS-positive, hyaline-like, amorphous material in the upper dermis with an associated patchy distribution surrounding blood vessels, sweat glands, and arrector pili muscles.

TREATMENT.—Lipoid proteinosis has a chronic but relatively benign course. Treatment is chiefly symptomatic and consists of surgical removal of laryngeal nodules, tracheostomy for laryngeal obstruction, and cosmetic measures such as dermabrasion or electrodesiccation and curettage for unappealing cutaneous lesions on the face or other exposed surfaces.

Focal Dermal Hypoplasia (Goltz syndrome)

Focal dermal hypoplasia (Goltz syndrome) is a rare hereditary disorder characterized by linear areas of dermal hypoplasia with herniation of underlying tissue, telangiectasia, linear or reticular areas of hyperpigmentation or hypopigmentation, localized superficial fatty deposits in the skin, red papillomas on mucous membranes or periorificial skin, and anomalies of the extremities including syndactyly, adactyly, and oligodactyly. Available family histories of patients with focal dermal hypoplasia suggest that this condition is caused by an X-linked dominant trait lethal to homozygous males.[23] The disorder generally occurs in females. When it occurs in males, it probably represents a new mutation.[24]

CLINICAL MANIFESTATIONS.—The cutaneous manifestations of focal dermal hypoplasia include (1) widely distributed linear areas of hypoplasia of the skin; (2) soft yellowish nodules, often in a linear distribution; and (3) large ulcers (due to congenital absence of skin) that gradually heal with atrophy. Additional abnormalities include lack of a digit which may be associated with syndactyly and "lobster-claw" deformities, colobomata of the eyes, and hypoplasia of hair, nails, or teeth[23] (Table 4–3).

Streaky pigmentation, atrophy, and telangiectasia are usually present at birth over the trunk and extremities. Yellowish-brown nodules of subcutaneous fat; red papillomatosis of the skin or mucosae of the oral, anal, or genital regions; hypohidrosis; and paper-thin nails have been associated with this syndrome. Other cutaneous abnormalities include sparseness of hair, lichenoid follicular hyperkeratotic papules and keratotic lesions on the

TABLE 4–3.—FOCAL DERMAL HYPOPLASIA
(GOLTZ SYNDROME)

1. X-linked dominant, lethal to homozygous males
2. Linear hypoplasia of skin, soft yellowish nodules in a linear distribution, large ulcers, syndactyly, "lobster-claw" deformities, colobomata of eyes, and hypoplasia of hair, nails, or teeth
3. Dx:
   a. Hypoplasia or absence of dermal tissue with upward extension of subcutaneous fat
   b. Osteopathia striata (striations in metaphyses of long bones or near epiphyseal junctions)

palms and soles. Skeletal anomalies include syndactyly, polydactyly, absence or hypoplasia of a digit or hand bone, clinodactyly, vertebral anomalies, scoliosis, spina bifida, and aplasia or hypoplasia of the clavicle. Other associated abnormalities include umbilical or inguinal hernia, strabismus, colobomata, microphthalmia, hypodontia and hypoplasia of the dental enamel and, in some affected individuals, microcephaly and mental retardation.

DIAGNOSIS.—Disorders included in the differential diagnosis of this condition include congenital ectodermal dysplasia, congenital poikiloderma (Rothmund-Thomson syndrome), incontentia pigmenti, linear scleroderma, and nevus lipomatosus cutaneous superficialis of Hoffman and Zurhelle (an extremely rare cutaneous nevus of localized groups of soft papules or nodules manifested in the newborn).

Virtually all cases of focal dermal hypoplasia reveal fine parallel linear striations in the metaphysis of long bones at or near the epiphyseal junctions on x-ray. Although striations can be seen with other bony abnormalities, this linear change in the metaphyseal regions of the long bones (termed *osteopathia striata*) is a very useful index for the diagnosis of this disorder.[25] When there is doubt, the diagnosis can be verified by biopsy of an affected area of the skin. Histopathologic features consist of absence or hypoplasia of dermal connective tissue with upward extension of the subcutaneous fat tissue almost to the normal epidermis.

TREATMENT.—Except for surgery for developmental defects such as syndactyly or polydactyly, very little can be done for patients with focal dermal hypoplasia.

Osteogenesis Imperfecta

The term osteogenesis imperfecta (OI) refers to a group of inherited connective tissue disorders characterized by osseous fragility, skeletal deformity, blue sclerae, impaired hearing, cutaneous fragility, hypermobility of the joints, and imperfect dentition. Along with Marfan syndrome, osteogenesis imperfecta ranks among the most common inherited disorders of connective tissue. A heterogeneous disorder, several clinical groups have been described. These include a congenital form, a tarda form that can be subdivided into a severe heterogeneous group and a mild autosomal dominant form, and a fourth type, autosomal dominant in nature, termed the dentogenesis imperfecta form[26] (Table 4–4). Abnormalities in the bone and other connective tissues of patients with the various forms of osteogenesis imperfecta suggest an abnormality of type I collagen synthesis and maturation with secondary effects combining to produce the defects seen in patients with the various forms of this disorder.[26–28]

SYSTEMIC MANIFESTATIONS.—In patients with the congenital form of os-

TABLE 4–4.—OSTEOGENESIS IMPERFECTA

GROUP	INHERITANCE	CLINICAL FEATURES
I Congenital (severe)	Autosomal recessive	Low birth weight, severe micromelia, bowing of limbs, and multiple fractures. Patients rarely survive.
II Tarda (severe)	Heterogeneous, sporadic	Normal birth weight, progressive deformities, growth failure, recurrent fractures, blue or normal sclerae, dentogenesis imperfecta usually present, deafness uncommon, frequent neonatal deaths.
III Tarda (mild)	Autosomal dominant	Fracture tendency mild (congenital fractures rare), blue sclerae, dentogenesis imperfecta usually absent, deafness and family history of deafness common.
IV Dentogenesis imperfecta	Autosomal dominant	Patients are mildly affected, occasional fractures, normal sclerae, dentogenesis imperfecta (cardinal feature), deafness not reported.

teogenesis imperfecta, fractures may occur in utero or during delivery. These patients are usually stillborn or die early. Generally of low birth weight, they have severe micromalia (abnormally small limbs) with bowing, and multiple fractures. Patients with the tarda variety often do not sustain fractures until later in life, generally when they are one or two years of age or older. Repeated fractures produce grotesque deformities (especially of the limbs, and, in many patients, shortened stature), and affected individuals have bluish to normal colored sclera. Patients with the dentogenesis imperfecta form have normal sclerae, mild to moderate osteoporosis, and only occasionally have fractures (Table 4–4).

The skin may be thin, atrophic, and somewhat translucent. Although wound healing may be normal, scars frequently are atrophic or hypertrophic. Widened fishmouth scars such as seen in patients with Ehlers-Danlos syndrome have been described. The teeth are susceptible to caries, break easily, and have an abnormal color ranging from amber yellow to bluish gray. China blue sclerae, when present, are a particularly distinctive feature of the disease and are seen in about 90% of patients. Caused by the choroid pigment showing through the thin sclera, several hues of blue have been described. Blue sclerae, however, also may be seen in patients with Marfan's and Ehlers-Danlos syndromes and therefore are not pathognomonic of osteogenesis imperfecta. Other features of OI include otosclerosis with hearing loss which may begin during the second or third decade of life, and cardiovascular lesions including mitral and aortic valve dilatation with regurgitation, floppy mitral valve syndrome and cystic medionecrosis of the aorta.[26]

DIAGNOSIS.—Diagnosis is dependent upon the clinical manifestations and at times family history. Affected bones show thinning of the cortex and trabeculae spongiosa, disorganization of collagen matrix and poor organic bone matrix. Histopathologic examination of the skin shows a reduction of normal adult collagen fibers and an increase in argyrophilic fibers.

TREATMENT.—The treatment of this disorder is difficult and frequently requires psychological as well as medical and surgical support. Since pregnancy presents a danger to an affected mother or infant, cesarean section is recommended in an effort to prevent fractures. Pinning and plating of fractures has been helpful but immobilization is to be avoided since this results in further decrease in bone matrix. Promising results have been achieved in some cases with synthetic salmon calcitonin (Calcimar), a compound that directly inhibits bone absorption and enhances bone formation. However, the efficacy of this therapy requires further confirmation.[29, 30]

Marfan Syndrome

The Marfan syndrome is a heritable disorder of connective tissue characterized by excessive length of long bones, ocular defects (particularly ectopia lentis), and cardiovascular defects. Inherited as an autosomal dominant trait with a high degree of penetrance and variable expressivity, it has an estimated prevalence of about 1.5 per 100,000 population. Although the nature of the basic defect is unknown, studies of collagen metabolism suggest abnormalities of collagen function and disorders of cross-link formation in type I collagen as factors in the biochemical etiology of this syndrome.[26, 31] Other investigations suggest alterations in the synthesis of hyaluronic acid.[32] Future investigations will need to focus on abnormalities in the structural aspects of collagen cross-link formation and on the relationships of collagen and proteoglycan metabolism. It now appears that several distinct biochemical abnormalities will eventually be found as factors in the etiology of this complex clinical syndrome.

CLINICAL MANIFESTATIONS.—The chief manifestations of the Marfan syndrome are skeletal, ocular, and cardiovascular (Table 4–5). Patients with this disorder are often tall and their extremities are long. The arm span characteristically is greater than the height, and after puberty the lower segment (pubis to sole) measurement is greater than that of the upper segment (vertex to pubis). Arachnodactyly, hyperextensible joints, kyphoscoliosis, pectus excavatus, and flat feet are commonly seen in patients with this disorder. At times the great toes are elongated out of proportion to the

TABLE 4–5.—Marfan Syndrome

1. Autosomal dominant (approximately 1.5/100,000)
2. A disorder of cross-link formation in type I collagen?
3. Skeletal manifestations (arachnodactyly, hyperextensible joints, dolichocephaly, kyphoscoliosis, pectus excavatus)
4. Ocular manifestations (ectopia lentis in 50% to 70%, myopia, heterochromia iridis, retinal detachment)
5. Cardiovascular manifestations (aortic insufficiency, mitral regurgitation, aneurysms of ascending aorta)

others; the skull and face are elongated; and dolichocephaly, frontal bossing, high arched palate, and large deformed ears are frequently seen.[33–35]

Ocular abnormalities consist of ectopia lentis (the hallmark of ocular involvement, seen in 50% to 70% of patients), myopia, heterochromia iridis, and retinal detachment. Cardiovascular defects, due to a defect in the media of the great vessels, consist of aneurysmal dilatation of the ascending aorta, dilatation of the aortic rings with aortic insufficiency, and dilatation of the mitral rings with mitral regurgitation. Contrary to previous emphasis, mental retardation is not a component of this syndrome. Studies suggest that Abraham Lincoln had Marfan syndrome, and investigation of some of his relatives revealed evidence of this disease or a form fruste of it.[36] Cutaneous changes in this disorder include a pronounced sparsity of subcutaneous fat, striae (particularly over the pectoral and deltoid regions, the thighs, and abdomen), and elastosis perforans serpiginosa.

Diagnosis.—Diagnosis of the Marfan syndrome presents little problem in the severely affected patient, the diagnosis being based on the presence of at least two of the following features: skeletal, ocular, cardiovascular, and genetic abnormalities.[33] Because of the heterogeneity of this disorder, however, diagnosis must occasionally remain tentative in some patients. Careful, long-term observations may be required before a definitive diagnosis can be established.

Treatment.—The prognosis of the Marfan syndrome depends upon the extent and severity of cardiovascular defects. Dissection of the aorta, a frequent cause of death in children as well as adults, is common during the first decade of life and is most commonly seen during the thirties. The average age at the time of death in a study of 72 patients was 32 years, and survival beyond the fifth decade is unusual.[37, 38]

Effective treatment depends upon proper diagnosis and awareness of possible clinical complications. Early ophthalmologic examination should be performed on all patients and relatives suspected of having the Marfan syndrome. Genetic counselling should include a discussion of the fact that an infected parent has a 50% chance of transmitting this disorder to progeny and that even mildly affected patients may produce severely affected offspring.

Although propranolol (Inderal) has been shown to decrease myocardial contractility and reduce the abruptness of ventricular ejection (thus limiting the progression of aortic dilatation), results to date have not been encouraging.[33] Surgical replacement of the aortic or mitral valve and excision of aortic aneurysms, however, have been successful for some patients.[37] Orthopedic surgery with casts and fusion have been helpful in the management of kyphoscoliosis, and aspiration techniques have been recommended when lens extraction is required for patients with glaucoma or serious visual impairment.

Disorders of Elastin

Cutis Laxa

Cutis laxa (generalized elastolysis) is an extremely rare disorder of the elastic tissue characterized by inelastic, loose, and pendulous skin, which results in a wrinkled, prematurely aged, bloodhound-like appearance. Although its pathogenesis is not well understood, current studies suggest a decrease in the amount of elastic tissue in the skin (and rest of the body) as a result of a defect in the synthesis of elastin or an increased destruction of elastic fibers, possibly caused by low levels of elastase inhibitor.[39] The disorder can be acquired or congenital in nature, with the genetic forms inherited as a severe autosomal variant, a less commonly observed, relatively benign, autosomal dominant form, or a rare, X-linked recessive disorder which shares some features with Ehlers-Danlos syndrome. Patients with this type of cutis laxa have a deficiency of the collagen and elastin cross-linking enzyme lysyl oxidase.[40, 41] The acquired form of cutis laxa has been associated with other generalized disorders and may follow a febrile illness, an allergic reaction, urticaria, drug eruption, or erythema multiforme. It also has been described in a patient with multiple myeloma and may occur as a manifestation of an autosomal recessive form of pseudoxanthoma elasticum or as an autosomal dominant form of amyloidosis[26, 39, 42] (Table 4–6).

CLINICAL MANIFESTATIONS.—Patients with cutis laxa present a striking picture of loose, inelastic redundant skin that sags and hangs in pendulous folds as if it were too large for the body. The dropping and ectropion of the eyelids together with the sagging facial skin and accentuation of the nasal, labial, and other facial folds help produce the "bloodhound" or aged appearance (Fig 4–4). Although frequently prominent and, at times, almost grotesque in appearance, as the children grow older they often grow into the skin abnormality and are not as severely affected in later life.

TABLE 4–6.—CUTIS LAXA

TYPE	DEFECT	CLINICAL FEATURES
Autosomal recessive	Abnormal collagen linkage with defect in lysyl oxidase	Relatively rare (more common in females); severe, skin changes; progressive; vascular and pulmonary abnormalities and early death
Autosomal dominant	Unknown	May appear at any age; loose sagging skin with few systemic abnormalities, normal growth and life expectancy
X-linked recessive	Diminished lysyl oxidase with a defect in copper metabolism	Relatively normal facies, mild cutaneous laxity, moderate hypermobility of joints (association with Ehlers-Danlos syndrome?)
Acquired	Unknown	Cutaneous changes mild to moderate; occasional systemic involvement

Systemic manifestations (caused by weakened support tissue) include aortic dilatation, pulmonary artery stenosis, pulmonary emphysema, diverticulae of the gastrointestinal tract or urinary bladder, uterine or rectal prolapse, and ventral, hiatal, or inguinal hernias.[45, 46]

In patients with the severe autosomal recessively inherited disease, the disorder is gradually progressive. Death from pulmonary complications re-

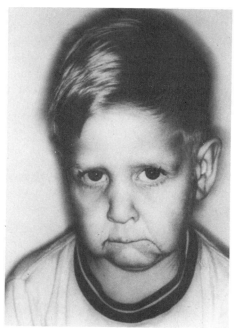

Fig 4–4.—Cutix laxa. Sagging cheeks and bloodhound-like facies. (From Klaus S., in Braverman I.M.: *Skin Signs of Systemic Diseases.* W.B. Saunders Co., Philadelphia, 1970. Used by permission.)

lated to emphysema may occur early in infancy. The autosomal dominant form may appear at any age and presents as a cosmetic problem with few systemic changes. In the X-linked variety, patients share features with Ehlers-Danlos syndrome (relatively normal facies, mild cutaneous laxity and moderate hypermobility of the joints). The acquired type has no genetic background. In some patients, the disorder may be preceded or accompanied by a cutaneous eruption consisting of urticaria, vesicles, or erythematous plaques. As a result of systemic complications, death may occur later in life.[22]

DIAGNOSIS.—The skin in cutis laxa is extensible but, in contrast to that of Ehlers-Danlos syndrome, does not spring back to place on release of tension. In Ehlers-Danlos syndrome, the hyperextensibility of the joints and pseudotumors of the skin with large atrophic scars are diagnostic. In pseudoxanthoma elasticum, the lax skin is covered with characteristic soft yellowish papules and plaques and in neurofibromatosis (von Recklinghausen's disease), the presence of café au lait spots, Lisch nodules and/or fibrous tumors indicate the true nature of the disorder.

Histopathologic examination of the skin in cases of cutis laxa without inflammatory infiltrate reveal a decrease in elastic fibers in the dermis. Those elastic fibers that are present may be thickened in their midportion and taper to a point at either end. Their borders may be indistinct and they may stain unevenly and show a granular appearance. In cases in which an inflammatory infiltrate is present, a nonspecific chronic inflammatory infiltrate of lymphocytes and histiocytes and at times neutrophils may be noted. If vesicles are present, they are subepidermal in location and may show papillary microabscesses composed of neutrophils and eosinophils, suggesting a diagnosis of dermatitis herpetiformis.[22]

TREATMENT.—The therapy of cutis laxa is limited and prognosis in general is poor. Management is based on the awareness of possible complications and affected individuals should be referred to appropriate specialists for evaluation. Family members should be examined for the presence of cutis laxa or other heritable connective tissue disorders. The determination of inheritance patterns, when possible, should guide genetic counseling. Surgery can correct diverticulae, rectal prolapse, or hernias; pulmonary function studies may aid in the early detection of emphysema; and plastic surgery is frequently beneficial with psychological improvement following surgical correction of cosmetic defects.[47]

Pseudoxanthoma Elasticum

Pseudoxanthoma elasticum (PXE) is a degenerative inherited disorder of elastic tissue that involves the skin, eyes, and cardiovascular system. It is characterized by soft yellowish papules and polygonal plaques on the neck, below the clavicles, and in the axillae, antecubital fossae, periumbilical areas, perineum, and thighs. Seen in at least 1 individual per 160,000 population (with a 2:1 predominance in females), there are two recessive and two dominant forms of this disorder. Most cases are autosomal recessive in nature.[48, 49] The pathogenesis remains controversial and appears to be related to an abnormal proliferation of elastic fibers that prematurely calcify and fragment.[49, 50]

CLINICAL MANIFESTATIONS.—Skin lesions are a hallmark of this disorder, with the sides of the neck, the axillae and groin being the most common sites of involvement. Lesions are yellowish in color and xanthoma-like (hence the name pseudoxanthoma), and vary from several papules to linear plaques resembling plucked chicken skin, morocco leather, or orange skin (peau d'orange) (Fig 4–5). As the skin in affected areas becomes relatively inelastic, it may hang in lax redundant folds. This is especially prominent on the neck where the affected skin appears loose and wrinkled. Although lesions may be seen in childhood, they are frequently overlooked because of their small size and lack of symptomatology. As a result, the diagnosis frequently does not become apparent until the patient reaches the second or third decade of life.

Eye changes of this disorder are particularly characteristic. They include reddish, orange-red or slate-gray to brown linear bands (angioid streaks), caused by tears in Bruch's membrane with subsequent fibrosis. Seen in 50% to 70% of cases, angioid streaks are uncommon in young children and usually appear in the second or third decades of life. The association of skin

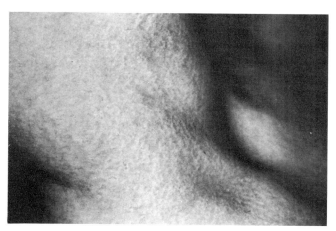

Fig 4–5.—Soft yellowish papules and polygonal plaques in the axilla of a patient with pseudoxanthoma elasticum. (From Hurwitz S.: *Clinical Pediatric Dermatology.* W.B. Saunders Co., Philadelphia, 1981. Used by permission.)

lesions with angioid streaks is known as the Grönblad-Strandberg syndrome. Loss of central vision is the most frequent disability and may develop in more than 70% of cases with this complication. These retinal changes, however, are not pathognomonic as they may also be found in patients with sickle cell anemia, idiopathic thrombocytopenic purpura, acromegaly, Ehlers-Danlos syndrome, lead poisoning, and Paget's disease of the bone.

Significant cardiovascular changes include peripheral artery disease with easy fatigability, intermittent claudication, hypertension, coronary artery involvement, and cerebral, gastrointestinal or uterine hemorrhage. Various authors have cited degeneration of either collagen or elastic tissue in the pathogenesis of mitral-valve prolapse. It is not surprising that patients with PXE have a high incidence of mitral-valve prolapse.[51]

Of the four varieties of pseudoxanthoma elasticum described to date, dominant type I PXE shows the classic "plucked chicken skin" lesions and is characterized by severe retinopathy with visual loss, severe vascular disease, and hypertension. Patients with the more common dominant type II variety exhibit major and minor forms of the eruption with a high incidence of blue sclerae, high arched palate, and loose jointedness. Vascular and ocular disorders in this group are mild. Recessive type I PXE (the classic form of the disorder) is characterized by flexural lesions in most patients, with moderate degrees of retinal and vascular disease. Recessive type II disease is extremely rare with only three cases described to date. These patients had universal involvement of their skin with a lax, loose-fitting appearance and no evidence of systemic involvement[52] (Table 4–7).

DIAGNOSIS.—The diagnosis of PXE is based on the clinical findings described above and histopathologic evidence of calcification of elastic tissue with basophilic degeneration of the elastic tissue in the middle and deeper zones of the dermis. Elastic tissue degeneration also affects connective tis-

TABLE 4–7.—PSEUDOXANTHOMA ELASTICUM

TYPE	CLINICAL FEATURES
Dominant type 1	Classic "plucked chicken skin" lesions; severe and early retinopathy with visual loss frequently leading to blindness; severe vascular disease with hypertension, uterine and gastrointestinal bleeding common
Dominant type 2	Clinical features less severe than dominant type 1; a high incidence of blue sclerae with myopia and mild retinopathy; vascular changes minimal; arched palate, loose jointedness, extensible skin and Marfanoid appearance common
Recessive type 1	Classic flexural lesions, hematemesis may occur but vascular and ocular changes only of moderate severity
Recessive type 2	Extremely rare; universal cutaneous involvement with lax, loose fitting appearance; no systemic involvement

sue elements of the aorta and medium-sized muscular arteries in the heart, kidneys, gastrointestinal tract and other organs.

TREATMENT.—There is no specific therapy for this disorder. Genetic counselling should be provided for patients and their family members. Patients should be advised to avoid contact sports such as boxing, soccer, football, and heavy straining (such as occurs during lifting of weights). Since the disabling aspects of PXE are slow but progressive, regular vascular examinations (including careful auscultation and echocardiographic evaluation in an effort to rule out mitral valve prolapse) and ophthalmologic surveys are important. Fluorescein angiography and stereoscopic ophthalmic examinations are particularly important since early laser beam photocoagulation may prevent progression of retinal tears. Antibacterial prophylaxis before dental work is recommended for patients with mitral-valve prolapse to reduce the possibility of bacterial endocarditis and, although surgical intervention may be necessary at times for gastrointestinal hemorrhage, this complication can generally be managed by a conservative medical approach. Removal of redundant skin by plastic surgery can improve the cosmetic appearance of affected individuals. Dietary restriction of calcium and phosphorus to a minimum daily requirement has been advocated. Although the efficacy of this dietary program is promising, prolonged patient follow-up is required before a thorough statistical analysis can be established for this mode of therapy.[53]

Elastosis Perforans Serpiginosa

Elastosis perforans serpiginosa (EPS, perforating elastoma) is a disorder of elastic tissue characterized by an annular, arciform or linear arrangement of keratotic papules with a predilection for the posterolateral aspects of the neck and occasionally the chin, cheeks, mandibular areas of the face, antecubital fossae, elbows, and knees. Predominantly affecting males, EPS appears to be a genetically determined disorder that frequently serves as a cutaneous marker for systemic disease. Up to 44% of the reported cases of elastosis perforans serpiginosa have been seen in association with disorders such as Down's syndrome, osteogenesis imperfecta, Ehlers-Danlos syndrome type IV, pseudoxanthoma elasticum, cutis laxa, Rothmund-Thomson syndrome, congenital berry aneurysms of the circle of Willis, acrogeria, the Marfan syndrome, morphea, and at times as a complication of penicillamine therapy[54-60] (Table 4-8).

CLINICAL MANIFESTATIONS.—Elastosis perforans serpiginosa usually affects young males, especially those in the second decade of life, and generally disappears spontaneously in five to ten years. Characteristic features consist of deep red conical papules, 2 to 4 mm in diameter, arranged in a linear, circinate, horseshoe, or serpiginous fashion, with an overall length

TABLE 4–8.—ELASTOSIS PERFORANS SERPIGINOSA

1. Annular, arciform, linear or serpiginous arrangement of keratotic papules
   a. Predilection for posterolateral neck
   b. Occasionally chin, cheeks, mandibular areas of face, antecubital fossae, elbows and knees
   c. Distinctive keratotic plugs generally cap individual papules
2. Association with systemic disease (in up to 44%)
3. Histopathology: elongated tortuous channels within epidermis perforated by degenerated elastic tissue

varying from 1.0 to 2.5 cm to as much as 15 to 20 cm (Fig 4–6). Individual papules are generally capped by a distinctive keratotic plug, which when forcibly dislodged, reveals a characteristic bleeding crateriform lesion. Although lesions usually are confined to one area, particularly the nape of the neck, the face, or upper extremities, they may also be widely disseminated.[55]

DIAGNOSIS.—Diagnosis is dependent upon recognition of the characteristic keratotic plug-topped conicle papules in an arciform or linear arrangement. The distinctive histopathologic features consist of elongated tortuous channels within the epidermis, perforated by abnormal and degenerated elastic tissue that is extruded from the dermis.[57]

The histology of penicillamine-induced elastosis perforans serpiginosa, when stained for elastic tissue, reveals less hyperplasia of elastic fibers (except in areas of active transepidermal elimination). In the middle and deep dermis, however, a greater number of hyperplastic elastic fibers with lat-

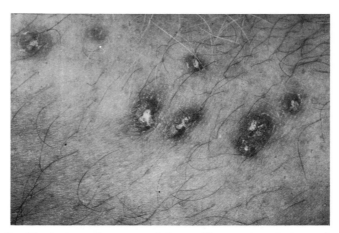

Fig 4–6.—Elastosis perforans serpiginosa. Deep red conical papules in a linear configuration. When forcibly dislodged, the distinctive keratotic plugs seen on individual papules reveal a characteristic bleeding crateriform lesion.

eral budding may be noted. These buds, arranged perpendicular to the principal fibers, have been described as having a characteristic serrated saw-toothed or bramble bush-like histologic appearance.[60]

TREATMENT.—Recognition of the high incidence of associated systemic diseases is crucial in the management of patients with this disorder. Although treatment is generally unsatisfactory and recurrences are common, stripping of the surface keratinous material by repeated application of Scotch tape has resulted in improvement of some lesions, and cryosurgical techniques may produce a satisfactory cosmetic result. Because of a high incidence of residual scar and keloid formation, however, electrodesiccation, curettage, and surgical excision are not recommended.[54]

REFERENCES

1. Byers T.H., Barsh G.S., Holbrook K.A.: Disorders of connective tissue metabolism as related to the skin, in Blandau R.J. (ed.): *Morphogenesis and Malformation of the Skin.* Alan R. Liss, Inc., New York, 1981, pp. 147–172.
2. Cupo L.N., Pyeritz R.E., Olson J.L., et al.: Ehlers-Danlos syndrome with abnormal collagen fibrils, sinus of Valsalva aneurysms, myocardial infarction, panacinar emphysema and cerebral heterotopias. *Am. J. Med.* 71:1051–1058, 1981.
3. Hashimoto K., diBella R.J.: Electron microscopic studies of normal and abnormal elastic fibers of the skin. *J. Invest. Dermatol.* 48:405–423, 1967.
4. Jansen L.H.: The structure of connective tissue, an explanation of symptoms of Ehlers-Danlos syndrome. *Dermatologica* 110:108–120, 1955.
5. McKusick V.A.: *Heritable Disorders of Connective Tissue,* ed. 4. C.V. Mosby Company, St. Louis, 1972.
6. Beighton P., Murdoch J.L., Votteler T.: Gastrointestinal complications of the Ehlers-Danlos syndrome. *Gut* 10:1004–1008, 1969.
7. Uitto J., Lichtenstein J.R.: Defects in the biochemistry of collagen in diseases of connective tissue (Review). *J. Invest. Dermatol.* 66:59–79, 1976.
8. Barabas A.P.: Vascular complications in the Ehlers-Danlos syndrome with special reference to the "arterial type" or Sack's syndrome. *J. Cardiovasc. Surg.* 13:160–167, 1972.
9. Prockop D.J., Kivirriko K.I., Tuderman L., et al.: Medical Progress. The biosynthesis of collagen and its disorders. *N. Engl. J. Med.* 301:13–23; 77–85, 1979.
10. Pope F.M., Martin G.R., McKusick V.A.: Inheritance of Ehlers-Danlos type IV syndrome. *J. Med. Genet.* 14:200–204, 1977.
11. Pope F.M., Martin G.R., Lichtenstein J.R., et al.: Patients with Ehlers-Danlos syndrome type IV lack type III collagen. *Proc. Natl. Acad. Sci., U.S.A.,* 72:1314–1316, 1975.
12. Pinnell S.R., Krane S.M., Kenzora J.E., et al.: A heritable disorder of connective tissue: hydroxylysine-deficient collagen disease. *N. Engl. J. Med.* 286:1013–1020, 1972.
13. Lichtenstein J.R., Martin G.R., Kohn L., et al.: Defect in conversion of procollagen to collagen in a form of Ehlers-Danlos syndrome. *Science* 182:298–300, 1973.

14. Nelson D.L., King R.A.: Ehlers-Danlos syndrome type VIII. *J. Am. Acad. Dermatol.* 5:297–303, 1981.

15. Arneson M.A., Hammerschmidt D.E., Furcht L.T., et al.: A new form of Ehlers-Danlos syndrome, I. Fibronectin corrects defective platelet function. *J.A.M.A.* 244:144–147, 1980.

16. Hammerschmidt D.E., Arneson M.A., Larson S.L., et al.: Maternal Ehlers-Danlos syndrome type X. Successful management of pregnancy and parturition. *J.A.M.A.* 248:2487–2488, 1982.

17. Sulica V.I., Cooper P.H., Pope M.F., et al.: Cutaneous histologic features in Ehlers-Danlos syndrome. Study of 21 patients. *Arch. Dermatol.* 115:40–42, 1979.

18. Elsas L.J., Miller R.L., Pinnell S.R.: Inherited human collagen lysyl hydroxylase deficiency: ascorbic acid response. *J. Pediatr.* 92:378–384, 1978.

19. Caplan R.M.: Visceral involvement in lipoid proteinosis. *Arch. Dermatol.* 95:149–155, 1967.

20. Hashimoto K., Klingmuller G., Rodermund O.E.: Hyalinosis cutis et mucosae. *Acta Dermatovener.* 52:179–195, 1972.

21. Shore R.N., Howard B.V., Howard W.J., et al.: Lipoid proteinosis. Demonstration of normal lipid metabolism in cultured cells. *Arch. Dermatol.* 110:591–594, 1974.

22. Lever W.F., Schaumburg-Lever G.: Congenital diseases (Genodermatoses) and Metabolic Diseases, in *Histopathology of the Skin*, ed. 6. J.P. Lippincott Co., Philadelphia, 1983, pp. 57–91, pp. 407–439.

23. Goltz R.W., Henderson R.R., Hitch J.M., et al.: Focal dermal hypoplasia syndrome: a review of the literature and report of two cases. *Arch. Dermatol.* 101:1–11, 1970.

24. Happle R., Lenz W.: Striation of bones in focal dermal hypoplasia: manifestation of functional mosaicism. *Br. J. Dermatol.* 96:113–138, 1977.

25. Howell J.B., Reynolds J.: Osteopathia Striata. *Trans. St. John's Hosp. Dermatol. Soc.* 60:178–182, 1974.

26. Freiberger H.L., Pinnell S.R.: Heritable disorders of connective tissue, in Moschella S.L. (Editor-in-Chief): *Dermatology Update*. Reviews for physicians. 1979 Edition, Elsevier, New York, pp. 221–253.

27. Sykes B., Francis M.J.O., Smith R.: Altered relation of two collagen types in osteogenesis imperfecta. *N. Engl. J. Med.* 296:1200–1203, 1977.

28. Trelstad R.L., Rubin D., Gross J.: Osteogenesis imperfecta congenita: evidence for a generalized molecular disorder of collagen. *Lab. Invest.* 36:501–508, 1977.

29. Zansi I., Wallach S., Ellis K.J., et al.: Long term treatment of osteogenesis imperfecta tarda in adults with salmon calciton and calcium. *Curr. Ther. Res.* 19:189–197, 1976.

30. Rosenberg E., Lang R., Boisseau V., et al.: Effect of long-term calcitonin therapy on the clinical course of osteogenesis imperfecta. *J. Clin. Endocrinol. Metabol.* 44:346–355, 1977.

31. Boucek R.J., Noble N.L., Gunja-Smith Z., et al.: Marfan syndrome: deficiency in chemically stable collagen cross-links. *N. Engl. J. Med.* 305:988–991, 1981.

32. Appel A., Horwitz A.L., Dorfman A.: Cell-free synthesis of hyaluronic acid in Marfan syndrome. *J. Biol. Chem.* 254:12199–12203, 1979.

33. Pyeritz R.E., McKusick V.A.: Current concepts: the Marfan syndrome—diagnosis and management. *N. Engl. J. Med.* 300:772–777, 1979.

34. Beals R.K., Hecht F.: Congenital contractural arachnodactyly: a heritable disorder of connective tissue. *J. Bone Joint Surg.* 534:987–993, 1971.
35. Walker B.A., Beighton P.H., Murdoch J.L.: The Marfanoid hypermobility syndrome. *Ann. Int. Med.* 71:349–352, 1969.
36. Gordon A.M.: Abraham Lincoln—a medical appraisal. *J. Kentucky Med. Assn.* 60:249–253, 1962.
37. Murdoch J.L., Walker B.A., Halpern B.L., et al.: Life expectancy and causes of death in the Marfan syndrome. *N. Engl. J. Med.* 206:804–808, 1972.
38. Gallotti R., Ross D.N.: The Marfan syndrome: surgical techniques and follow-up in 50 patients. *Ann. Thorac. Surg.* 29:428–433, 1980.
39. Goltz R.W., Hult A.M., Goldfarb M., et al.: Cutis laxa: manifestations of generalized elastolysis. *Arch. Dermatol.* 92:373–387, 1965.
40. Gorlin R.J., Pindborg J.J., Cohen M.M., Jr.: *Syndromes of the Head and Neck,* ed. 2, McGraw-Hill, New York, 1976.
41. Sakati N.O., Nyhan W.L.: Congenital cutis laxa and osteoporosis. *Am. J. Dis. Child.* 137:452–454, 1983.
42. Marchase P., Holbrook, K., Pinnell, S.R.: A familial cutis laxa syndrome with ultrastructural abnormalities of collagen and elastin. *J. Invest. Dermatol.* 75:399–403, 1980.
43. Harris R.V., Hearphy M.R., Perry H.O.: Generalized elastolysis (cutis laxa). *Am. J. Med.* 68:815–822, 1978.
44. Beighton P.: The dominant and recessive forms of cutis laxa. *J. Med. Genet.* 9:216–221, 1972.
45. Mehregan A.H., Lee S.C., Nabai H.: Cutis laxa (generalized elastolysis). *J. Cutan. Pathol.* 5:116–126, 1978.
46. Maxwell E., Esterly N.B.: Cutis laxa. *Am. J. Dis. Child.* 117:479–482, 1969.
47. McKusick V.A.: *Heritable Disorders of Connective Tissue,* ed. 4. C.V. Mosby Co., St. Louis, 1972.
48. Pope F.M.: Two types of autosomal recessive pseudoxanthoma elasticum. *Arch. Dermatol.* 110:209–212, 1974.
49. Pope F.M.: Historical evidence for the genetic heterogeneity of pseudoxanthoma elasticum. *Br. J. Dermatol.* 92:493–509, 1975.
50. Goodman R.M., Smith E.W., Paton D., et al.: Pseudoxanthoma elasticum: a clinical and histopathological study. *Medicine* 42:297–334, 1963.
51. Lebwohl M.G., DiStefano D., Prioleau P.G., et al.: Pseudoxanthoma elasticum and mitral-valve prolapse. *N. Engl. J. Med.* 307:228–231, 1982.
52. Eddy D.D., Farber E.M.: Pseudoxanthoma elasticum. Internal manifestations with a report of cases and a statistical review of the literature. *Arch. Dermatol.* 86:729–740, 1962.
53. Neldner K.H.: Pseudoxanthoma elasticum, in Maddin S. (editor): *Current Dermatologic Therapy,* W.B. Saunders Publishing Co., Philadelphia, 1982, pp. 387–391.
54. Christianson H.B.: Elastosis perforans serpiginosa: association with congenital anomalies: Report of 2 cases. *Southern Med. J.* 59:15–19, 1966.
55. Barr R.J.: Elastosis perforans serpiginosa associated with morphea. *J. Amer. Acad. Dermatol.* 3:19, 1980.
56. Rasmussen J.E.: Disseminated elastosis perforans serpiginosa in four mongoloids. *Br. J. Dermatol.* 86:9–12, 1972.
57. Mehregan H.M.: Elastosis perforans. A review of the literature and report of 11 cases. *Arch. Dermatol.* 97:381–393, 1968.

58. Pass F., Goldfischer S., Sternlieb I., et al.: Elastosis perforans serpiginosa during pencillamine therapy for Wilson disease. *Arch. Dermatol.* 108:713–715, 1973.
59. Kirsch N., Hukill P.B.: Elastosis perforans serpiginosa induced by penicillamine. *Arch. Dermatol.* 113:630–635, 1977.
60. Hashimoto K., McEvoy B., Belcher R.: Ultrastructure of penicillinamine-induced skin lesions. *J. Am. Acad. Dermatol.* 4:300–315, 1981.

5 / The Collagen Vascular Disorders

THE COLLAGEN VASCULAR DISORDERS represent a group of diseases characterized by inflammatory changes of the connective tissue in various parts of the body. Of these, lupus erythematosus, dermatomyositis, scleroderma, eosinophilic fasciitis, rheumatoid arthritis, mixed connective tissue disease, and Sjögren's syndrome exhibit a variety of cutaneous findings that help indicate the presence of connective tissue disease.[1]

Lupus Erythematosus

Lupus erythematosus is a chronic inflammatory disorder that may affect the skin as well as most other organ systems. Although the etiology is unknown, current evidence suggests an autoimmune basis to the disorder. Current studies and reports of familial cases of lupus erythematosus suggest a strong genetic component with altered cellular immunity (reduction in circulating immune complexes of the DNA-anti-DNA type resulting in tissue inflammation and injury) in genetically predisposed individuals as factors in the pathogenesis of this disorder.[2, 3]

Typically a disease of young women, the disorder is seen in all age groups. Up to one-fourth (15% to 20%) of all cases of systemic lupus erythematosus (SLE) occur within the first two decades of life.[4] The onset in adults is usually during the third and fourth decades of life; in childhood the disorder usually begins in those over eight years of age, and the peak incidence occurs between the 11th and 13th years. Systemic lupus in children is generally more acute and severe than in adults. Although several cases have been described in newborns, except for neonatal lupus, the disorder rarely is seen before the age of three years.[5]

Clinically, two types of lupus erythematosus are generally described, but division into only two forms represents an oversimplification of this multifaceted disease complex. Cutaneous, often referred to as *discoid lupus erythematosus* (DLE), is a cutaneous disorder without systemic manifestations seen at the benign end of the LE spectrum; *systemic lupus erythematosus* (SLE) is a chronic multisystem disease. In addition, two intermediate types have been described. These have been termed *disseminated discoid lupus erythematosus* (disseminated DLE), which shows widespread discoid lesions and usually mild systemic involvement, and *subacute lupus erythematosus*, a subset used to describe individuals who manifest widespread erythematosus, confluent, often annular or polycyclic nonscarring cutaneous lesions, severe photosensitivity, diffuse nonscarring alopecia, and mild systemic disease (namely musculoskeletal [arthritis or arthralgia]) and serologic abnormalities without serious renal or CNS disease.[6]

Females with SLE outnumber males by a ratio of 8 to 1 in all age groups, except in prepubertal patients in whom the sex incidence seems to be about equal.[7] Cutaneous or discoid LE is rare in children, and most childhood cases have been systemic in nature, with widespread involvement of multiple organ systems.[8] Although it has been stated that SLE appears to have a greater severity in children than in adults (the younger the patient, the more acute the disorder), a recent review suggests that patterns and prognosis of this disorder in children may indeed be similar to those of adults.[9]

CLINICAL MANIFESTATIONS.—Although the incidence of cutaneous (discoid) lupus erythematosus is less common in childhood, the cutaneous lesions of discoid LE in children and adults are similar. About 80% of patients with systemic lupus erythematosus have cutaneous involvement at some time and in up to 25% of patients, cutaneous lesions are the initial presenting sign of the disorder. A butterfly rash often appears over the cheeks and bridge of the nose. This so-called malar or "butterfly" rash,

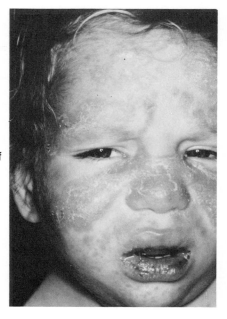

Fig 5–1.—Lupus erythematosus. Scaly erythematous urticarial plaques on the face, with scaling and crusting of the lips in a 2-year-old boy with systemic lupus erythematosus.

seen in 30% to 60% of patients with systemic lupus erythematosus is neither a specific nor the most frequent sign of lupus erythematosus.[1]

The classic discoid lesion of LE is a well-circumscribed, elevated, indurated red to purplish plaque with adherent scale (Fig 5–1), fine telangiectasia, and areas of atrophy. Discoid lesions can be asymmetrical on the head and face, scalp, arms, legs, hands, fingers, back, chest, or abdomen. At times the openings of hair follicles are dilated and plugged by an overlying scale. If the scale is thick enough, it can be lifted off in one piece. The undersurface then reveals follicular projections that resemble carpet tacks, a characteristic sign of lupus erythematosus.[1]

Another common lesion of LE is the reddish-purple urticarial plaque, which is relatively fixed in shape and does not undergo atrophy or scaling. This lesion, often associated with photosensitivity, usually occurs on the face of other exposed areas of the body (Fig 5–2). Although cutaneous lesions and photosensitivity are of diagnostic and cosmetic significance, photosensitivity reactions have also been known to precipitate fatal exacerbations of the disease. Untreated lesions may develop permanent areas of hyper- or hypopigmentation with atrophy—another common cutaneous manifestation of lupus erythematosus.

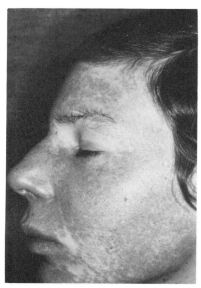
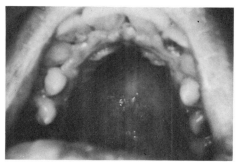

Fig 5–2 (left).—Reddish-purple plaques on the face following sun exposure in a 17-year-old patient with systemic lupus erythematosus.

Fig 5–3 (right).—Ulcerated mucosal lesions on the palate of a 16-year-old girl with lupus erythematosus.

Mucous membrane lesions (gingivitis, mucosal hemorrhage, erosions, and small ulcerations) (Fig 5–3) occur in 3% of patients with cutaneous LE and in from 10% to 15% of patients with the systemic form of the disorder. A silvery whitening of the vermilion border of the lips is highly characteristic and pathognomonic of lupus erythematosus. The lips are often involved, with slight thickening, roughness, and redness, with or without superficial ulceration and crusting. One must never neglect to examine the nose and mouth of patients for evidence of silvery-white scaling and ulcerations. The gingivae may also appear red, edematous, friable, and eroded, or they may exhibit silvery-white changes similar to those on the nasal or buccal mucosa.

Scarring alopecia, another important marker of lupus erythematosus, may be seen as single or multiple well-demarcated patches that exhibit erythema, scaling, telangiectasia, atrophy, and plugging (the classic changes of LE). Increased fragility of the hair in LE may produce broken hairs several millimeters from the roots, resulting in a receding hairline with an unruly appearance due to the short broken hairs ("lupus hair").

Livedo reticularis, a peculiar blotchy bluish-red discoloration of the skin due to vasospasm of the arterioles, although often normal in young children, may be the earliest sign of lupus erythematosus, rheumatoid arthritis, rheumatic fever, or scleroderma. It can also be seen in patients with leukemia, idiopathic thrombocytopenia, periarteritis nodosa, cryoglobulinemia, or neurologic abnormalities, or in those on immunosuppressive therapy. Aggravated by exposure to cold, the area becomes livid or cyanotic when the arterial supply is reduced. Livedo reticularis, when it affects the entire trunk or limbs in a continuous manner, is often a normal phenomenon. When it develops in a blotchy interrupted configuration, however, it is frequently a sign of systemic disease.

Other vascular phenomena associated with lupus erythematosus include Raynaud's phenomenon and urticaria. Raynaud's phenomenon, seen in 10% to 30% of patients with LE, as in scleroderma may precede the onset of disease by months or years.[1] This phenomenon is described in more detail in the section on scleroderma.

Chronic urticaria-like lesions associated with a leukocytoclastic vasculitis may also be the first sign of LE. The extent of hives, seen at some time in 7% to 22% of patients with lupus erythematosus, frequently reflects the activity of the disease and, at times, may serve as a useful guide to therapy.[1, 9] Generally persisting for a more prolonged period of time than classic urticaria, urticaria seen in association with lupus erythematosus tends to be chronic and is often associated with hypocomplementemia. Probably a manifestation of immune complex deposition, it generally occurs in patients demonstrating clinical or serologic evidence of systemic disease activity.[10]

Telangiectases represent another characteristic vascular marker of connective tissue disease. Distinctive findings here include papular telangiectasia of the palms and fingers (Fig 5–4) and linear telangiectasia of the cuticles and periungual skin (with or without thromboses). Cuticular telangiectasia is not specific for LE; it is also seen in patients with dermatomyositis and scleroderma, and in about 5% of patients with rheumatoid arthritis. Diffuse angitis, with or without ulceration, also occurs in about 10% of patients with lupus erythematosus.

Chilblains or perniosis may also be seen in patients with systemic lupus erythematosus. Seen as slightly tender cyanotic to reddish-blue nodules on the fingers or toes of some patients with SLE, the disorder represents cold-induced chronic vasospasm of digital vessels. Seen in up to 12% of patients with discoid lupus erythematosus, chilblain lupus may occur some years after lesions of DLE or may precede the onset of discoid or systemic LE.[11]

Lupus profundus (lupus erythematosus panniculitis), an uncommon subtype of chronic cutaneous lupus erythematosus characterized by deep dermal and subcutaneous inflammatory involvement, occurs in approximately

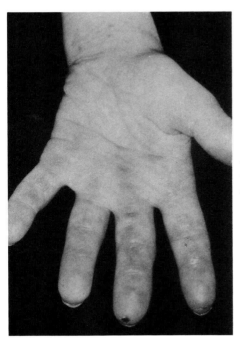

Fig 5–4.—Erythema and papular telangiectasia on the palms and fingers of a child with lupus erythematosus.

2% of patients with cutaneous or systemic LE (1). About 50% of patients with lupus profundus eventually develop systemic involvement. Lesions are seen as firm asymptomatic or tender sharply defined rubbery dermal and subcutaneous nodules with a predilection for the forehead, cheeks, upper arms, breasts, thighs and buttocks. Although the overlying skin usually appears normal, it may be drawn inward with cup-shaped depressions, and attachment to the underlying nodules and ulcerations may occur. Histologically lupus profundus is characterized by a perivascular lymphocytic infiltration in the deep dermis and subcutaneous fat without accompanying fat necrosis. Hyalinization of the connective tissue separating the fat lobules may result in broad septa subdividing the subcutaneous fat and in some cases mucinous changes and foci of calcification may be seen.

SYSTEMIC MANIFESTATIONS.—The systemic manifestations of SLE include fever, malaise, weight loss, fatigue, arthralgia (the most common symptom of the disorder), pleurisy and cardiac complications (pericarditis, endocarditis and extra- and intramural coronary arteritis),[12] ischemic necrosis of bone,[13] renal involvement, and, in 25% of patients, ocular complications (cotton wool patches, perivasculitis and edema of the optic disc). Lymphadenopathy, although common in adults, is relatively rare in children with SLE. Lupus nephritis (diffuse proliferative glomerulonephritis) is seen at the most severe end of the LE spectrum. Characterized by the abrupt appearance of polyarthritis, leukopenia, alopecia, severe proteinuria and an evanescent butterfly rash, it may be seen in 50% to 85% of children at the onset of their systemic lupus erythematosus. Anti-DNA antibody is a serologic marker for this complication (the most common cause of mortality for patients with SLE).[14]

DIAGNOSIS.—The diagnosis of lupus erythematosus is chiefly clinical and is based on the presence of typical cutaneous lesions, systemic manifestations, and confirmatory laboratory tests. A person is said to have SLE if four or more of the following criteria are present: (1) malar rash, (2) discoid rash, (3) photosensitivity, (4) oral ulcers, (5) arthritis, (6) serositis, (7) renal disorder, (8) neurologic disorder, (9) hematologic disorder, (10) immunologic disorder, (11) abnormal antinuclear antibody titer[15] (Table 5–1).

In most instances, a histopathologic diagnosis of lupus erythematosus can be established by a combination of histologic findings. These include hyperkeratosis with keratotic plugging; atrophy of the stratum malpighii; liquefactive degeneration of basal cells; a patchy, chiefly lymphoid cell infiltrate with a tendency to arrangement about the cutaneous appendages; and edema, vasodilation and extravasation of erythrocytes in the upper dermis. However, all five changes are not present in every patient. Of these, focal liquefaction degeneration of the basal layer represents perhaps the most significant histologic change in lupus erythematosus. In its absence, a his-

TABLE 5–1.—CRITERIA FOR CLASSIFICATION OF SYSTEMIC LUPUS
ERYTHEMATOSUS*

CRITERION	DEFINITION
1. Malar rash	Fixed erythema, flat or raised, over the malar eminences (tending to spare the nasolabial folds)
2. Discoid rash	Erythematous raised patches with adherent keratotic scaling and follicular plugging; atrophic scarring may occur in old lesions
3. Photosensitivity	A cutaneous rash following exposure to sunlight (by history or observation)
4. Oral ulcers	Oral or nasopharyngeal ulceration
5. Arthritis	Nonerosive arthritis (characterized by tenderness, swelling, or effusion) involving two or more peripheral joints
6. Serositis	Pleuritis (history of pleuritic pain or rub heard by a physician, or evidence of pleural effusion) *or* Pericarditis (by ECG, pericardial rub or evidence of pericardial effusion)
7. Renal disorder	Persistent proteinuria greater than 0.5 grams/day (greater than 3+ if quantitation not performed) *or* Cellular casts
8. Neurologic disorder	Seizures in the absence of offending drugs or known metabolic derangements *or* Psychosis (in the absence of offending drugs or known metabolic derangements)
9. Hematologic disorder	Hemolytic anemia with reticulocytosis *or* Leukopenia less than 4,000/mm^3 on two or more occasions *or* Lymphopenia less than 1,500/mm^3 on two or more occasions *or* Thrombocytopenia less than 100,000/mm^3 (in the absence of offending drugs)
10. Immunologic disorder	Positive LE cell preparation *or* Anti-DNA antibody to native DNA in abnormal titer *or* Anti-Sm (presence of antibody to Sm nuclear antigen) *or* Chronic false positive serologic test for syphilis, positive for at least six months (confirmed by *Treponema palladum* immobilization or fluorescent treponemal antibody absorption test)
11. Antinuclear antibody	An abnormal titer of antinuclear antibody by immunofluorescence or equivalent assay in the absence of drugs known to be associated with "drug-induced lupus" syndrome

*A person is said to have systemic lupus erythematosus if any 4 or more of the above 11 criteria are present, serially or simultaneously, during any interval of observation. (Modified from Tan, E.M., et al.[15])

tologic diagnosis is difficult and often impossible. Histopathologic findings of oral lesions consist of parakeratosis, hydropic degeneration of the stratum germinativum, and perivascular lymphocytic infiltration.[16]

Laboratory features include antinuclear antibodies, anti-DNA antibodies, low complement levels, and deposits of immunoglobulin and complement at the dermoepidermal junction. Leukopenia of less than 5,000 frequently occurs. Anemia and thrombocytopenia are frequently noted in patients with systemic LE, and serum globulins are elevated in about 80% of patients. In patients with active disease, a reduced serum complement level may be frequently noted. The erythrocyte sedimentation rate is elevated in all but an occasional patient during periods of clinical activity.

Of all the tests available, the antinuclear antibody (ANA) determination employing standard immunofluorescent techniques is the most valuable screening test for SLE, with approximately 90% of patients with systemic disease displaying a positive ANA titer when mouse liver is used as a substrate for nuclear antigens. Detection of antibodies against DNA have been found to be extremely valuable in the evaluation of patients with SLE. Patients with anti-DNA antibodies appear to be at risk for the development of renal disease.[17] Native DNA antibodies can also be detected, employing a *Crithidia lucillia* immunofluorescent technique, with a modification of this technique demonstrating good correlation between complement-fixing anti-nDNA antibodies, renal disease, and disease activity in patients with SLE.[18] Since the test for anti-nDNA is as sensitive and specific as the LE cell test, and has the advantage of being less time-consuming and easier to read, it is frequently used to replace the traditional LE test.

Direct immunofluorescence has also been utilized for the diagnosis of lupus erythematosus. In patients with SLE, the lupus band test (the demonstration of immunoglobulin at the dermo-epidermal junction) may be demonstrated by the direct method of testing for immunofluorescence at the dermal-epidermal junction of clinically involved and uninvolved skin. When involved skin is tested, immunoglobulins (most commonly IgG and IgM) and complement are found in over 90% of specimens of both SLE and DLE. Thus, direct immunofluorescence testing of involved skin is more sensitive and specific than routine histologic studies of biopsy specimens. When uninvolved sun-exposed skin (taken from the dorsal surface of the forearm) is tested, the lupus band test is positive in over 80% of untreated patients with SLE and is almost always negative in those with DLE. When uninvolved sun-protected skin is tested (taken from the volar aspect of the forearm or from the buttock area), there is a correlation between the incidence of a lupus band and the severity of renal disease. The incidence of a lupus band in sun-protected skin of patients with SLE is about 50%; in patients with diffuse renal disease, it is positive in slightly more than 80%; and in those with no renal disease, the test is positive in approximately 20% of patients.[19]

TREATMENT.—Our understanding of lupus erythematosus has improved substantially over the past 30 years. Recent statistics reveal that patients with cutaneous lupus erythematosus have an excellent prognosis, with about 5% going on to develop systemic disease.[1, 20] Patients with systemic lupus erythematosus currently have a ten-year survival rate of 85%.[21] The main causes of death in children are renal failure; arteritis and phlebitis of the central nervous system leading to convulsions, psychoses, coma, and paralysis; and cardiac failure. Although previous reports suggested that children had a worse prognosis than adults with SLE,[22, 23] a recent study of 46 children with systemic disease revealed that children with milder disease are now recognized. Although those with renal involvement are indeed seriously ill, SLE in childhood is not always associated with a poor prognosis.[4]

The therapy of lupus erythematosus depends upon the extent of local and systemic involvement. Avoidance of sun exposure and daylight fluorescent light (by hats and appropriate sun-screen preparations) is essential. Although only 30% to 40% of patients with lupus erythematosus are photosensitive, particularly those with disseminated or systemic lupus and those with circulating antibodies, ultraviolet light may induce or exacerbate cutaneous lesions or produce a fatal deterioration of systemic disease. It is generally the ultraviolet (290-320nm) portion of the spectrum that is most damaging, but infrared exposure and heat or trauma may also precipitate exacerbations.[1] Fatigue is also a problem in patients with SLE and is often the last symptom to respond to therapy. SLE patients do not need to give up schooling, employment or recreation, but they should adjust their schedules to allow for intervals of rest between periods of activity.[21]

Patients with mild disease without nephritis should be treated with salicylates or other nonsteroidal agents for symptomatic relief of arthritis or other discomforts.[7] Topical corticosteroid preparations are effective for most cutaneous lesions, and antimalarial therapy is beneficial for long-term suppression of the disease. When antimalarials are utilized, they should be closely monitored since deposition of the drug in the pigmented portion of the retina can produce an irreversible retinopathy following long-term usage. Many reviews have mentioned a special sensitivity of children to antimalarial drugs. Fatal reactions were usually related to the ability of antimalarials to depress myocardial excitability. Reports of fatal reaction were invariably associated with overdosage of the medication.[24] The average dosage of hydroxychloroquine (Plaquenil) for adults is 400 mg one or two times a day initially with a maintenance dose of 200 to 400 mg/day; the dosage for children is 5 to 7 mg/kg/24 hrs.

Systemic lupus erythematosus should be considered a lifelong, controllable, but incurable disease. Although children with mild lupus erythematosus may respond well to mere bed rest, aspirin, and the avoidance of excessive sun exposure, they should be carefully evaluated for major organ involvement, particularly for the presence of nephritis (the major cause of death in individuals with this disorder).[25–27] In severe cases, hospitalization may be necessary for diagnostic evaluation as well as for definitive therapy of systemic LE and prednisone (in dosages of 1 to 2 mg per kg per 24 hours) may be lifesaving for patients with renal complication, pericarditis, neurologic involvement, or hemolytic anemia. Once remission is induced, a minimal corticosteroid maintenance dose, preferably alternate-day therapy, is advisable. Although it appears that steroid therapy has increased the survival rate, the possibility of complications such as widespread tuberculosis, viral and bacterial pneumonia, bacterial (especially gram-negative) sepsis and systemic fungal disease must be considered.

Since immunosuppressive agents are beneficial (but carry an increased risk of neoplasia, aplastic anemia, and sepsis), when renal disease is present, the patient is best referred to a center where immunosuppressive therapy is available. The recommended pediatric dosage for azathioprine (Imuran) is 100 to 200 mg per day; for 6-mercaptopurine, 50 to 100 mg per day; for cyclophosphamide (Cytoxan), 50 mg per day; and for chlorambucil (Leukeran), 0.1 mg per kg per day, with appropriate modification depending on the size and weight of small children.[27–29]

Two new therapeutic regimens also deserve mention. Intravenous pulse steroid therapy with Solu-Medrol (methylprednisolone) (30 mg/kg/dose), given as a bolus for three days, has been reported to reverse rapid renal deterioration and is frequently beneficial in other acute situations. Some patients can be managed on an intermittent weekly or biweekly schedule, thus avoiding daily use of steroids and their potential side effects. Plasmapharesis is another experimental therapy that modifies the disease. Although experience is limited, in profoundly ill SLE patients, this form of therapy may prove beneficial. In addition, renal transplantation has been beneficial for patients with end stage renal disease.[21]

Neonatal Lupus Erythematosus

Neonatal lupus erythematosus (NLE) is a unique variant of lupus erythematosus found in infants born to mothers with systemic LE, rheumatoid arthritis, or undifferentiated connective tissue disease before, during, or after the pregnancy (Table 5–2).[30–32] Affected infants have a lupus-like rash, lupus-associated hematologic and serologic abnormalities and, in 15% to 30% of patients, congenital atrioventricular heartblock.[31] A relatively rare syndrome, with slightly over 100 cases reported to date, neonatal lu-

TABLE 5–2.—NEONATAL LUPUS ERYTHEMATOSUS

1. Seen in infants born to mothers with SLE, rheumatoid arthritis, or undifferentiated connective tissue disease.
2. Lupus-like rash, often in areas of sun exposure; diffuse erythema of face; and oval atrophic hypopigmented discoid lesions with telangiectasia
3. Associated with anti-Ro(SSA) and anti-La(SSB) antibodies
4. Congenital a-v heart block in 15% to 30%

pus erythematosus is probably much more common than stated in the literature. Systemic manifestations, especially complete heart block, may be present even in the absence of cutaneous lesions.[34, 35]

ETIOLOGY.—Infants born to mothers with disseminated LE are usually normal but occasionally have some manifestations of neonatal lupus. Some believe that maternal IgG antibodies, which readily cross placental barriers, play a major role in the pathogenesis of neonatal lupus and that the disorder is associated with immune complexes formed by transplacental passage of maternal antibodies. Autoantibodies to soluble tissue ribonucleoprotein antigens Ro(SSA) and La(SSB) have had a strong association with neonatal lupus erythematosus, suggesting a role for these antibodies in the pathogenesis of NLE.[36–38] An increased frequency of histocompatability antigens HLA-DR2 and DR3 has been reported in patients with SLE, and an unusual frequency of HLA-B8 and DR3 may occur in mothers of infants with congenital heart block.[35, 39] While genetics are important, a report of an infant with neonatal lupus and congenital heart block who shared antibody to SS-A and SS-B with her mother but failed to inherit the chromosome containing HLA-DR3 suggests that the HLA system may not be the sole factor determining susceptibility to neonatal LE.[32]

CLINICAL FEATURES.—The majority of infants with neonatal lupus erythematosus are female with a ratio thought to be similar to that of adults with systemic lupus erythematosus. Cutaneous lesions appear from the time of birth (in two-thirds of patients) until about 12 weeks of age,[34] and the majority of infants have spontaneous resolution by the age of 6 to 12 months. In a few patients, however, the eruption has lasted for a period of up to 20 months.[30, 36–41] The cutaneous lesions of neonatal lupus erythematosus generally appear on the head and neck, the extensor surfaces of the arms and, less frequently, on the trunk and other areas of the extremities (including the palms and soles).[42] They are manifested as a diffuse erythema of the face (especially the forehead and periorbital regions) (Figs 5–5, 5–6), scaly atrophic discoid lesions and, at times, hypopigmented atrophic plaques with telangiectasia. Although occurring predominantly in areas of sun exposure, particularly following intense sun exposure or sunburn, lesions may also occur in sun-protected areas of the skin.[36, 43]

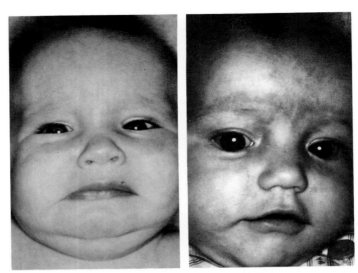

Fig 5–5 (left).—Neonatal lupus erythematosus. Diffuse erythema of the forehand and periorbital regions of the face of a 5-month-old infant following sun exposure.
Fig 5–6 (right).—Erythematous patches on the scalp, forehead, and periorbital region seen in a 3½-month-old infant with neonatal lupus erythematosus.

Neonatal lupus erythematosus was originally thought to be a transient disease, but it is now apparent that systemic involvement may also occur. Cardiac involvement, the most serious complication, occurs in 75% of cases[34] and congenital heart block occurs in 15% to 30% of affected patients. Unlike other complications of NLE, congenital heart block is irreversible and infants with this complication have a mortality rate of 20% to 30%, with the greatest risk occurring in the first few months of life. Death may also result from congestive heart failure or other associated complications such as septal defects and endocardial fibroelastosis. Other systemic complications include hepatomegaly (in 30%), splenomegaly (in 40%), lymphadenopathy (in 7%), leukopenia, thrombocytopenia, Coombs' positive hemolytic anemia and anemia with or without a positive Coombs' test.[34] Brustein has described a family in which two infants of a mother with cutaneous LE developed neonatal lupus[43] and other infants with neonatal lupus erythematosus eventually developed systemic lupus erythematosus (SLE) at later ages.[44, 45] It is essential that all children with cutaneous neonatal LE be investigated for the possibility of congenital atrioventricular block and that they be followed for signs of active or recurring disease. Furthermore, since neonatal LE can develop in subsequent pregnancies of mothers with previously affected babies, infants born to mothers with previously affected children should be evaluated for the possibility of this disorder.

DIAGNOSIS.—The diagnosis of neonatal lupus erythematosus is aided by the presence of typical cutaneous lesions, systemic manifestations, and confirmatory laboratory studies (positive LE preparations, lymphocyte tuboreticular inclusions, leukopenia, thrombocytopenia, and Coombs' test-positive hemolytic anemia) in infants born to mothers with LE, rheumatoid arthritis, or undifferentiated connective tissue disease.[43-46] Since antibodies to the nuclear antigens Ro(SSA) and La(SSB) have been demonstrated as markers of this disorder, all infants with discoid skin lesions or congenital heart block should have their serums and their mother's serums examined for these antibodies.[31, 36, 37]

Cutaneous biopsy of skin lesions of affected infants generally demonstrate the histopathologic features of lupus erythematosus with injury to the basal epidermal cells as a prominent feature. Although immunofluorescent studies have been performed in a relatively low percentage of affected cases, positive immunofluorescence of skin lesions has been demonstrated as immunoreactants of C_3, IgG, or IgM at the dermal-epidermal junction of infants with this disorder. Fluorescent tests of affected infants for antinuclear antibodies have been shown to be positive with speckled patterns.

TREATMENT.—Although the natural course of cutaneous lesions suggests spontaneous resolution in most instances, appropriate treatment of neonatal lupus erythematosus suggests avoidance of sun exposure and the topical use of midpotency glucocorticosteroids on cutaneous lesions. Since 20% to 30% of infants with congenital A-V block may die during the first year of life,[47] pacemakers should be utilized and inasmuch as this block may persist, pacemakers may have to be continued throughout the lifetime of the child. Children who have cutaneous neonatal LE must be investigated for the possibility of congenital atrioventricular block and be monitored for signs of active or recurring disease.

Dermatomyositis

Dermatomyositis is an inflammatory disorder of unknown etiology that primarily affects the skin, striated muscles, and occasionally other internal organs in children as well as adults (Table 5–3). In cases in which cutaneous changes are absent or insignificant, the term *polymyositis* is used. Since the clinical and pathological features of involved skin and muscles are similar, dermatomyositis and polymyositis are believed to be variants of the same disease process.

ETIOLOGY.—The etiology of dermatomyositis is unknown. Recent studies suggest that the pathogenesis involves an immunologic reaction di-

TABLE 5–3.—DERMATOMYOSITIS

1. An inflammatory disorder of unknown etiology primarily affecting the skin and striated muscles (other organs rarely involved)
2. Erythematous red to purplish heliotrope edematous patches on face (especially eyelids, forehead, cheeks and temples), extensor surfaces of arms, shoulders, elbows, knees, and dorsal interphalangeal joints
3. Gottron's papules pathognomonic
4. Association with malignancy in 15% to 20% of adults (but not in children)
5. Cutaneous calcinosis generally a favorable prognostic sign in children

rected at blood vessels and skeletal muscle. Although vascular deposits of immunoglobulins and complement have been demonstrated in blood vessel walls of skeletal muscle of involved children and it has been suggested that they are antigen-antibody complexes, their pathogenic role remains uncertain.[48] In adults, an abnormal cellular immunity has been hypothesized. In children, however, more than one mechanism may be involved. An immune complex mechanism producing vasculitis appears to be more important than cell-mediated immunity.[49, 50] A febrile illness occasionally precedes the onset of childhood dermatomyositis, suggesting an infectious origin.[51, 52] Preliminary reports of increased frequency of HLA-B8/DR3 in children and HLA-B14 in adults with dermatomyositis suggest the possibility of a genetic predisposition to the disorder.[53–55] These hypotheses, however, require further evaluation.

CLINICAL MANIFESTATIONS.—The onset of dermatomyositis is usually insidious, with muscle weakness and fatigue as prominent features. Children often present with fever. Characteristic cutaneous lesions include a violaceous erythema of the upper eyelids and extensor joint surface (Figs 5–7,

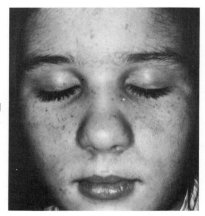

Fig 5–7.—Edema and purplish-red heliotrope erythema on the cheeks and eyelids of a child with dermatomyositis.

5–8, 5–9). They may appear after polymyositis or may precede muscle disease by an interval of a few weeks to three years. When skin markings precede the development of polymyositis, the interval is generally between three and six months.

The disorder occurs twice as frequently in females as in males and, although it may occur at any age, it rarely begins before the second year of life. At least 15% of cases are seen in children less than 15. About 25% of those afflicted are less than 18 years of age at the time of onset.[56] In adults the disorder occurs most commonly between the ages of 50 and 70. In childhood, however, the highest incidence is between 5 and 12 years, and the youngest case reported to date was that of a 4-month-old infant.

The course of dermatomyositis is different in children than it is in adults.[57, 58] Malignancy is associated with adult dermatomyositis in 15% to 20% of cases, and is more common in dermatomyositis than pure polymyositis (1). In children, although malignancy has been reported three times, there appears to be no relationship between this disorder and malignancy.[56, 59–62] In addition, children rarely have Raynaud's phenomenon; they tend to have more inflammation and necrosis of muscle, and, in con-

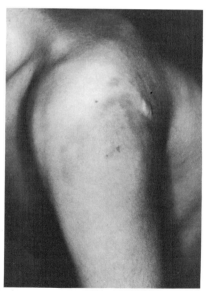
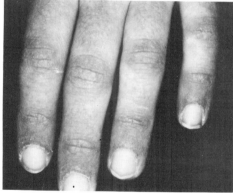

Fig 5–8 (left).—Heliotrope eruption on the shoulder and upper arm of an 11-year-old boy with dermatomyositis.

Fig 5–9 (right).—Erythema and violaceous flat-topped papules (Gottron's papules) on the dorsal interphalangeal joints, and cuticular erythema and telangiectasia in a patient with dermatomyositis.

trast to adults, a respiratory illness often precedes the onset of the dermatomyositis and the mortality is lower.[52]

A variety of cutaneous findings may be noted in dermatomyositis. The dermatitis may be the most striking feature of the illness, or it may be so minor as to be easily overlooked. In most cases the rash is distinctive and highly suggestive, but not necessarily pathognomonic. A purplish-red erythema occurs on the face, especially on the eyelids, upper cheeks (Fig 5–7), forehead, and temples. Frequently associated with photosensitivity, it is often described as a heliotrope erythema, from the flower of the reddish-purple plant bearing this name. When present, this color is highly distinctive and often diagnostic. Sometimes the facial lesions are very edematous, leading to a periorbital edema with the reddish or purplish heliotrope color. Within a few weeks a confluent, violaceous, often edematous erythema with fine scaling may also appear over the hairline of the scalp, nape of the neck, extensor surfaces of the arms and shoulders (Fig 5–8), elbows, knees, and dorsal interphalangeal joints (often suggesting a diagnosis of contact dermatitis or photosensitivity).

In almost every case, there is erythema of the cuticles at the base of the nails, with accompanying cuticular linear telangiectasia (Fig 5–9). At times, the cuticles may also be thickened, hyperkeratotic, and irregular, giving an appearance of overzealous or excessive picking or manicuring.[63] Hypertrichosis and hyperpigmentation, independent of corticosteroid therapy, may also complicate previously involved skin, particularly in children and ulcerations of the fingertips, probably associated with angiitis, and may be seen in acute forms of this disorder.

A pathognomonic diagnostic sign of dermatomyositis is the *Gottron papule*, a violaceous flat-topped lesion over the dorsal interphalangeal joints (Fig 5–9), which usually occurs late in the disease (in about one-third of patients). When the papule resolves, atrophy, telangiectasia, or hypopigmentation may persist. Other cutaneous features include cutaneous atrophy, a tight glossy appearance over involved extremities and poikiloderma. In long-standing disease, there may be cutaneous atrophy, and the skin is frequently bound down to underlying structures.

The mucous membranes may also be involved in dermatomyositis. Erythema of the palate and buccal mucosa (with or without ulceration), erythema of the gum margin, and whitish patches on the tongue and buccal mucosa have been observed.

A sequel to the inflammatory phase of the disease is the occurrence of calcinosis. Cutaneous calcinosis, more characteristic of juvenile rather than adult-onset dermatomyositis, is seen in 44% to 70% of children as compared to 20% of adults with dermatomyositis.[59] Most commonly seen on the buttocks and about the shoulders and elbows, subcutaneous calcium deposits may produce local pain, and can be extruded, leading to ulcers, sinuses, or cellulitis. Calcinosis, although often resulting in impaired function, is associated with a longer survival time and, accordingly, is viewed as a favorable prognostic sign.[64] Sometimes patients may present with widespread calcification without apparent preceding illness. In such cases, it is suspected that calcinosis may be the result of an old dermatomyositis.

DIAGNOSIS.—The diagnosis of dermatomyositis is made on clinical grounds and depends upon the typical cutaneous manifestations and evidence of muscle involvement. It is confirmed by electromyography, elevated serum enzyme levels (serum aldolase, serum glutamic oxaloacetic transaminase, lactic dehydrogenase and serum creatine phosphokinase) and biopsy from a muscle of the shoulder or pelvic girdle (preferably a muscle that is tender).

Five diagnostic criteria have been suggested for dermatomyositis and polymyositis. These include: (1) symmetrical weakness of the limb-girdle muscles and anterior neck flexors, with or without dysphagia or respiratory weakness; (2) muscle biopsy evidence of degeneration, regeneration, necrosis, phagocytosis, and a mononuclear cellular infiltrate of the involved muscles; (3) elevation in the serum of skeletal muscle enzymes, particularly creatinine phosphokinase, but also the transaminases, LDH, and aldolase; (4) electromyographic evidence of myopathy; and (5) the typical skin rash of dermatomyositis. A diagnosis of dermatomyositis can be made when three to four of the above criteria (plus the rash) are present; a diagnosis of polymyositis can be established with four of the criteria (without the rash). A probable diagnosis of dermatomyositis requires two of the above criteria (plus the rash).[65–67]

TREATMENT.—The course of dermatomyositis is highly variable. Without specific treatment, about one-third of affected children recover completely, usually within one year of onset of the disorder.[68] Although the mortality in untreated cases is about 33% to 40%, with modern steroid management, the death rate has been reduced to less than 10%.[69] Long-term follow-up of chronically affected children indicates that in most instances the disease subsides after about three years, leaving various degrees of disability. If the children can be kept alive for three to five years, although calcinosis and mild manifestations of the disease may persist, medication can often be discontinued.

Hospitalization is advisable in the acute stages, as the disease processes may involve the muscles of respiration or deglutition and necessitate tracheotomy or the use of a mechanical respirator. A physical therapy program aimed at prevention of deformities and increasing muscle strength should be initiated early. Physical rest is extremely important during active phases of dermatomyositis and may permit control on much lower steroid dosages than otherwise would be possible. When palatorespiratory muscles are affected, great care is required to prevent aspiration and to ensure adequate respiration.

Severe dermatomyositis may be accompanied by diffuse cardiomyopathy. Although this is a rare complication, nonspecific electrocardiographic abnormalities are found in about 20% of cases. In severely affected patients, respiratory insufficiency must be carefully watched for. When direct measurements of ventilation or arterial pCO_2 indicate that this is occurring, it is usually necessary to perform a tracheostomy. Tube feedings or intravenous maintenance may be required when dysphagia is present. In those instances in which prompt vigorous therapy is begun, palatal-respiratory function is monitored, adequate physical therapy is actively pursued, and meticulous long-term follow-up is maintained, successful outcomes occur in over two-thirds of the cases.

Most childhood forms of dermatomyositis require high-dosage corticosteroid therapy. The initial dose of prednisone is 1.5 to 2.5 mg per kg of body weight per day, usually a dose of 60 mg of prednisone or its equivalent (up to 90 to 100 mg every day if that proves insufficient). As soon as a response is attained, as judged by muscle enzyme levels, the dosage may be reduced by decrements of about 15% (at intervals of about two weeks) over a period of 10 to 12 months.

Some patients may fail to respond to even very large doses of corticosteroids. Cytotoxic agents such as azathioprine (Imuran) in dosages of 1 to 3 mg per kg of body weight (up to 200 mg a day) or biweekly injections of methotrexate (2 to 3 mg per kg per dose) may be used as ancillary therapeutic agents in severe life-threatening forms of dermatomyositis, or when the disease cannot be adequately managed with prednisone alone.[70, 71]

Although areas of calcinosis frequently disappear spontaneously, disodium etidronate (EHDP) or a diet low in phosphorus and calcium in conjunction with aluminum hydroxide gels (15 ml to 30 ml 4 times a day) may help to lower serum phosphorus and aid in the resolution of cutaneous calcification.[72, 73]

During the active phase of dermatomyositis, children are particularly at risk for sudden, overwhelming gram-negative sepsis secondary to aspiration due to weak palatal-respiratory function or perforation of a viscus. The risk is intensified by the masking effects of corticosteroids. A high index of suspicion must be maintained for these complications, and early, aggressive therapy must be instituted when necessary.

Scleroderma

Scleroderma, a chronic inflammatory disorder of connective tissue, can be classified into two categories: a variety limited to the skin (morphea and linear scleroderma) and the multisystem disease, systemic scleroderma (progressive systemic sclerosis). Although the etiology of scleroderma is unknown, the pathogenesis of progressive systemic sclerosis is thought to be related to genetic factors, immunologic abnormalities, generalized vascular disease, and a dysfunction in collagen metabolism. Of major importance are the vasospastic phenomena with endothelial damage that precede the stage of pulmonary and cutaneous fibrosis, cell-mediated abnormalities that facilitate the proliferation of fibroblasts and collagen synthesis, and decreased levels of collagenase resulting in the firm hidebound appearance of sclerodermatous tissue.[74–76] On rare occasions, morphea and systemic scleroderma occur in the same patients. The relationship between morphea and systemic scleroderma, however, is controversial and not well understood. Most authorities feel that morphea is essentially a benign disease that, particularly in children, resolves spontaneously. If a transition from morphea to scleroderma does indeed occur, it is extremely rare.[77–79]

CLINICAL MANIFESTATIONS.—Systemic scleroderma (progressive systemic sclerosis) is a generalized disorder of connective tissue affecting the skin, lungs, heart, gastrointestinal tract, joints, and kidneys (Table 5–4). Seen in all age groups, although relatively uncommon in childhood, it has been reported in children as young as two years of age[80] and, as in adults, the disorder occurs three times more frequently in women than in men.[81–83]

Initially, systemic scleroderma was divided into two forms (acrosclerosis and diffuse scleroderma). Diffuse scleroderma begins with cutaneous sclerosis over the central portion of the body and gradually spreads to the extremities. Raynaud's phenomenon is invariably absent and sex distribution is equal. Acrosclerosis accounts for 95% of all cases of scleroderma and is characterized by cutaneous sclerosis of the digits (sclerodactyly) (Fig 5–10) and Raynaud's phenomenon. It was initially thought that diffuse scleroderma was rapidly fatal and that acrosclerosis generally had a long and

TABLE 5–4.—CLINICAL FEATURES OF SYSTEMIC
SCLEROSIS

---

1. Acrosclerosis (in 95%)
   a. Cutaneous sclerosis of digits (sclerodactyly)
   b. Raynaud's phenomenon
2. Subcutaneous calcification and/or ulceration
3. Telangiectatic mats, cuticular telangiectasia
4. Characteristic facies (tight skin, fixed stare, pinched nose and perpetual grimace)
5. Variable degrees of internal organ involvement
   a. Polymyositis
   b. Esophageal and g.i. pathology
   c. Cardiovascular, pulmonary, or renal abnormalities

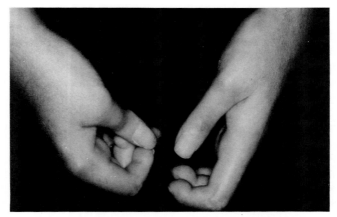

Fig 5–10.—Acrosclerosis. Cutaneous sclerosis (sclerodactyly) with flexion contractures in a young woman with scleroderma.

benign course. This concept now appears to be incorrect. The only value of this classification is that it describes the mode of onset and distribution of lesions.

Raynaud's phenomenon, although extremely uncommon in childhood, is frequently the first sign of systemic scleroderma in this age group. Precipitated by cold or emotional stress, this disorder is characterized by a triphasic reaction of pallor, cyanosis and hyperemia with pain, burning, numbness, tingling, swelling and hyperhidrosis of the affected fingers or toes and, at times, the nose, lips, tongue, cheeks, ears and chest. This disorder is present in almost all patients with systemic scleroderma, in 10% to 30% of patients with systemic lupus erythematosus, in some cases of dermatomyositis, mixed connective tissue disease, and in other individuals as an idiopathic disorder of variable severity.[1]

Even in the prepuberal years, systemic scleroderma has a preponderance of female patients. The appearance of the face is characteristic. The forehead is smooth and cannot be wrinkled, and atrophy and tightening of the skin give a characteristic appearance due to a fixed stare, pinched nose, prominent teeth, pursed lips, and perpetual grimace (Fig 5–11). The hands become shiny, with tapered finger ends and restricted movements. Subcutaneous calcification and ulceration may be seen as well as telangiectases and hypo- and hyperpigmentation (common cutaneous signs of scleroderma).

Three varieties of telangiectasia are characteristic of scleroderma. These include linear telangiectasia of the cuticles similar to that seen in other connective tissue disorders, sharply defined telangiectatic macules of linear, oval, square, and multiangular configurations that vary in size from 1 to 6 mm in diameter (telangiectatic mats) (see Fig 5–11), and in a very small percentage of patients, telangiectasia similar to that seen in patients with Rendu-Osler Weber disease.[1]

The names CRST syndrome (calcinosis, Raynaud's phenomenon, sclerodactyly, and telangiectasia) or CREST syndrome (this acronym includes the feature of esophageal dysfunction) have been used to describe various combinations of features seen in patients with systemic scleroderma. These are not separate disorders. They merely represent clinical variants of the disorder and do not connote any prognostic or therapeutic significance for affected individuals.

Polymyositis and involvement of the esophagus probably are the most common extracutaneous sites of sclerotic change in scleroderma. Other gastrointestinal disturbances include constipation, regurgitation, weight loss, and malabsorption. Although cardiovascular, respiratory, and renal involvement have been described, these do not appear to be prominent in childhood forms of this disorder.

DIAGNOSIS.—The diagnosis of systemic scleroderma is easily established when cutaneous sclerosis of the face and hands are present, particularly when they are associated with Raynaud's phenomenon, telangiectasia and visceral involvement. Symptoms or signs of dysphagia or gastroesophageal reflux (or radiologic demonstration of an aperistaltic dilated esophagus) help confirm the diagnosis. Although patients with visceral scleroderma without apparent cutaneous involvement have been described,[84, 85] it has been suggested that in such cases cutaneous features (Raynaud's phenomenon with telangiectasia) may indeed have been present but were not unappreciated at the time the initial diagnosis was made.[1]

The histologic appearance of the skin in systemic scleroderma is often

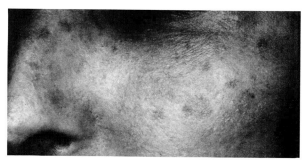

Fig 5–11.—Scleroderma. Smooth atrophic skin, pinched nose, and telangiectatic mats on the face of a young woman with scleroderma. The disorder started when she was 20 years of age.

similar to that seen in morphea, so that a histologic differentiation of the two types is frequently difficult. Lesions of systemic scleroderma, however, show more pronounced degenerative changes in the collagen bundles and vessel walls in the later stages; the epidermis may show epidermal atrophy with a disappearance of rete ridges in areas of involvement; and the marked inflammatory changes seen in the active borders of morphea do not occur in active lesions of systemic scleroderma.

TREATMENT.—No specific therapy is available, and management of progressive systemic sclerosis is mainly supportive. General measures include avoidance of factors producing vasospasm (tension, fatigue, stress, and cold weather) and minimizing trauma to the hands. Rest is important and, if polyarthritis is present, salicylates may be beneficial. Nifedipine (Procardia; Pfizer), a drug used in the treatment of vasospastic angina, has recently been recommended in a dosage of 10 to 20 mg three times a day for the treatment of Raynaud's phenomenon. This preparation is not recommended for the treatment of Raynaud's phenomenon in the Physicians' Desk Reference. Its use and dosage in children is not defined, and further studies are required to corroborate the efficacy of this preparation in this disorder.[86] Treatment of gastrointestinal symptoms includes small frequent feedings, with elevation of the head of the bed, bland diet, and antacids. Corticosteroids, because of complications from long-term therapy, should be reserved for those with debilitating arthritis not controlled by aspirin and for patients with extensive cutaneous edema with severe recurring digital ulcerations and acute toxic phases of the disease. Corticosteroids do not appear to help the sclerodermatous process and, according to many authorities, in many cases may even be harmful.

Eosinophilic Fasciitis

Eosinophilic fasciitis (fasciitis with eosinophilia) is a recently described scleroderma-like disease characterized by diffuse infiltration of the skin of the extremities and trunk without visceral involvement or Raynaud's phenomenon (Table 5–5). First described by Shulman in 1974, the disorder is characterized by a sudden onset following strenuous physical activity; pain-

TABLE 5–5.—EOSINOPHILIC FASCIITIS

1. A variant of scleroderma? (still controversial)
2. Painful swelling and induration of skin and subcutaneous tissue (sudden onset following trauma, stress, or strenuous physical activity)
3. Eosinophilia
4. Absence of visceral involvement or Raynaud's phenomenon
5. Good response to systemic steroids

ful swelling, induration, and scleroderma-like changes of the extremities; marked thickening of the subcutaneous fascia; absence of systemic changes; transient peripheral eosinophilia early in the disease; hypergammaglobulinemia; an elevated sedimentation rate; and a good response to systemic corticosteroids.[86-88] Since the pathologic findings are restricted to the deep fascia between the subcutaneous tissue and muscle, Shulman suggested the term "diffuse fasciitis" for this apparently new disease or syndrome. Rodnan and his associates, noting the presence of eosinophils in the involved fascia, suggested the term "eosinophilic fasciitis" for this disorder.[89]

A disease initially recognized in adults and only occasionally encountered in children,[90] it has been suggested that eosinophilic fasciitis may merely represent a variant of morphea or scleroderma.[91] The high male preponderance of eosinophilic fasciitis (a male to female ratio 3:1), its lack of visceral involvement, a low incidence of serologic abnormalities, and prompt response to systemic corticosteroids suggest that it actually represents a separate and distinct disorder. Features favoring its relationship to morphea and scleroderma include histologic features (inflammation and fibrosis of the fascia), blood eosinophilia and hypergammaglobulinemia.[88]

Shulman has proposed an immunologically mediated mechanism for eosinophilic fasciitis. Suggestive evidence includes the presence of hypergammaglobulinemia (usually IgG), deposition of IgG and complement in the fascia of some patients, and occasional bone marrow plasmacytosis.[87] He also hypothesized that exercise (or other trauma) and subsequent tissue damage in a susceptible host might release an antigen which could then initiate a hypersensitivity reaction leading to the fasciitis seen in individuals with this disorder.[87]

CLINICAL MANIFESTATIONS.—In the majority of patients, the onset of eosinophilic fasciitis follows trauma or excessive physical exertion and is marked by the occurrence of pain, swelling, and tenderness of the hands, forearms, feet and legs, followed by the development of severe induration of the skin and subcutaneous tissues, and, at times, carpal tunnel syndrome, with flexion contractures of the fingers and marked limitation of motion of the hands and feet.[89-92] Primarily affecting the skin of the arms and legs, and occasionally that of the trunk, hands, and feet, the cutaneous features consist of a cobblestone or puckered appearance with a yellowish or erythematous color. The skin is indurated, taut, and bound down without pigmentary change. Although the extremities usually are the areas of initial involvement, the disease may progress to the trunk and face.

DIAGNOSIS.—Most patients with eosinophilic fasciitis are young to middle-aged males. In most patients, the disease symmetrically involves the subcutaneous tissue of the arms and legs. The appearance of the cobblestone or puckered skin without significant color change following strenuous physical activity or trauma is highly suggestive of the diagnosis. Eosinophilia and hypergammaglobulinemia in the form of elevated IgG are commonly observed laboratory findings, but antinuclear antibody reactions remain negative.

Histopathologic examination of cutaneous lesions of early lesions of eosinophilic fasciitis are characterized by edema of the lower subcutis and deep fascia with infiltration by lymphocytes, plasma cells, histiocytes, and intravascular or perivascular eosinophils in the trabeculae of the subcutaneous tissue. As the illness progresses, these structures and the dermis become collagenized, thickened and sclerotic, and focal or diffuse eosinophilia may be observed in the fascia, lower subcutis, or both.[92–97]

TREATMENT.—Although eosinophilic fasciitis frequently resolves spontaneously, or with physiotherapy alone, systemic corticosteroids seem to hasten resolution. Once the patient responds, corticosteroids should be tapered to an alternate-day regimen. The length of time required for improvement varies, however, with individual patients. It is not uncommon for affected individuals to be on systemic corticosteroids for years with relapses occurring following the termination of steroid therapy.

Juvenile Rheumatoid Arthritis

Juvenile rheumatoid arthritis (JRA) is a common generalized systemic disease of unknown etiology that may occur at any age in childhood (Table 5–6). The disorder occurs almost twice as frequently in females as in males. The most common age of onset is between two and four years, with another peak in frequency in girls during adolescence. Although the age of onset is rarely under one year, it has been reported as early as the first week of life.[98] First described in the English literature by George Still in 1897, it probably encompasses several subgroups. The term *Still's disease* is used

TABLE 5–6.—JUVENILE RHEUMATOID ARTHRITIS

1. Cutaneous eruption (in 20% to 50%)
   a. Often with fever, lymphadenopathy and splenomegaly
   b. Flat to slightly elevated macules, papules or urticarial lesions
2. Spindling of fingers (in 50%)
3. Subcutaneous nodules (in 6% to 10%)
   a. Barely palpable to several cm in size (deep in dermis or subcutaneous tissue)
   b. Near olecranon process on dorsal aspect of hands, knees, ears, and pressure areas (scapulae, sacrum, buttocks and heels)
4. 80%–85% survive without serious disability (10% have severe crippling arthritis)

to describe the disorder in young children when the onset is abrupt and the patient has systemic as well as joint symptoms.

The etiology of juvenile rheumatoid arthritis remains unknown. Infectious agents, immunologic abnormalities, physical trauma to joints, psychological trauma, and allergy or reactions to drugs, foods, or toxins have been proposed as antecedent causes of JRA. Whether any epidemiologic meaning can be attributed to these hypotheses, however, requires further investigation and verification.[99]

CLINICAL MANIFESTATIONS.—Juvenile rheumatoid arthritis is not a rare disease; it has been estimated that there are a quarter of a million affected children in the United States. About 5% of all cases of rheumatoid arthritis begin in childhood. The onset of juvenile rheumatoid arthritis may be sudden and fulminating, with a high spiking fever (which may last for weeks or months), adenopathy, splenomegaly, and anemia, with or without arthralgia: or it may begin slowly, with insidious involvement of a single joint for weeks or months before other joints are affected. The type of onset, to a considerable extent, is related to the age of the patient—the younger the patient, generally the more prominent the systemic manifestations. In adults there is thought to be a seasonal difference in onset of rheumatoid arthritis, with more cases occurring between October and April; in children, however, there appears to be no significant difference in the month or season of onset.

A highly characteristic rash may be the first clue to the diagnosis of juvenile rheumatoid arthritis. Seen in 25% to 50% of patients, it may precede other manifestations by up to three years. The eruption, generally seen at the height of fever, appears as flat to slightly elevated macules or papules that measure from 2 to 6 mm in diameter. Lesions vary in color from salmon-pink to red and display a characteristic slightly irregular or serpiginous margin (Fig 5–12).[100–102] Some lesions may be slightly raised, edematous, and urticarial in nature, but unlike true urticaria, they do not itch, migrate, or change in shape. They are often surrounded by a zone of pallor, and larger lesions frequently have a pale center.

The eruption is usually intermittent, is often evanescent, and frequently subsides during periods of remission. The rash may appear at any time during the course of the disease and is associated with spikes in fever, splenomegaly, and lymphadenopathy. Accentuated by local heat or trauma, it may be precipitated by emotional, infectious, or surgical stress. Individual lesions often coalesce to form large plaques 8 to 9 cm in diameter and, in severely affected individuals, the eruption may persist for periods of one week to several years.

Children with juvenile rheumatoid arthritis characteristically have an anxious or worried facial expression and an intense desire to be left alone,

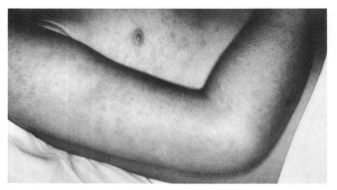

Fig 5–12.—Rheumatoid arthritis. A salmon-pink to red maculopapular eruption with irregular serpiginous margins seen in a child with juvenile rheumatoid arthritis (Still's disease). (From Hurwitz S.: *Clinical Pediatric Dermatology.* W.B. Saunders Co., Philadelphia, 1981. Used by permission.).

perhaps owing to their extreme discomfort and an attempt to guard their joints against movement. Thirty percent to 50% of affected children have involvement of only one joint for a time, usually the knee or ankle, but eventually almost all manifest polyarthritis.[103] When multiple joint involvement occurs, it usually is symmetrical and may involve any synovial joint in the body (with the possible exception of joints of the lumbothoracic spine). Joints of the lower extremities are usually affected first, especially the knee joint, which is involved in 90% of patients. Finger joints are involved in approximately 75% and the ankles and wrists in approximately two-thirds of all patients. There is limitation of motion, usually due to pain; the joints may be warm but not tender; and redness is not marked. The skin, especially over the affected joint of the extremity, becomes atrophic, smooth, and glossy. The thenar and hypothenar eminences may be red; the palms, however, usually remain cold and damp.

Morning stiffness in adult patients with rheumatoid arthritis is a well-known symptom and frequently is helpful in diagnosis of the disease. This is most common early in the morning and is not the result of pain and, with activity, completely disappears during the day. Children frequently have the same experience after periods of inactivity or sleep, sometimes to the point that they are unable to rise from bed spontaneously. After a few minutes in a tub with moist heat and activity, however, the stiffness disappears and the child is able to move about more freely. Whether inactivity or pain is responsible for morning stiffness is difficult to determine, but the stiffness proves to be a useful clinical manifestation in the diagnosis of this disorder.

Spindling of the fingers, one of the earliest objective signs of joint involvement, is seen in more than 50% of children with juvenile rheumatoid arthritis. The spindle-shaped deformity of the fingers develops because the proximal interphalangeal joints are affected more severely than the distal joints. This finding, rarely seen in other childhood disease, may also be seen in Kawasaki disease but is highly characteristic of juvenile rheumatoid arthritis or mixed connective tissue disease.

Subcutaneous nodules are seen in 6% to 10% of children with rheumatoid arthritis at some time during the course of the disease. Barely palpable to several centimeters in size, they may be the first presenting sign of juvenile rheumatoid arthritis. Their most common location is near the olecranon process on the ulnar border of the forearm. They occur less commonly on the dorsal aspect of the hands, on the knees and ears, and over pressure areas such as the scapulae, sacrum, buttocks, and heels. In the areas of fingers and toes, subcutaneous nodules are only a few millimeters in size. They are firm and nontender, and may be attached to the periarticular capsules of the fingers. In contrast to lesions of granuloma annulare, they may be deep in the dermis or in the subcutaneous tissue. Subcutaneous nodules are associated with severe exacerbation of the disease but are not related to prognosis.

Approximately 5% of patients with rheumatoid arthritis have cuticular telangiectases, a characteristic sign of connective tissue disease also seen in patients with lupus erythematosus, scleroderma, and dermatomyositis. This finding is seen as linear wiry vessels perpendicular to the base of the nail in the overlying cuticular and periungual skin. Cuticular telangiectases are usually bright red; not caused by trauma; and when thrombosed, appear to be black. Cuticular telangiectases are rarely seen in normal healthy individuals and accordingly are particularly helpful in the diagnosis of connective tissue disease.

The natural course of juvenile rheumatoid arthritis is variable. The disease may end after a few months and never recur, or it may recur after months or years of remission. The active process often improves by puberty. Although about 10% of patients are severely crippled by this disorder, 75% to 80% of children can be expected to survive without serious disability.[103]

DIAGNOSIS.—The diagnosis of juvenile rheumatoid arthritis is based upon the clinical features with a history of arthritis (effusion or pain and limitation of motion in at least one joint), lasting for at least six weeks with appropriate studies to exclude other causes of arthritis. Although a number of laboratory tests are helpful, none is diagnostic of JRA or any other disease.[99] Approximately 80% of patients have a positive rheumatoid factor by latex fixation. Other less specific laboratory tests include an elevated erythrocyte sedimentation rate, leukocytosis, anemia, hyperglobulinemia and hypoalbuminemia. IgG elevations are seen in 25%, IgA in 17%, IgM in 10%, and ANA is elevated in 4% of affected individuals.

Histologic examination of the cutaneous eruption, although not diagnostic, is characterized by edematous collagen fibers and perivascular cell infiltrate in the upper portion of the corium, with polymorphonuclear leukocytes and, to a lesser extent, plasma cells and histiocytes.[98]

TREATMENT.—There is no specific or curative treatment for juvenile rheumatoid arthritis. Aspirin (acetylsalicylic acid) is the drug of choice for early treatment, with an attempt to maintain serum salicylate levels between 20 and 30 mg per 100 ml. Such blood levels can be achieved by doses of 100 mg/kg daily for children of 25 kg or less and total daily doses of 40 to 60 grains for heavier children. Once active disease is suppressed, aspirin must be continued for months, sometimes years, before it is gradually withdrawn. Corticosteroids (0.5 to 1.0 mg per kg of prednisone or its equivalent) are indicated only for the seriously ill child or when disease threatens life or sight. Corticosteroids are vital for patients with protracted iridocylitis and vasculitis, and intrasynovial steroid injections are helpful for patients with severe joint involvement.

Gold therapy, with weekly doses of 1 mg per kg of the salt for a total of 500 mgm, may be useful for patients with nonresponsive polyarthritis. Careful examination, however, for leukopenia, thrombocytopenia, eosinophilia, proteinuria, hematuria, severe pruritus, or cutaneous eruption, particularly exfoliative dermatitis, should be performed at frequent intervals. Corticosteroid drops in association with mydriatics are helpful in the management of iridocyclitis. Appropriate rest, splinting, exercise, and physical therapy are important for the prevention and correction of deformity. Although severe deformities can be corrected by surgery, surgical treatment (synovectomy for removal of granulation tissue) should be considered only after a fair trial of medical therapy has been undertaken. Children six years of age or younger are poor surgical risks, however, because of their inability to cooperate effectively with postoperative measures.[104]

Sjögren's Syndrome

Sjögren's syndrome is a chronic autoimmune disorder of unknown etiology characterized by keratoconjunctivitis sicca (inflammation of the cornea and the conjunctiva with dryness and atrophy), xerostomia (dryness of the mouth from lack of normal secretion), enlargement of the salivary glands (as a result of lymphocytic infiltration) and a connective tissue disease (rheumatoid arthritis in at least 50% of cases, SLE, dermatomyositis, or scleroderma) (Table 5–7). Other disorders associated with Sjögren's syndrome include chronic hepatobiliary disease, Hashimoto's thyroiditis, pan-

TABLE 5–7.—SJÖGREN'S SYNDROME

1. Major clinical features
   a. Keratoconjunctivitis sicca (dryness and atrophy of cornea and conjunctiva)
   b. Xerostomia (dryness of mouth)
   c. Chronic enlargement of salivary glands
   d. Association with CT disease
      (1) Usually rheumatoid arthritis
      (2) Occasionally SLE, DM, or scleroderma
2. Cutaneous features
   a. Dryness and scaling of skin (with partial or complete loss of perspiration)
   b. Sparse dry brittle hair
   c. Purpura (usually lower extremities)
   d. Raynaud's phenomenon and telangiectasia of fingers and lips

arteritis, and interstitial pulmonary fibrosis. Although rarely seen in childhood,[105] the presence of chronic parotid enlargement and chronically dry mouth or eyes should suggest the possibility of Sjögren's syndrome.[106–107]

CLINICAL MANIFESTATIONS.—More than 90% of patients with Sjögren's syndrome are female. Although it has been reported in children, the disease generally begins after the patient has reached the age of 40 (in the fourth, fifth and sixth decades). The most prominent dermatologic manifestations are associated with dryness of the gingiva and mucous membranes of the mouth. The tongue may become smooth, red, and dry and in severe cases there may be difficulty in swallowing dry food. The lips may be cracked, fissured, or ulcerated, particularly at the corners of the mouth, and the teeth frequently undergo rapid and severe decay.[106]

Fatigue is a prominent symptom. Other clinical manifestations include arthritis or other connective tissue disease; dryness of the skin (seen in about 50% of affected patients); scaling of the skin; sparse, dry, and brittle hair; purpura, especially on the lower extremities (the most common cutaneous manifestation); telangiectasias of the lips and fingers; Raynaud's phenomenon; hoarseness; epistaxis; atrophic rhinitis; recurrent upper respiratory infection and otitis media. Dryness may also involve the conjunctivae, nose, pharynx, larynx, lower respiratory tract, and vagina. The eyes may be reddened and moist, and thick, tenacious secretions forming ropy mucous strands in the inner canthi may be noted (particularly when the patient arises in the morning). Other ocular manifestations include a burning sensation as when a foreign body is present in the eye, and an inability to produce tears in response to either irritants or emotion.

DIAGNOSIS.—The diagnosis of Sjögren's syndrome can be made when any two of the three major features (keratoconjunctivitis sicca, xerostomia, and rheumatoid arthritis or another connective tissue disorder) are present.

Diagnostic studies include scintigraphy (a determination of uptake, concentration, and excretion of intravenously injected radioactive material by major salivary glands); demonstration of decreased salivary flow by secretory sialography; biopsy of minor salivary glands of the lips; careful examination of the eyes, including Schirmer's test (less than 5 mm wetting of a strip of filter paper inserted under the lower eyelid); conjunctival staining with Rose Bengal solution; filamentary keratitis on slit lamp examination; and serological workup for autoimmune disease.[105]

Among the hematologic and serologic changes in Sjögren's syndrome are leukopenia (with or without an accompanying splenomegaly), a relative lymphocytosis, eosinophilia, hypergammaglobulinemia, positive tests for rheumatoid factor, antinuclear factor, antithyroglobulin factor, anti-Ro (SS-A), and other nonspecific antitissue antibodies.[108]

TREATMENT.—The management of Sjögren's syndrome includes treatment of the keratoconjunctivitis, xerostomia, and associated connective tissue or lymphoproliferative disorders. Since children with Sjögren syndrome may also be at risk for extraglandular diseases (such as other autoimmune disease and lymphoma), long-term follow-up is indicated.[109] Burning and irritation of the eyes may be treated by the installation of 0.5% methyl cellulose drops or artificial tear substitutes. Ophthalmologic consultation should be obtained for patients with ophthalmologic problems, and appropriate antibiotics should be utilized for the staphylococcal infections which are common in patients with keratoconjunctivitis sicca. Since such individuals are susceptible to bacterial and fungal infections, the danger of repeated eye infections should be emphasized. Affected patients should be cautioned to practice strict personal hygiene, including the use of separate face cloths and towels, and the avoidance of eye bath cups and solutions. Although systemic corticosteroids are capable of reducing the swelling of the salivary glands, they usually do not improve the function of affected glands. Side effects outweigh the benefits of the form of therapy. If the accompanying systemic disease is severe, however, treatment with systemic corticosteroids, immunosuppressive drugs, or both may be helpful.

Mixed Connective Tissue Disease

Mixed connective tissue disease (MCTD, Sharp's syndrome) is a recently defined clinical entity characterized by the combination of clinical features and laboratory data seen in systemic lupus erythematosus, dermatomyositis, polymyositis, rheumatoid arthritis and/or Sjögren's disease (Table 5–8). Originally described by Sharp in 1972, the disorder is characterized by high serum titers of RNAase-sensitive extractable nuclear antigen (ENA) and a high titer of speckled ANA staining on direct immunofluorescence of normal skin.[110–116]

TABLE 5–8.—MIXED CONNECTIVE TISSUE DISEASE

1. A combination of clinical features and laboratory data of
   a. Systemic lupus erythematosus
   b. Polymyositis
   c. And/or Sjögren's disease
2. Cutaneous features
   a. Cutaneous photosensitivity
   b. A heliotrope rash over eyelids
   c. Alopecia
   d. Malar telangiectasia and/or erythema
   e. Cutaneous lesions of LE
   f. Hyper- and/or hypopigmentation
   g. Periungual erythema
   h. Livedo reticularis
   i. Mucosal dryness
   j. Arthritis or arthralgia
   k. Tapered or sausage-shaped fingers
3. Laboratory features
   a. Anti-RNP titer greater than 1:1000
   b. Speckled distribution of IgG in epidermal nuclei on direct immunofluorescence

CLINICAL MANIFESTATIONS.—The cutaneous features of MCTD include cutaneous photosensitivity, a heliotrope rash over the eyelids, alopecia, malar telangiectasia or erythema or both, cutaneous lesions of lupus erythematosus, hyperpigmentation, hypopigmentation, periungual erythema, livedo reticularis, mucosal dryness, arthritis or arthralgia, sclerodactyly, puffy fingers with cutaneous sclerosis, and a tapered or sausage appearance of the fingers. The most common presenting features are joint complaints, Raynaud's phenomenon, or cutaneous lupus erythematosus.[106] Although some patients with MCTD have deforming arthritis, the most common symptom is an evanescent nonerosive nondeforming polyarthritis similar to that seen in patients with systemic lupus erythematosus.

The most important diagnostic features of MCTD are Raynaud's phenomenon, periungual telangiectasia, swelling of the hands with a tapered sausage appearance to the fingers, abnormal pulmonary function tests, myositis, disturbances of esophageal motility, joint pain, alopecia, and lesions of cutaneous lupus erythematosus (lupus-like rashes of the face may be found in 50% of untreated MCTD patients). Cine-esophagogram and monometric studies of the esophagus reveal abnormalities (even in the absence of symptoms) in 70% to 80% of patients. Up to 80% of patients have evidence of pulmonary disease on the basis of pulmonary function, roentgenographic measurements, or both. Proximal muscle weakness is common, with or without tenderness or elevated levels of serum creatine phosphokinase (CPK) and aldolase; nearly all patients have polyarthralgia and three-fourths of them have frank arthritis. Approximately two-thirds of children with MCTD have cardiac involvement, including pericarditis, myocarditis, congestive heart failure, and aortic insufficiency; about 10% have renal disease and about 10% of affected individuals have neurologic abnormalities (trigeminal sensory neuropathy, "vascular" headaches, seizures, multiple peripheral neuropathies, and cerebral infarction or hemorrhage).[114]

When MCTD was first described, it was thought to have a better prognosis than SLE and to be readily amenable to corticosteroid therapy. Although corticosteroid therapy does produce symptomatic improvement in many patients, and although life-threatening disease manifestations are not as common as in SLE, mixed connective tissue disease is at times much more severe than originally suggested. When MCTD occurs in childhood, it may mimic juvenile rheumatoid arthritis. Distinct differences, however, frequently exist between adult and childhood forms of mixed connective tissue disease. Severe thrombocytopenia appears to be limited to childhood forms, and the incidence of renal and cardiac involvement is higher in children than in adults.[115, 116]

DIAGNOSIS.—Characteristically, mixed connective tissue disease has overlapping features of two or even three connective tissue diseases (rheumatoid arthritis, systemic lupus erythematosus, dermatomyositis or polymyositis, Sjögren's syndrome or systemic scleroderma).[117–120] Common presenting features include arthritis, Raynaud's phenomenon, myositis, abnormal esophageal mobility, swollen hands, and lymphadenopathy (the most suggestive clinical features are the presence of Raynaud's phenomenon and swollen hands). A physician, therefore, should hesitate to make a diagnosis of MCTD in a patient in whom Raynaud's phenomenon is not present.[113]

The most distinguishing laboratory marker for this disease is the demonstration of serum antibody specific for ribonucleoprotein (RNP), a ribonuclease-sensitive component of extractable nuclear antigen (ENA). An anti-RNP titer greater than 1:1000 in patients with overlapping features of connective tissue disease, therefore, will generally serve to confirm the diagnosis.[1] In addition, most patients with MCTD have high serum titers of antinuclear antibody (ANA) in a speckled pattern, and a high titer of rheumatoid factor is present in up to 50% of patients.[121] LE cells may also be found in up to one-third of patients with MCTD, indicating the close association of these two disorders. In contrast with most cases of SLE, however, patients with MCTD lack antibodies to DNA. The deposition of IgG in epidermal nuclei in a speckled (particulate) pattern on direct immunofluorescence of normal skin is also strongly suggestive of MCTD. This finding, however, is not pathognomonic since SLE patients with high titers of Sm antibodies may show identical changes.[113]

TREATMENT.—The prognosis of mixed connective tissue disease in children is not as good as originally suggested. Although most patients have a relatively benign disease, the course frequently may be one of remission and relapse, similar to that observed in patients with SLE. Recent studies suggest significant morbidity and mortality from pulmonary or renal involvement, or both. Patients should be treated according to the particular systems of involvement, with high doses of steroids and, when necessary, immunosuppressive agents similar to those required in the management of patients with severe systemic lupus erythematosus.

REFERENCES

1. Braverman I.M.: Connective tissue (rheumatic) diseases, in *Skin Signs of Systemic Disease*, ed. 2. 1981, W.B. Saunders Co., Philadelphia, pp. 255–376.
2. Block S.R., Winfield J.B., Lockshin M.D., et al.: Studies of twins with systemic lupus erythematosus. A review of the literature and presentation of 12 additional sets. *Am. J. Med.* 59:533–552, 1975.
3. Cleland L.G., Bell D.A., Willans M., et al.: Familial lupus. Family studies of HLA and serologic findings. *Arthritis Rheum.* 21:183–191, 1978.
4. Fish A.J., Blau E.B., Westberg G., et al.: Systemic lupus erythematosus within the first two decades of life. *Am. J. Med.* 62:99–117, 1977.
5. Peterson R.D.A., Vernier R.L., Good R.A.: Lupus erythematosus. *Pediatr. Clin. North Am.* 10:941–978, 1963.
6. Sontheimer R.D., Thomas J.R., Gilliam J.N.: Subacute cutaneous lupus erythematosus: a cutaneous marker for a distinct lupus erythematosus subset. *Arch. Dermatol.* 115:1409–1415, 1979.
7. Schaller J.G., Wedgewood R.J.: Rheumatic diseases of childhood, in Behrman R.E., Vaughn V.C. III: *Nelson's Textbook of Pediatrics*, ed. 12. 1983, W.B. Saunders Co., Philadelphia, pp. 561–588.
8. Winkelmann R.K.: Chronic discoid lupus erythematosus in children. *J.A.M.A.* 205:675–678, 1968.
9. O'Laughlin S., Schroeter A.L., Jordon R.E.: Chronic urticaria-like lesions in systemic lupus erythematosus. A review of 12 cases. *Arch. Dermatol.* 114:879–883, 1978.
10. Provost T.T., Zone J.J., Synkowski D., et al. Unusual cutaneous manifestations of systemic lupus erythematosus. 1. urticaria-like lesions, correlation with clinical and serologic abnormalities. *J. Invest. Dermatol.* 75:495–499, 1980.
11. Millard L.G., Rowell N.R.: Chilblain lupus erythematosus (Hutchinson): a clinical and laboratory study of 17 patients. *Br. J. Dermatol.* 98:497–506, 1978.
12. Englund J.A., Lucas R.V., Jr.: Cardiac complications in children with systemic lupus erythematosus. *Pediatrics* 72:724–730, 1983.
13. Zizic T.M., Hungerford D.S., Stevens M.B.: Ischemic bone necrosis in systemic lupus erythematosus. *Med.* 59:134–142, 1980.
14. Caeiro F., Michielson F.M.C., Bernstein R., et al.: Systemic lupus erythematosus in childhood. *Ann. Rheum. Dis.* 40:325–331, 1981.
15. Tan E.M., Cohen A.S., Fries J., et al.: The 1982 revised criteria for the

classification of systemic lupus erythematosus. *Arthritis Rheum.* 25:1271–1277, 1982.

16. Shklar G.: Histopathology of oral lesions of discoid lupus erythematosus. *Arch. Dermatol.* 114:1031–1035, 1978.
17. Synkowski D.R., Mogavero H.S., Provost T.T.: Lupus erythematosus. Laboratory testing and clinical subsets in the evaluation of patients, in Callen J.P. (editor): *Cutaneous Signs of Systemic Disease.* Med. Clin. No. Am. 64:921–940, 1980.
18. Huber O., Greenberg M.L., Huber J.: Complement fixing anti-double stranded DNA with the Crithidia method. *J. Lab. Clin. Med.* 93:32–39, 1979.
19. Lever W.F., Schaumburg-Lever G.: Connective Tissue Diseases, in *Histopathology of the Skin.* J.P. Lippincott Co., Philadelphia, ed. 6. 1983, pp. 445–471.
20. Millard L.G., Rowell N.R.: Abnormal laboratory test results and their relationship to prognosis in discoid lupus erythematosus. *Arch. Dermatol.* 115:1055–1058, 1979.
21. Hollister J.R.: Connective Tissue, in Gellis S.S., Kagan B.M. (Eds.): *Current Pediatric Therapy,* ed. 10. W.B. Saunders Co., Philadelphia, 1982, pp. 342–346.
22. Meislin A.G., Rothfield N.: Systemic lupus erythematosus in childhood. *Pediatrics* 42:37–49, 1968.
23. Walvarens P.A., Chase P.: The prognosis of childhood systemic lupus erythematosus. *Am. J. Dis. Child.* 130:929–933, 1976.
24. Rasmussen J.E.: Antimalarials—are they safe to use in children? *Pediat. Dermatol.* 1:89–91, 1983.
25. Korter-King K., Kornreich H.K., Bernstein B.H., et al.: The clinical spectrum of SLE in childhood. *Arthritis Rheumatism 20(Suppl.)*:287–294, 1977.
26. Wallace D.J., Podell T., Weiner J., et al.: Systemic lupus erythematosus-survival pattern. Experience with 609 patients. *J.A.M.A.* 245:934–938, 1981.
27. Tejani A., Nicastri A.D., Chen C., et al.: Lupus nephritis in black and hispanic children. *Am. J. Dis. Child.* 137:481–483, 1983.
28. Ehrlich G.E.: Trends in therapy: systemic lupus erythematosus. *J.A.M.A.* 232:1361–1364, 1975.
29. Urman J.D., Rothfield N.F.: Corticosteroid treatment in systemic lupus erythematosus—survival studies. *J.A.M.A.* 238:2272–2276, 1977.
30. Vonderheid E.C., Koblenzer P.J., Ming P.M.L., et al.: Neonatal lupus erythematosus. *Arch. Dermatol.* 112:698–705, 1976.
31. Draznin T.H., Esterly N.B., Furey N.L., et al.: Neonatal lupus erythematosus. *J. Am. Acad. Dermatol.* 1:437–442, 1979.
32. Lockshin M.D., Gibofsky A., Peebles C.L., et al.: Neonatal lupus erythematosus with heart block: family study of a patient with anti-SS-A and SS-B antibodies. *Arthritis and Rheumatism* 26:210–213, 1983.
33. Chamiedes L., Truex R.C., Vetter V., et al.: Association of maternal lupus erythematosus with congenital complete heart block. *N. Engl. J. Med.* 297:1204–1207, 1977.
34. Korkij W., Soltani K.: Neonatal lupus erythematosus: a review. *Pediatric Dermatol.* Vol. 1, No. 3, 189–195, 1984.
35. Lee L.A., Weston W.L.: New findings in neonatal lupus syndrome. *Am. J. Dis. Child.* 138:233–236, 1984.

36. Kephart D.C., Hood A.F., Provost T.T.: Lupus erythematosus. New serological findings. *J. Invest. Dermatol.* 77:331–333, 1981.

37. Weston W.L., Harmon C., Peebles C., et al.: A serological marker for neonatal lupus. *Br. J. Dermatol.* 107:377–382, 1982.

38. Scott J.S., Maddison P.J., Taylor P.V., et al.: Connective tissue disease, antibodies to ribonucleoprotein, and congenital heart block. *N. Engl. J. Med.* 309:209–212, 1983.

39. Vasquez-Rodriguez J.J., Garcia-Seoane J., Gial-Aguado A., et al.: Complete heart block and the HLA system (letter). *Ann. Int. Med.* 96:126, 1982.

40. Epstein H.C., Litt J.Z.: Discoid lupus erythematosus in a newborn infant. *N. Engl. J. Med.* 265:1106–1107, 1961.

41. Soltani K., Pacernick L.J., Lorincz A.L.: Lupus erythematosus-like lesions in newborn infants. *Arch. Dermatol.* 110:435–437, 1974.

42. Klippel J.H., Grimley P.M., Decker J.L.: Lymphocyte inclusions in newborns of mothers with systemic lupus erythematosus. *N. Engl. J. Med.* 290:96–97, 1974.

43. Brustein D., Rodriguez J.M., Minkin W., et al.: Familial lupus erythematosus. *J.A.M.A.* 238:2294–2296, 1977.

44. Jackson R., Gulliver M.: Neonatal lupus erythematosus progressing into systemic lupus erythematosus. *Br. J. Dermatol.* 101:81–86, 1979.

45. Fox R.J., Jr., McCuistion H.B., Schoch E.P., Jr.: Systemic lupus erythematosus: association with previous neonatal lupus erythematosus. *Arch. Dermatol.* 115:340, 1979.

46. Levy S.B., Goldsmith L.A., Morohashi M., et al.: Tubuloreticular inclusions in neonatal lupus erythematosus. *J.A.M.A.* 235:2743–2744, 1976.

47. Vetter V.L., Rashkind W.J.: Editorial. Congenital complete heart block and connective tissue disease. *N. Engl. J. Med.* 309:236–237, 1983.

48. Dawkins R.E., Mastiglia F.L.: Cell-mediated cytotoxicity in polymyositis. *N. Engl. J. Med.* 288:434–438, 1973.

49. Banker B.Q., Victor M.: Dermatomyositis (systemic angiopathy) of childhood. *Medicine* 45:261–288, 1966.

50. Pachman L.M., Cooke N.: Juvenile dermatomyositis: a clinical and immunologic study. *J. Pediatr.* 96:226–234, 1980.

51. Travers R.L., Hughes G.R.V., Cambridge G., et al.: Coxsackie B neutralization titres in polymyositis/dermatomyositis. *Lancet* 1:1268, 1977.

52. Koch M.J., Brody J.A., Gillespie M.M.: Childhood polymyositis: a case-control study. *Am. J. Epidemiol.* 104:627–631, 1976.

53. Pachman L.M., Jonasson L.M., O'Cannon R.A., et al.: Increased frequency of HLA-B8 in juvenile dermatomyositis. *Lancet* 2:1238, 1977.

54. Friedman J.M., Packman L.M., Maryowski M.L., et al.: Immunogenetic studies of juvenile dermatomyositis: HLA or antigen frequencies. *Arthritis and Rheum.* 26(2):214–216, 1983.

55. Behan W.M.H., Behan P.O., Dick H.A.: HLA-B8 in polymyositis. *N. Engl. J. Med.* 298:1260–1261, 1978.

56. Everett M.A., Curtis A.C.: Dermatomyositis: A review of nineteen cases in adolescents and children. *Arch. Int. Med.* 100:70–76, 1967.

57. Goel K.M., Shanks R.A.: Some skin manifestations of connective tissue disorders in childhood. *Dermatology Digest,* 14–19, January, 1977.

58. Winkelmann R.K.: Dermatomyositis in childhood. *JCE Dermatology* 18:13–21, 1979.

59. Cook D.C., Rosen F.S., Banker B.Q.: Dermatomyositis and focal scleroderma. *Pediatr. Clin. N. Am.* 10:979–1016, 1963.
60. Lell M.E., Swerdlow M.L.: Dermatomyositis of childhood. *Pediatr. Ann.* 6:203–211, 1977.
61. Sunde H.: Dermatomyositis in children. *Acta Paediatr.* 37:287–308, 1949.
62. Sheldon J.H., Young F., Dyke S.C.: Acute dermatomyositis associated with reticulo-endotheliosis. *Lancet* 1:82–84, 1939.
63. Samitz M.H.: Cuticular changes in dermatomyositis. *Arch. Dermatol.* 110:866–867, 1974.
64. Muller S.A., Winkelmann R.K., Brunsting L.A.: Calcinosis in dermatomyositis. Observations on the course of the disease in children and adults. *Arch. Dermatol.* 76:669–673, 1959.
65. Bohan A., Peter J.B.: Polymyositis and dermatomyositis. *N. Engl. J. Med.* 292:344–347, 1975.
66. Bohan A., Peter J.B., Bowman R.L., et al.: Computer-assisted analysis of 153 patients with polymyositis and dermatomyositis. *Medicine* 56:255–286, 1977.
67. Caro I.: Dermatomyositis, in Maddin S. (editor): *Current Dermatologic Therapy.* W.B. Saunders Co., 1982, pp. 123–125.
68. Bitnum S., Daeschner C.W., Jr., Travis L.B., et al.: Dermatomyositis. *J. Pediatr.* 64:101–131, 1964.
69. Sullivan D.B., Cassidy J.T., Petty R.E., et al.: Prognosis in childhood dermatomyositis. *J. Pediatr.* 80:555–563, 1972.
70. Jacobs J.C.: Methotrexate and azathioprine treatment of childhood dermatomyositis. *Pediatrics* 59:212–217, 1977.
71. Fischer T.J., Rachelefsky G.S., Klein R.B., et al.: Childhood dermatomyositis and polymyositis. Treatment with methotrexate and prednisone. *Am. J. Dis. Child.* 133:386–389, 1979.
72. Nassim J.M., Connolly C.K.: Treatment of calcinosis universalis with aluminum hydroxide. *Arch. Dis. Child.* 45:118–121, 1970.
73. Mazzafarin G., Lafferty F.W., Pearson O.H.: Treatment of calcinosis with phosphorus deprivation. *Ann. Int. Med.* 77:741–745, 1972.
74. Brady A.H.: Collagenase in scleroderma. *J. Clin. Invest.* 56:1175–1180, 1975.
75. Bauer E.A., Eisen A.Z.: Scleroderma: increased biosynthesis of triple-helical type I and type III procollagens associated with unaltered expression of collagenase by skin fibroblasts in culture. *J. Clin. Invest.* 64:921–930, 1979.
76. Buckingham R.B., Prince R.K., Rodnan G.P., et al.: Increased collagen accumulation in dermal fibroblast cultures from patients with progressive systemic sclerosis (scleroderma). *J. Lab. Clin. Med.* 92:5–21, 1978.
77. Kass H., Hanson V., Patrick J.: Scleroderma in childhood. *J. Pediatr.* 68:243–256, 1966.
78. Curtis A.C., Jansen T.G.: The prognosis of localized scleroderma. *Arch. Dermatol.* 78:749–757, 1958.
79. Chazen E., Cook C.D., Cohen J.: Focal scleroderma. Report of 19 cases in children. *J. Pediatr.* 60:385–393, 1962.
80. Goel K.M., Shanks R.A.: Scleroderma in childhood. *Arch. Dis. Child.* 49:861–865, 1974.
81. Jaffe M.O., Winklemann R.K.: Generalized scleroderma in children. *Arch. Dermatol.* 83:402–413, 1961.
82. Sullivan D.B., Cassidy J.T.: Scleroderma in the child. *J. Pediatr.* 85:770–775, 1974.

83. Larrègue M., Canuel C., Bazex J., et al.: Systemic scleroderma in childhood: report of 5 cases of review of literature. *Ann. Dermatol. Venerol.* 110:317–326, 1983.

84. Crown S.: Visceral scleroderma without skin involvement. *Br. Med. J.* 2:1541–1543, 1961.

85. Rodnan G.P., Fennell R.H., Jr.: Progressive systemic sclerosis *sine* scleroderma. *J.A.M.A.* 180:665–670, 1962.

86. Rodeheffer R.J., Rommer J.A., Wrigley F., et al.: Controlled double-blind trial of nifedipine in the treatment of Raynaud's phenomenon. *N. Engl. J. Med.* 308:880–883, 1983.

87. Shulman L.E.: Diffuse fasciitis with eosinophilia: a new syndrome? *Trans. Assoc. Am. Physicians.* 88:70–86, 1975.

88. Fleischmajer R., Jacotot A.B., Shore S., et al.: Scleroderma, eosinophilia, and diffuse fasciitis. *Arch. Dermatol.* 114:1320–1325, 1978.

89. Rodnan G.P., DiBartholomeo A., Medsger T.A., Jr., et al.: Eosinophilia fasciitis. Report of seven cases of a newly recognized scleroderma-like syndrome. *Arthritis Rheum.* 18:422–423, 1975.

90. Patrone N.A., Kredich D.W.: Eosinophilic faciitis in a child. *Am. J. Dis. Child.* 138:363–365, 1984.

91. Caperton E.M., Hathaway D.E., Dehner L.P.: Morphea, fasciitis and scleroderma with eosinophilia: a broad spectrum of disease. *Arthritis Rheum.* 19:792, 1976.

92. Michet C.J., Jr., Doyle J.A., Ginsburg W.W.: Eosinophilic fasciitis: report of fifteen cases. *Mayo Clinic Proceedings* 56:27–34, 1981.

93. Barnes L., Rodnan G., Medsger T.A., Jr., et al.: Eosinophilic fasciitis: a pathological study of twenty cases. *Am. J. Pathol.* 96:493–518, 1979.

94. Moutsopoulos H.M., Webber B.L., Pavlidis M.A., et al.: Diffuse fasciitis with eosinophilia: clinical pathologic study. *Am. J. Med.* 68:701–709, 1980.

95. Shewmake S.W., Lopez A., McGlammory J.C.: The Shulman syndrome. *Arch. Dermatol.* 114:556–559, 1978.

96. Jarratt M.: Eosinophilic fasciitis. *J. Am. Acad. Dermatol.* 1:221–226, 1979.

97. Golitz L.E.: Fasciitis with eosinophilia: the Shulman syndrome. *Int. J. Dermatol.* 19:552–555, 1980.

98. Brewer E.J., Jr.: *Major Problems in Clinical Pediatrics, VI, Juvenile Rheumatoid Arthritis.* W.B. Saunders Co., Philadelphia, 1970.

99. Schaller J.G.: Juvenile rheumatoid arthritis. *Pediatrics in Review* 2:163–174, 1980–1981.

100. Isdale I.C., Bywaters E.G.L.: The rash of rheumatoid arthritis in Still's disease. *Quart. J. Med. New Series XXV*, No. 99:377–387, 1956.

101. Calabro J.J., Marchesano J.M.: Rash associated with juvenile rheumatoid arthritis. *J. Pediatr.* 72:611–619, 1968.

102. Jorizzo J.C., Daniels J.C.: Dermatological conditions reported in patients with rheumatoid arthritis. *J. Am. Acad. Derm.* 8:439–457, 1983.

103. Schlesinger B.E., Forsyth C.C., White R.H.R., et al.: Observations on the clinical course and treatment of one hundred cases of Still's disease. *Arch. Dis. Child.* 36:65–76, 1961.

104. Calabro J.J.: Diseases of connective tissue, in Gellis S.S., Kagen B.M. (Eds.): *Current Pediatric Therapy*, ed. 6. W.B. Saunders Co., Philadelphia, 1973, pp. 377–381.

105. Athreya B.H., Norman M.E., Myers A.R., et al.: Sjögren's syndrome in children. *Pediatrics* 59:931–937, 1977.

106. Chudwin D.S., Daniels T.E., Wara D.W., et al.: Spectrum of Sjögren syndrome in children. *J. Pediatr.* 98:213–217, 1981.
107. Bernstein B., Korter-King K., Singsen B., et al.: Sjögren's syndrome in childhood. *Arthritis Rheum.* 20(Suppl): 361–362, 1977.
108. Talal N.: Sjögren's syndrome, in Demis D.J., Dobson R.L., McGuire J.: *Clinical Dermatology*, ed. 10. Harper & Row Publishers, Philadelphia, 1983, 5–5:104.
109. Kassan S.S., Thomas T.L., Moutsopoulos H.M., et al.: Increased risk of lymphoma in sicca syndrome. *Ann. Int. Med.* 89:888–892, 1978.
110. Sharp G.C., Irvin W.S., Tan E.M., et al.: Mixed connective tissue disease: An apparently distinct rheumatic disease syndrome associated with a specific antibody to extractable nuclear antigen (ENA). *Am. J. Med.* 52:148–159, 1972.
111. Fraga A., Gudino J., Ramos-Niembro F., et al.: Mixed connective tissue disease in childhood. Relationship with Sjögren's syndrome. *Am. J. Dis. Child.* 132:263–265, 1978.
112. Gilliam J.N., Prystkowsky S.D.: Mixed connective tissue disease syndrome. Cutaneous manifestations of patients with epidermal nuclear staining and high titer serum antibody to ribonuclease-sensitive extractable nuclear antigen. *Arch. Dermatol.* 113:583–586, 1977.
113. Gilliam J.M., Prystkowsky S.D.: Mixed connective tissue disease. In Moschella S.L., (Ed.): *Dermatology Update. Review for Physicians.* Elsevier Publishing Company, New York, 1979, pp. 173–193.
114. Sharp G.C., Anderson D.C.: Current concepts in the classification of connective tissue disease. Overlapping syndromes and mixed connective tissue disease (MCTD). *J. Am. Acad. Dermatol.* 2:269–279, 1980.
115. Sanders D.H., Huntley C.C., Sharp G.C.: Mixed connective tissue disease in a child. *J. Pediatr.* 83:642–645, 1973.
116. Singsen B.H., Bernstein B.H., Kornreich H.K., et al.: Mixed connective tissue disease in childhood, clinical and serological survey. *J. Pediatr.* 90:893–900, 1977.
117. Oetgen W.J., Boise J.A., Lawless O.J.: Mixed connective tissue disease in children and adolescents. *Pediatrics* 67:333–337, 1981.
118. Prystkowsky S.D., Tuffanelli D.L.: Speckled (particulate) epidermal nuclear IgG deposition in normal skin—correlation of clinical features and laboratory findings in 46 patients with a subset of connective tissue disease characterized by antibody to extractable nuclear antigen. *Arch. Dermatol.* 114:705–710, 1978.
119. Bentley-Phillips C.D., Geake T.M.S.: Mixed connective tissue disease characterized by speckled epidermal nuclear IgG deposition in normal skin. *Br. J. Dermatol.* 102:529–533, 1980.
120. Kish L.S., Steck W.D.: Mixed connective tissue disease in identical twins. A sclerodermoid variant with concurrent psoriasis. *Cleve. Clin. Q.* 50:205–207, Summer, 1983.
121. Black C.: Mixed connective tissue disease. *Br. J. Dermatol.* 104:713–719, 1981.

6 / Endocrine Disorders

ENDOCRINE DISEASES FREQUENTLY DISPLAY cutaneous features that provide rewarding clues to the physician asked to diagnose or assist in the management of unusual dermatoses or systemic disorders of patients in the pediatric age group. This chapter will review some of these conditions and their dermatologic features, clinical manifestations and therapy.

Thyroid Disorders

The spectrum of thyroid disease in pediatric patients is broad and may manifest as hypothyroidism (congenital or acquired), hyperthyroidism, tumors of the thyroid, and acute, subacute or chronic thyroiditis. Of these, thyroiditis is probably the most common endocrine disease in pediatrics. This section includes a discussion of hypothyroidism, hyperthyroidism, and the multiple mucosal neuroma syndrome (multiple endocrine adematosis III, multiple endocrine neoplasia type 2b or 3), all of which present striking dermatologic features. Thyroiditis, the most common cause of thyroid disease in children and adolescents, accounts for many of the enlarged thyroids formerly designated as "adolescent" goiter. Also the most common cause of juvenile hypothyroidism (with or without goiter), its incidence may be as high as 1% in children.[1] Most children affected with thyroiditis are clinically euthyroid and asymptomatic (some may merely present with symptoms of pressure in the neck). Those with clinical signs of hypothyroidism or hyperthyroidism will be described under the respective disorders.

Hypothyroidism

The term *hypothyroidism* refers to a group of clinical disorders that result from inadequate production of thyroid hormone. Congenital or acquired in nature, hypothyroidism in the first two or three years of life may result in irreversible damage to the nervous system. Beyond this age, however, most effects of hypothyroidism are reversible.[1]

Congenital hypothyroidism, a disorder of thyroid deficiency present from birth or early infancy, may develop as a result of agenesis or dysgenesis of the thyroid gland; by defective synthesis of thyroid hormone caused by an enzymatic defect; by the presence of antithyroid antibodies in a pregnant mother; by lack of maternal iodine during pregnancy (endemic goiter); or by the ingestion of antithyroid medications such as propylthyouracil or methimazole (Tapazole, Lilly) by pregnant women being treated for thyrotoxicosis. Of these, thyroid dysgenesis is the most common cause of congenital hypothyroidism (Table 6–1). Although "cretinism" is often used synonymously with congenital hypothyroidism, current texts suggest the avoidance of the uncomplimentary term.

CLINICAL MANIFESTATIONS.—Congenital hypothyroidism is estimated to occur in 1 in 2500 to 1 in 7000 newborns.[2, 3] The classic clinical features include puffy myxematous facies; depressed nasal bridge; hypertelorism; a large protruding tongue; thick lips; coarse brittle hair; short neck; large fontanels with wide cranial sutures; hoarse cry; abdominal distention; umbilical hernia; goiter; hypotonia; cold, mottled or jaundiced skin; a sallow complexion; translucent "alabaster"-like ears; stunted growth; delayed and defective dentition; poor weight gain; poor peripheral circulation with subnormal body temperature and intolerance to cold; inactivity; broad hands; stubby fingers; seborrhea of the scalp; purpura; prolonged relaxation phase of tendon reflexes; mental retardation; and delayed motor development with neurologic damage such as lack of coordination and ataxia[1–4] (Table 6–2).

DIAGNOSIS.—Although congenital hypothyroidism may present in the newborn with no clinical signs, most infants manifest a constellation of clinical features which include general sluggishness, failure to gain weight, constipation, weak hoarse cry, large protruding tongue, wide anterior fontanel, short stubby fingers, umbilical hernia, short lower extremities, an otherwise unexplained heart murmur, and, in some cases, myxedema. Radiological examination in a term infant may reveal absence of the distal femoral epiphyses and laboratory findings of a low serum thyroxine (T_4) and triiodothyronine (T_3) resin uptake, and elevated thyroid-stimulating hormone (TSH). Since triiodothyronine (T_3) levels may be normal or low, they

TABLE 6–1.—ETIOLOGY OF CHILDHOOD HYPOTHYROIDISM

1. *Congenital hypothyroidism*
   a. Thyroid agenesis or dysgenesis (over 80%)
   b. Inborn defect of thyroid hormone synthesis
   c. Maternal causes
      1. Maternal antithyroid antibodies
      2. Endemic goiter (maternal iodine deficiency)
      3. Ingestion of goitrogenic (antithyroid agents) or radioactive iodine therapy
2. *Acquired hypothyroidism*
   a. Hashimoto's (chronic lymphocytic) thyroiditis
   b. Thyroid dysgenesis (with delayed failure of thyroid remnants)
   c. Inborn defect in synthesis of thyroid hormone
   d. Thyroidectomy or radioactive thyroid ablation
3. Antithyroid ingestion

TABLE 6–2.—CLINICAL FEATURES
OF CONGENITAL HYPOTHYROIDISM

Puffy (myxedematous) facies
Sallow complexion
Large fontanels and wide sutures
Macroglossia and thick lips
Hypertelorism, depressed nasal bridge
Coarse, brittle hair
Hoarse cry
Translucent ("alabaster") ears
Umbilical hernia and abdominal distension
Hypotonia and slow reflexes
Stubby fingers and broad hands
Seborrhea of scalp
Purpura
Cold, mottled or jaundiced skin
Sluggishness and inactivity
Delayed motor development, mental retardation
Lack of coordination and ataxia
Poor weight gain, stunted growth
Subnormal body temperature, poor circulation and intolerance to cold
Delayed/defective dentition

are generally not very useful. A rapid radioimmunoassay measurement of serum T_4 and TSH levels on filter paper, heel-stick or cord blood samples in the first few days of life are helpful as an early screening procedure for newborn infants.[2, 5]

Acquired hypothyroidism in children below the age of five or six years is usually caused by a delayed failure of thyroid remnants (with thyroid dysgenesis). It can also develop as a result of inborn defects of thyroid hormone synthesis, ingestion of antithyroid agents, thyroidectomy or ablation following radiation, and chronic thyroiditis or hypothalamic-pituitary disease. After the age of 5 or 6, although the same etiologies may be involved, chronic lymphocytic thyroiditis (Hashimoto's disease) appears to be the most common cause of this disorder (Table 6–1).

CLINICAL MANIFESTATIONS.—The clinical manifestations of acquired hypothyroidism depend upon the age of the child at onset and upon the extent of the dysfunction. Seen in approximately 1 in 500 to 1 in 1000 children (with a female to male ratio of 6:1), the later in life that acquired hypothyroidism occurs, the less the impairment of growth and development. Acquired hypothyroidism caused by Hashimoto's disease is often insidious in onset with the most common presentation being a decrease in growth rate with or without an accompanying goiter. This emphasizes the value of carefully kept growth records on the part of the physician.[1]

The onset of acquired hypothyroidism is often insidious. Clinical signs are frequently subtle, with a decrease in growth rate, delayed dentition, mild obesity (with myxedema), an increase in upper to lower body segment ratio, delayed puberty, developmental delay and a decreased quality in school performance. If the hypothyroidism persists without therapy, the classic features of hypothyroidism become apparent. Symptoms include generalized puffiness, with thick lips and puffiness about the eyes, nose and cheeks producing a typical dull expressionless facies (Fig 6–1); lethargy; poor appetite; constipation; short stature; bradycardia; decreased blood pressure with narrow pulse pressure; goiter; protruberant abdomen and buttocks; pale thick cool skin with sallow appearance; coarse hair; hypertrichosis (Fig 6–2); flabby pseudohypertrophic muscles; and delayed deep tendon reflexes. Although hypothyroidism usually delays the onset of puberty, some children will develop a paradoxical precocious puberty with elevated serum gonadotropin concentrations (Table 6–3).

Patients with hypothyroidism complain of cold intolerance and frequently require a sweater or jacket when everybody else is comfortably warm. The hair typically disappears from the outer part of the eyebrows and becomes sparse, dry and thin. Nails are brittle and show longitudinal and transverse striations. The tongue and oral mucous membranes become thickened, and speech becomes slow and labored. As a result of deposition of mucin, the hands and feet frequently become puffy, the skin becomes rough and dry, and purpura and ecchymoses may be present.[6]

Children with acquired hypothyroidism have a pleasant disposition but

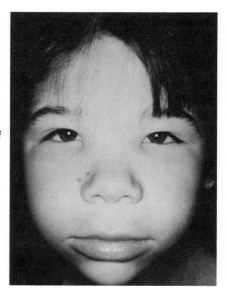

Fig 6–1.—Typical expressionless facies with thick lips and puffiness of the eyes, nose and cheeks in a 10-year-old girl with acquired hypothyroidism.

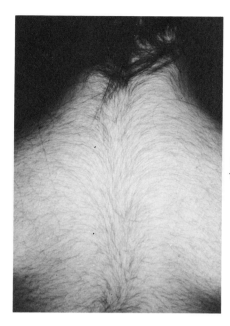

Fig 6–2.—Acquired hypothyroidism. Hypertrichosis and rough dry skin on the upper back of 10-year-old girl.

do poorly scholastically. Unfortunately, because they are usually placid, quiet, and good natured, teachers frequently fail to recognize their intellectual deficiency and think of them as ideal students. Such children may continue to present satisfactory scholastic records despite their obvious intellectual deficiency.[4]

DIAGNOSIS.—The same diagnostic tests are utilized in acquired as in congenital hypothyroidism. The diagnosis of primary hypothyroidism is confirmed by a low T4 and T3 resin uptake and an elevated serum TSH concentration. In cases of long duration, a lateral x-ray of the skull may reveal enlargement of the sella turcica, and roentgenologic examination of long bones may reveal delayed appearance of ossification centers. Besides epiphyseal degenesis, a decrease in the anteroposterior diameter and breaking of the vertebral body (similar to that seen in patients with Hurler's disease) may be noted. Other laboratory features include an elevated serum cholesterol level and, since untreated children with hypothyroidism do not grow, a low serum alkaline phosphatase level may help establish the diagnosis.

TREATMENT.—The treatment of choice for children with hypothyroidism is oral sodium-L-thyroxine (Synthroid; Flint), with dosage adjustments according to the individual's age and clinical and biochemical response. The dosage should be adjusted at two- to 4-week intervals to a level that main-

TABLE 6–3.—CLINICAL FEATURES
OF ACQUIRED HYPOTHYROIDISM

Generalized puffiness (thick lips and puffiness around
   eyes) with a dull expressionless facies
Mild obesity, myxedema
Decreased growth rate and short stature (increase in
   upper to lower body segment ratio)
Delayed development
Poor scholastic performance
Placid disposition
Poor appetite
Lethargy
Constipation
Bradycardia, decreased blood pressure
Thick pale cool skin (with sallow appearance)
Hypertrichosis with coarse hair
Flabby pseudohypertrophic muscles
Delayed deep tendon reflexes
Cold intolerance
Goiter
Rough dry skin, brittle nails (with longitudinal striations)
Slow labored speech
Puffy hands and feet
Purpura or ecchymoses
Delayed or precocious puberty

---

tains the serum T4 concentration in the mid-range of normal, with normal
T3 and TSH concentrations. Fortunately, in contrast to patients with congenital hypothyroidism, irreversible brain damage is usually not a problem
when the child acquired hypothyroidism after the age of 2 to 3 years.

The suggested dosage of thyroxine for infants under 1 year of age is 6 to
12 micrograms/kg/24 hrs (usually 30 to 50 micrograms a day during the first
six months of age) administered in one daily dose for infants.[7] Older children require a dosage of about 4 micrograms/kg/day with individualization
of dosage according to the biochemical (T_4, TSH and on occasion T_3 levels)
and clinical response. Weight gain in infants should be monitored daily and
is probably the most sensitive indicator. Overtreatment may result in clinical signs of hyperthyroidism (diarrhea, hyperirritability, disturbed sleep
patterns, and tachycardia). Since cardiac deaths have been reported in the
early phases of thyroid replacement, it is strongly recommended that children with congenital hypothyroidism be referred to a pediatric endocrinol-
ogist and be hospitalized for careful monitoring, particularly during the
early phases of therapy.[4]

The treatment of acquired hypothyroidism may at times lead to temporary periods of personality upheaval characterized by argumentativeness
and the loss of the patient's previous docile personality. School performance may deteriorate as the child adjusts to a resurgence of energy and

a loss of interest in scholastic achievements. In such instances, parents and teachers need to be supportive, and appropriate guidance and counseling may be required. Fortunately, this period of adjustment generally lasts only for a few months.

Hyperthyroidism

Hyperthyroidism, a relatively uncommon disorder of childhood, occurs most frequently in the 11– to 16-year-old age group and is five or six times more common in girls than in boys. Only one-fifth as common as hypothyroidism in childhood, about 5% of all patients with hyperthyroidism are under 15 years of age. Thyrotoxicosis can also occur in the newborn period, and in infants as young as two days to two months of age, it can be life-threatening. This disorder, termed neonatal thyrotoxicosis or transient neonatal hyperthyroidism, is often transient and may last for about six months, or it may persist indefinitely. Neonatal thyrotoxicosis is characterized by irritability, flushing, tachycardia, exophthalmos, goiter, weight loss, voracious appetite, and other features of Graves' disease. Affected infants invariably are offspring of women who have or have had thyrotoxicosis caused by long-acting thyroid stimulator (LATS) transferred from the mother to the infant during pregnancy.[13]

Although most other cases of hyperthyroidism in children are associated with autoimmune thyroid disease (diffuse toxic goiter [Graves' disease]), it may also be associated with chronic lymphocytic thyroiditis (Hashimoto's thyroiditis), hyperfunctioning thyroid nodules, or hypersecretion of thyroid-stimulating hormone (TSH) (Table 6–4). Despite the fact that a number of immunologic reactions have been demonstrated in Graves' disease, the events that precipitate these immune reactions remain obscure.

CLINICAL MANIFESTATIONS.—The clinical features of hyperthyroidism include nervousness, emotional lability, tachycardia and palpitation, heat intolerance, weakness, fatigue, tremors, hyperactivity, increased appetite, weight loss, increased systolic and pulse pressure, accelerated growth, sleep disturbances, school problems, vomiting, diarrhea, thyroid gland enlargement, and, at times, exophthalmos (Table 6–5).

The skin of the hyperthyroid patient is warm, soft, smooth and velvety. Flushing of the face, increased sweating (particularly of the palms and

TABLE 6–4.—CAUSES OF HYPERTHYROIDISM
(THYROTOXICOSIS) IN CHILDREN

Diffuse toxic goiter (Graves' disease)
Hashimoto's thyroiditis
Hyperfunctioning thyroid nodules (functional adenoma)
Thyroid cancer
Hypersecretion of TSH

TABLE 6–5.—CLINICAL FEATURES
OF HYPERTHYROIDISM (THYROTOXICOSIS)

Thyroid gland enlargement
Exophthalmos
Nervousness, emotional lability
Tachycardia and palpitation
Increased systolic and pulse pressure
Heat intolerance
Weakness, fatigue
Hyperactivity and tremors
Increased appetite and accelerated growth
Sleep disturbances
Vomiting and diarrhea
Warm soft smooth skin
Flushing of face
Rapidly growing shiny nails, onycholysis with upward
    curvature (Plummer's nails)
Pruritus, chronic urticaria
Addisonian pigmentation
Pretibial myxedema and thyroid acropachy

soles) and palmar erythema are common. The nails grow rapidly, are shiny, and may have onycholysis (separation or loosening of the nail plate from the nail bed) with distal upward curvature (Plummer's nails). Chronic urticaria and generalized pruritus are uncommon manifestations of thyrotoxicosis. Chronic, active hyperthyroidism can be complicated by Addisonian hyperpigmentation. The latter feature, thought to be caused by increased "MSH" secretion from the pituitary, is probably not as common today since most patients with hyperthyroidism are now treated earlier. Patients with hyperthyroidism have an increased incidence of alopecia areata and/or vitiligo, and about one-third have a history or clinical features of atopic dermatitis.

Other cutaneous features of hyperthyroidism include pretibial myxedema and thyroid acropachy. *Pretibial myxedema* is a localized form of myxedema characterized by flesh-colored, pink, or purplish-brown to yellow asymptomatic or pruritic plaques or nodules on the anterolateral aspect of the legs, at times extending to the dorsal aspect of the feet.[9] The overlying epidermis is thin with a waxy and at times translucent quality with prominent hair follicles. The hypertrichosis with dilated hair follicles and accentuation of coarse hairs may be responsible for the orange peel (peau d'orange) or pigskin-like appearance of lesions in these areas.

Thyrotropin (TSH), long-acting thyroid stimulator (LATS), and 7S gamma globulin have been implicated as the cause of acid mucopolysaccharides in the skin of patients with pretibial myxedema. But a recent study has shown that the serum of patients with this disorder contain a nonimmunoglobulin protein that stimulates the skin fibroblasts to produce mucin and proteins.[10] The pathogenesis of the skin lesions in pretibial myxedema appears to be distinct and unrelated to the mechanisms proposed for the other clinical and biochemical features of Graves' disease, Hashimoto's thyroiditis, and hypothyroidism.

The clinical features of *thyroid acropachy* are clubbing of the digits, diaphyseal periosteal proliferation of distal bones, and thickening of the soft tissues over the distal extremities. Reported to occur in up to 1% of patients with Graves' disease, it is usually found in patients with a combination of exophthalmos and pretibial or localized myxedema. Diagnostic signs include reduced temperature without obvious abnormality over areas of localized myxedema and increased width of the diaphysis of distal short bones (especially the mid-diaphyseal areas of the metacarpals, metatarsals, and phalanges and, in severe cases, the distal long bones [radius, ulna, tibia, and fibula]). Typical physical findings include drumstick-like clubbing, enlargement of the hands and feet, and radiographic changes (fluffy, spiculated or homogeneous subperiosteal thickening with new bone formation and spicules perpendicular to the long axis of the bone).[9, 11–13] Seen in patients with localized pretibial myxedema, exophthalmos, and past or present hyperthyroidism, thyroid acropachy appears to be related to LATS (long–acting thyroid stimulator) in the serum of affected patients.

DIAGNOSIS.—In patients with clinical signs and symptoms suggestive of hyperthyroidism, careful physical examination will usually demonstrate the presence of enlargement of the thyroid gland. To confirm the clinical suspicion, increased serum levels of T4 and T3 can be determined by radioimmunoassay (RIA), and TSH measured by RIA will identify those few cases caused by TSH hypersecretion. If there is a question of pretibial myxedema, the demonstration of edema and large bluish deposits of mucin, with splitting up of collagen bundles extending down to the subcutaneous tissue, on histopathologic examination of cutaneous biopsy specimens help confirm this clinical feature of thyrotoxicosis.

TREATMENT.—Treatment of hyperthyroidism in children may be accomplished by the use of antithyroid drugs such as propylthiouracil (5 to 7 mg/kg/per day) or methimazole (Tapazole, Lilly) 0.5 to 0.7 mg/kg/day in three divided doses; thyroidectomy; or radioiodine ablation. In patients with severe disease or distressing cardiovascular symptoms, propranolol is a useful adjunctive form of therapy. Potassium iodide (2 to 4 mg/kg/day) given as a strong iodine solution, or saturated solution of potassium iodide, potentiates the action of thionamide drugs and inhibits thyroid hormone secretion. The effect of potassium, however, is transient. This drug, therefore, is seldom used except for short-term treatment of severe disease or for preoperative preparation of patients for surgery.[6]

In patients where the goiter is three or more times greater than normal size, once euthyroidism has been produced by appropriate antithyroid therapy, subtotal thyroidectomy has been recommended. In patients where the goiter appears to be larger than 60 gm at surgery, however, near-total thyroidectomy is suggested.[14]

Multiple Endocrine Adenomatosis Syndromes

The multiple endocrine adenomatosis (MEA) syndromes are familial disorders characterized by hyperplasia or tumors involving more than one endocrine gland. The clinical manifestations are variable and reflect the variable involvement of hormone-producing tissues. Although the pathogenesis of the multiple syndromes are unknown, they are inherited in an autosomal dominant pattern with variable expressivity and high penetrance.[1]

The *mucosal neuroma syndrome*, a prototype of these syndromes, is a term used to describe a group of disorders characterized by the association of multiple mucosal neuromas, intestinal ganglioneuromatosis, medullary thyroid carcinoma, parathyroid adenoma and/or hyperplasia and pheochromocytoma. Other terms used to denote variations of this combination include multiple mucosal neuroma syndrome, medullary thyroid carcinoma syndrome, oral mucosal neuroma-medullary thyroid carcinoma syndrome, multiple endocrine adenomatosis III (MEA III), and multiple endocrine neoplasia (MEN) type 2b or 3.[15, 16] Although variations of the above features may occur sporadically (perhaps as the result of new mutations), most cases of the mucosal neuroma syndrome are transmitted as an autosomal dominant trait.[15]

A relationship between carcinoma of the thyroid and pheochromocytoma was first described by Eisenberg in 1932, but it was not until almost 30 years later (1961) that Sipple reported a patient with this combination of findings.[16] Since then, reports of this assoication with other findings such as parathyroid hyperplasia and multiple mucosal neuromas have frequently been known as the Sipple syndrome (MEA II or MEN 2a). Endocrine neoplasias may occur singly or in various clinical patterns. *MEN type 1* (multiple endocrine adenomatosis) is characterized by tumors of the pituitary gland, pancreatic islets, adrenal cortex, and parathyroid glands; *MEN type 2* by neoplasia of the C cells of the thyroid (medullary carcinoma), adrenal medulla (pheochromocytoma) and parathyroid glands (chief cell hyperplasia or adenoma); and *MEN type 3* (sometimes termed type 2b or the mucosal neuroma syndrome) is characterized by the association of multiple mucosal neuromas, medullary thyroid carcinoma, and pheochromocytoma (Table 6–6).

CLINICAL MANIFESTATIONS.—Mucosal neuromas (seen in 80% of patients with the mucosal neuroma syndrome) may present at multiple sites (the lips, tongue, eyes, and gastrointestinal tract) and represent the hall-

TABLE 6–6.—Multiple Endocrine Adenomatosis Syndromes

1. Multiple endocrine adenomatosis I (MEA I)
   (Wermer's syndrome, multiple endocrine neoplasia type 1)
   a. Simultaneous or successive tumors of the anterior pituitary, islet cells of the pancreas, parathyroids, and adenomas of the thyroid and adrenal cortex
   b. Lipomas, bronchial and intestinal carcinoid tumors; schwannomas and thymomas (less common)
2. Multiple endocrine adenomatosis II (MEA II)
   (Sipple's syndrome, multiple endocrine neoplasia type 2a)
   a. Medullary carcinoma of the thyroid, pheochromocytoma and parathyroid tumor or hyperplasia
   b. Medullary carcinomas of the thyroid is inherited as an autosomal dominant trait (pheochromocytoma and parathyroid disease have lower degree of penetrance)
3. Multiple endocrine adenomatosis III (MEA III)
   (mucosal neuroma syndrome, multiple endocrine neoplasia type 2b or 3)
   a. Major components include multiple neuromas, medullary thyroid carcinoma and pheochromocytoma
   b. Other features include characteristic facies, skeletal abnormalities and ganglioneuromatosis of lips and g.i. tract

mark of this disorder.[15–19] Labial involvement results in diffusely enlarged lips with a characteristic fleshy, blubbery, or Negroid appearance (Fig 6–3). Lingual neuromas, generally limited to the anterior third of the tongue, appear as pink, sessile, or pedunculated nodules. These may be congenital or may be noted in the first few years of life and often represent the first markers heralding this syndrome (Fig 6–4). Nasal, laryngeal, and gingival neuromas may be present, and cutaneous involvement has also been seen on rare occasions. Neuromas may also be seen at the limbus of the conjunctivae and at the margins of the eyelids, with thickening of the margin and displacement of the cilia (Fig 6–5).

Intestinal ganglioneuromatosis may commonly be seen as another form of mucosal neuroma in this disorder. Here, failure to thrive, constipation, or diarrhea may lead to further evaluation and eventual demonstration of the full abnormality.[20]

Physical features of patients with MEA III (the mucosal neuroma syndrome) include a marfanoid appearance with long slender limbs and fingers (Fig 6–3), poor muscular development with very little subcutaneous fat, and skeletal defects such as kyphoscoliosis, pectus excavatum (funnel chest), and pectus carinatum (pigeon breast). Other abnormalities, such as a high-arched palate and pes cavus, may also be seen.

Medullary carcinoma of the thyroid, a malignancy seen in only 5% to 10% of all thyroid cancers, is the major endocrine tumor of this syndrome. Here the perifollicular cells of the thyroid (termed "C" cells because of their secretion of calcitonin, the calcium-lowering polypeptide hormone)

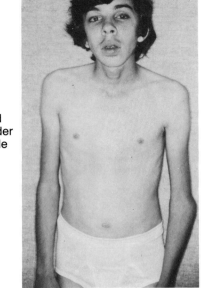

Fig 6–3.—Characteristic facies and marfanoid appearance with long slender limbs in a 16-year-old boy with multiple mucosal neuroma syndrome.

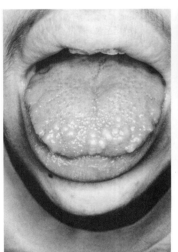

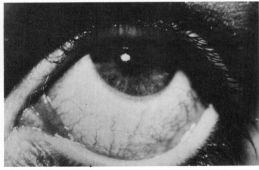

Fig 6–4 (left).—Multiple mucosal neuroma syndrome. Lingual neuromas and protuberant fleshy lips are highly characteristic of this disorder.

Fig 6–5 (right).—Multiple mucosal neuroma syndrome. Neuromas of the limbus of the conjunctiva and margins of the eyelids. The latter results in thickening of the margins and displacement of the cilia of the eyelids.

may be the source of other humoral substances such as prostaglandin and serotonin in some patients. Histopathologic examination of medullary carcinoma of the thyroid reveals sheets of rather uniform, round to spindle-shaped cells, often binucleated, with eosinophilic cytoplasm. The increased calcitonin released by these cells lowers serum calcium, thus stimulating a compensatory parathyroid response resulting in hyperparathyroidism or parathyroid adenoma. Parathyroid abnormalities represent a secondary response and are not the direct result of genetic aberration.

Pheochromocytoma may be present in 38% of patients with MEN type 2a (MEA II, the Sipple syndrome). In two-thirds of those affected, they are bilateral.[21, 22] Here the chromaffin cells of the adrenal medulla and sympathetic nerves and ganglia, also derived from primitive neural crest ectoderm, synthesize catecholamines, norepinephrine, and epinephrine, with resultant hypertension, tachycardia, anxiety, hyperhidrosis, weight loss, and/or fatigue.

DIAGNOSIS.—Patients with mucosal neuroma syndrome have a characteristic facies with diffusely enlarged, slightly everted lips and a characteristic fleshy, blubbery, or Negroid appearance, the upper lip being more affected than the lower. The distinctive facies and neuromas, generally appearing as pink, sessile, or pedunculated nodules on the tip and anterior third or half of the tongue, are often present at birth or in the first few years of life. These characteristic markers of the syndrome are distinctive and appear early in the disorder (in one patient they appeared at four weeks of age)[25] and, when recognized, can lead to early diagnosis, before the other features of the syndrome become apparent.

Since medullary thyroid carcinoma and pheochromocytoma will develop in a high percentage of patients with the mucosal neuroma syndrome,[18, 20, 24] calcitonin levels should be followed and patients with mucosal neuromas and facies characteristic of this syndrome should be evaluated for evidence of thyroid cancer and pheochromocytoma.[19, 23, 25]

TREATMENT.—Early recognition and removal of medullary carcinoma of the thyroid gives the best chance for survival. Unfortunately, most patients with medullary carcinoma expire in their early twenties or thirties. Adequate therapy includes thyroidectomy and a search for parathyroid hyperplasia, hypercalcinosis and nephrocalcinosis. Pheochromocytomas and eye lesions should be sought, and since this syndrome appears to be genetic in origin, all relatives should be examined and appropriately counseled.[20, 23, 25]

Parathyroid Disorders and the Skin

Disorders of the parathyroid glands (hyper- and hypoparathyroidism) affect the skin in various ways and often present significant cutaneous features than can assist the primary or consulting physician in the diagnosis and management of affected individuals. Although primary parathyroid disease is uncommon in children, the parathyroids play a major role in the regulation of calcium and phosphorus metabolism, and associated abnormalities manifest distinctive clinical patterns.

Hyperparathyroidism

Primary hyperparathyroidism, one of the least common endocrine disorders of infancy and childhood, is rarely diagnosed in childhood. It is usually due to a familial, genetically determined hyperplasia of the parathyroid, as a malignant neoplasm of the parathyroid, as secondary reaction to some other disease such as seen in patients with mucosal neuroma syndrome or chronic renal insufficiency,[26] or as autosomal dominantly inherited cases of parathyroid hyperplasia associated with other endocrinopathies involving the thyroid, pancreas, and adrenal glands (multiple endocrine neoplasia type 1).

CLINICAL MANIFESTATIONS.—The clinical features of hyperparathyroidism include systemic effects of hypercalcemia: failure to thrive, muscular weakness, lethargy, anorexia, vomiting, fever, headache, constipation, weight loss, polydipsia, polyuria, mental retardation, metastatic calcification, and, with marked hypercalcemia, stupor or death. Of these, cutaneous metastatic calcification is the most common cutaneous manifestation. Hypercalcemia may also produce the ophthalmologic finding known as *band keratopathy*. A result of calcium and phosphate deposition beneath Bowman's capsule, band keratopathy appears as a superficial corneal opacity resembling frosted or ground glass in a bandlike configuration with white flecks or "holes" in the band resulting in a "Swiss cheese"-like appearance. Concentric with the limbus of the cornea but separated from it by a margin of uninvolved cornea, this finding is not specific for hyperparathyroidism since it may also be seen as a manifestation of hypercalcemia secondary to vitamin D intoxication, uremia or sarcoidosis.[27]

Hyperparathyroidism secondary to chronic renal failure may also produce cutaneous manifestations. The skin of the uremic patient may be dry, scaly, sallow, and hyperpigmented; the sallow appearance is partially due to anemia, and the hyperpigmentation appears to be the result of decreased renal clearance of melanocyte-stimulating hormone (MSH).[28] Hyperphosphatemia caused by decreased renal clearance may also produce a secondary calcification of the arteries, skin, subcutaneous fat, and, at times, muscle. This may be manifested as infarcted and ecchymotic areas or as plaques of calcinosis with periodic extrusion of calcium. Pruritus is a major cutaneous complaint of patients with chronic renal disease. This manifestation is caused by xerosis and, as a result of excessive levels of parathyroid hormone, the proliferation of mast cells in the skin of uremic patients.

DIAGNOSIS.—The diagnosis of hyperparathyroidism is established by consistent elevations of total serum calcium above 12 mg/dl, the reduction of serum phosphorus below 4 mg/dl and elevated levels of parathyroid hormone. High alkaline phosphatase levels usually indicate bone disease. This complication of hyperparathyroidism may be demonstrated roentgenographically by generalized demineralization of bones, destructive changes at the growing ends of long bones, subperiosteal erosions (particularly in the phalanges, metacarpals and lateral portions of the clavicle), and in more advanced disease, generalized rarefaction, cysts, tumors, fractures, and deformities. Roentgenograms of the abdomen may reveal renal calculi or nephrocalcinosis. In infants with parathyroid hyperplasia, cupping and fraying at the ends of long bones and ribs may suggest rickets, severe demineralization and pathologic fractures are common.

TREATMENT.—The treatment of hyperparathyroidism requires subtotal or complete parathyroidectomy with careful postoperative management of calcium levels. A compromise procedure is the removal of all of the parathyroids with autotransplantation of the parathyroid tissue in the muscles of the patient's forearm. If the grafted tissue becomes hyperplastic causing a recurrence of hypercalcemia, it is easy to remove. The treatment of hypercalcemia requires maintenance of hydration and production of calciuresis and natriuresis by a sodium-losing diuretic such as furosemide (1 mgm/kg every six hours) or ethacrynic acid, with replacement of the sodium and potassium lost in the urine. The diet should be low in calcium, sources of vitamin D should be eliminated, and patients should not be exposed to sunshine during the period of hypercalcemia.

Isotonic saline (at 2 to 4 times the normal maintenance rate) combined with thiazide diuretics or furosemide is generally helpful and, in patients resistant to therapy, calcitonin available as Calcimar (salmon calcitonin) as an intramuscular injection is frequently beneficial. A satisfactory starting dose of Calcimar is 4 MRC units/kg administered as an intramuscular injection. If results are not satisfactory within a period of 24 to 48 hours, the dosage may be increased to a maximum of 8 MRC units/kg.[29] Uremic pruritus may respond to phototherapy with ultraviolet light in the UVB (290–320 mm) range, given cautiously, so as not to stimulate excessive vitamin D production of calcium.[30–32]

Hypoparathyroidism

Hypoparathyroidism in childhood may develop as a congenital idiopathic disorder that may occur in adults as late as the third or fourth decades of life, but usually appears in the neonatal period or in later infancy or childhood, or as an acute condition following inadvertent removal or damage of the parathyroid glands during neck thyroid surgery. Congenital hypoparathyroidism may occur alone or it may be seen as an autoimmune disorder where it may occur alone or with other endocrine disorders, or as a hereditary condition associated with an increased familial incidence of other endocrinologic disorders (Addison's disease, pernicious anemia, and Hashimoto's thyroiditis), candidiasis, and/or vitiligo.[9] When associated with hypoplasia of the thymus and immunologic defects, the condition is known as the DiGeorge syndrome.

CLINICAL MANIFESTATIONS.—Idiopathic or congenital hypoparathyroidism usually is first manifested by tetany or seizure and, in 25% to 50% of patients, ectodermal defects. The skin of affected individuals is rough, dry, thick and scaly; the hair and eyebrows are sparse; and the nails are short and thin with brittleness and crumbling of the distal half or, in less severe cases, longitudinal grooves in the proximal nail plate or irregular longitudinal cracking along the distal nail edge.[9] When hypoparapituitorism occurs while the teeth are developing, pitting, ridging, absence of dental enamel and absence or hypoplasia of the permanent teeth may result. Other clinical manifestations of congenital hypoparathyroidism include tetany, convulsions, carpopedal spasm, muscle cramps and twitching, numbness of tingling of the extremities, laryngeal stridor, exfoliative dermatitis, mental retardation, chronic diarrhea (especially in infants), photophobia, keratoconjunctivitis, blepharospasm, and, in 50% of affected patients, cataracts.

Mucocutaneous candidiasis is also seen as a complication in 15% of patients with idiopathic hypoparathyroidism (but not in those with postsurgical hypoparathyroidism). In addition, one-third to one-half of infants and young children who manifest mucocutaneous candidiasis have an associated endocrinopathy.[26] The candidal infection occurs most frequently on the lips, in the mouth, on the perineum, in the vagina, and less frequently, on the nails. Although reasons for this predisposition to candidiasis are unknown, the hair, nail and skin abnormalities appear to be related to a defect in cell-mediated immunity and an ectodermal defect seen in patients with this disorder.[9]

The clinical manifestations of hypoparathyroidism associated with surgical injury or removal of the parathyroid glands differ from those seen in patients with idiopathic or congenital hypoparathyroidism. These include thinning or loss of hair, the development of horizontal grooves (Beau's lines) in the nails, or a complete loss of nails following episodes of tetany (these abnormalities revert to normal when hypocalcemia is controlled). Hyperpigmentation (predominantly on the face and distal extremities resembling chloasma, pellagra or Addisonian pigmentation) may also occur in cases of postthyroidectomy hypoparathyroidism. Although cutaneous calcification has been noted it is uncommon.

Pseudohypoparathyroidism and pseudo-pseudohypoparathyroidism.— Pseudohypoparathyroidism is a hereditary disorder in which there is an abnormal response in the receptor tissues, particularly of the kidney and skeleton, to parathyroid hormone (rather than a parahormone deficiency). This causes a hypocalcemia and hyperphosphatemia which mimics idiopathic hypoparathyroidism in every way except for the presence of candidiasis.[9] Children with pseudohypoparathyroidism are short and stocky and have a round face, plethoric cheeks, short pudgy hands and feet, and stunted growth (probably a result of premature closure of the epiphyses). The most striking abnormality is growth failure of the fourth and fifth metacarpals and metatarsals and, at times, proximal phalanges causing the fourth and fifth fingers and toes to be strikingly short. The index finger is longer than the middle finger. When patients with this disorder make a fist, a depression is present where the knuckles should be. Most patients with pseudohypoparathyroidism have some degree of mental retardation and intracranial calcification. Ectopic subcutaneous and periarticular calcification and ectopic bone formation are frequently present.

Pseudopseudohypoparathyroidism is a congenital variant of pseudohypopothyroidism in which serum calcium and phosphate levels are normal. Although patients with pseudopseudohypoparathyroidism and psudohypoparathyroidism are physically indistinguishable, those with pseudopseudohypoparathyroidism do not develop hypocalcemia and tetany.[9]

The DiGeorge syndrome.—The DiGeorge syndrome is a disorder that develops as a result of faulty embryologic development of both the thymus and the parathyroid glands (a congenital malformation of the third and fourth pharyngeal pouch). Oral candidiasis is an almost constant finding in patients with this disorder. Overwhelming fungal, viral or bacterial infection usually leads to death early in infancy. In these patients the thymus is absent or hypoplastic. Affected individuals demonstrate parathyroid deficiency (with lack of parathormone), T cell dysfunction and, in some cases, coexisting congenital defects of the heart and great vessels. Features of this disorder include hypocalcemia and tetany at an early age, chronic diarrhea, interstitial pneumonia, failure to thrive, micrognathia, hypertelorism, low-set ears, bifid uvula, a shortened lip philtrum, bowed mouth, chronic rhinitis, maculopapular eruptions, mental retardation, calcification of the central nervous system, nephrocalcinosis, cardiac malformations and at times hyperthyroidism.[32]

TREATMENT.—The treatment of hypoparathyroidism is dependent on the restoration of normal serum levels of calcium and phosphate, while avoiding the deleterious effects of hypercalcemia. Although large doses of vitamin D used to be the mainstay of therapy, dihydrotachysterol (DHT) and 1,25-Dihydroxyvitamin D_3 (calcitriol) appear to be safer. The usual daily dose of calcitriol is 0.25 to 1.0 microgram, or approximately 0.015 to

.025 microgram/kg/24 hr; that for dihydrotachysterol (DHT) is 0.1 to 0.5 mg for infants and young children; for older children and adults it is 0.5 to 1.0 mg (0.01 to 0.02 mg/kg/24 hr). Patients who do not respond to treatment with DHT or 1,25-dihydroxyvitamin D_3 may benefit from additional calcium, either as calcium lactate or gluconate, in doses of 5 to 10 grams daily.[29]

The treatment of pseudohypoparathyroidism requires restriction of dietary phosphate and, in some cases, administration of vitamin D or its derivatives similar to that of patients with idiopathic hypoparathyroidism. The management of the DiGeorge syndrome is directed toward control of the hypoparathyroidism, treatment of recurrent infection, and surgical correction of the congenital heart disease whenever possible. If a cellular immune defect is documented, thymic transplantation has been successful in the treatment of the DiGeorge syndrome. An alternate to thymic transplantation is the injection of the thymic humoral factors contained in thymosin fraction V.[33]

Disorders of the Adrenal Glands

Adrenal gland dysfunction may result in a variety of systemic disorders with significant cutaneous manifestations. Those of particular interest to the pediatric dermatologist are Addison's disease, Cushing's syndrome and the adrenogenital syndrome.

Addison's Disease

Deficient production of cortisol and/or aldosterone may result from a variety of congenital or acquired lesions of the hypothalamus, pituitary, or adrenal cortex. Addison's disease, a metabolic disorder caused by a deficient production of adrenocorticol hormones, is characterized by weakness, anorexia, hypotension, loss of body hair, low values of serum sodium and chloride, high levels of serum potassium, and melanin hyperpigmentation of the skin (Fig 6–6) and mucous membranes (Fig 6–7). Relatively uncommon in children, most cases occur during the third through fifth decades. Until recently, tuberculosis of the adrenal glands was the most frequent etiologic factor, but histoplasmosis, coccidiomycosis, cryptococcosis, amyloidosis, metastatic malignancies and mycosis fungoides have now been identified as frequent causative agents in adults. In children, however, most instances of Addison's disease appear to be idiopathic. About half of the patients with idiopathic Addison's disease demonstrate antibodies against adrenal tissue, suggesting autoimmunity as a basis for the disorder. This form of Addison's disease (particularly when seen in association with other autoimmunities) often occurs in siblings, suggesting an autosomal recessive cause in some children with this disorder.[34]

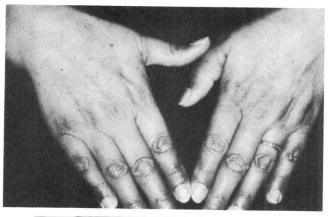

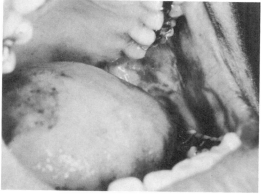

Fig 6–6 (top).—Hyperpigmentation of the skin of the hands (Addison's disease).

Fig 6–7 (bottom).—Addison's disease. Hyperpigmentation of the mucous membranes of the mouth.

CLINICAL MANIFESTATIONS.—Hyperpigmentation, the most prominent cutaneous feature of Addison's disease (Fig 6–6), appears to be the result of increased production of melanocyte stimulating hormone (MSH) by the pituitary gland (a compensatory phenomenon associated with decreased cortisol production by the adrenals).[35] Seen in 92% of patients, the hyperpigmentation is most intense in the flexures, at sites of pressure and friction, in creases of the palms and soles, in sunexposed areas, and in normally pigmented areas such as the genitalia and areolae. Pigmentation of the conjuctivae and vaginal mucous membranes is common, and pigmentary changes of the oral mucosae include spotty or streaked blue-black to brown hyperpigmentation of the gingivae, tongue, hard palate, and buccal mucosa (Fig 6–7).

Vitiligo also occurs in up to 15% of patients with Addison's disease. When seen together with the hyperpigmentation of Addison's disease, this combination produces a striking picture of hypo-and hyperpigmentation. In addition to the pigmentary changes, calcification and fibrosis of the pinna of the ear may also occur. Since calcinosis of the cartilage of the ear may also be seen in patients with acromegaly, hypopituitarism, hyperthyroidism, diabetes, sarcoidosis, ochronosis, trauma, frostbite, and bacterial chondritis, it cannot be considered diagnostic of Addison's disease.[9]

DIAGNOSIS.—The diagnosis of chronic adrenocortical insufficiency is suggested by its clinical features and may be confirmed by serum electrolyte studies and cortisol level determinations following stimulation by ACTH (the ACTH-stimulating test).

TREATMENT.—The treatment of Addison's disease requires replacement with glucocorticoid and mineralocorticoid hormones, the usual maintenance dose of hydrocortisone ranging from 12 to 20 mg/m^2/day administered in two or three divided doses and fludrocortisone 0.05 to 0.1 mg/day.

Cushing's Syndrome

Cushing's syndrome is a term used to describe a disease state characterized by obesity and hypertension caused by abnormally high blood levels of glucocorticoid hormones. It may be exogenous in origin (caused by administration of systemic corticosteroids and, at times, cutaneous absorption following long-term use of topical steroids), or it may be endogenous in nature. The term Cushing's disease refers to instances of Cushingism resulting from endogenous sources (bilateral adrenal hyperplasia resulting from ACTH secretion by the pituitary gland, or by a primary adenoma or carcinoma of the adrenal gland). Previously considered an uncommon disorder in infancy and childhood, Cushing's syndrome is currently being detected more frequently in the pediatric age group. In infants and early childhood, most cases of this disorder are caused by adrenocorticol tumors (usually a malignant carcinoma or occasionally a benign adenoma). Primary adrenocortical nodular hyperplasia is increasingly recognized as another cause of Cushing syndrome in infants. In children over age 7, the disorder is usually associated with bilateral adrenal hyperplasia (this is termed *Cushing's disease*). In children over the age of 8 years, as in adults, the majority of cases (50% to 80%) of Cushing's syndrome are caused by exogenous corticosteroid administration (this is referred to as a cushingoid syndrome).[36]

CLINICAL MANIFESTATIONS.—Cushing's syndrome is rare in childhood but may occur at any age, even in early infancy. The cutaneous manifestations include a characteristic plethoric "moon" facies, with telangiectasia

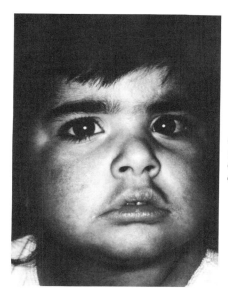

Fig 6–8.—Cushing's syndrome. A characteristic "moon" facies with plethora and telangiectasia of the cheeks in a 3-year-old girl on systemic corticosteroids.

over the cheeks (Fig 6–8); Addisonian hyperpigmentation; patchy cyanosis over the upper arms, breast, abdomen, buttocks, thighs, and legs; an increased amount of fine lanugo hair on the face and extremities; fatty deposits over the back of the neck ("buffalo hump"); increased fat deposits on the torso with a contrasting thinning of the arms and legs; purplish atrophic striae at points of tension such as the lower abdomen, thighs, buttocks, upper arms, and breasts; fragility of dermal blood vessels with increased tendency to bruisability and ecchymoses at sites of slight trauma; poor wound healing; frequent fungal infection (predominantly *T. rubrum* and *P. orbiculare*); frequent and recurrent pyoderma; and steroid acne (dull red, smooth, dome-shaped papules or small pustules seen primarily on the upper trunk, arms, neck, and to a lesser degree, the face). The latter complication is usually manifested in older children and adults.

DIAGNOSIS.—The diagnosis of Cushing's syndrome is suggested by the presence of weakness and muscle wasting, truncal obesity, osteoporosis, diabetes mellitus and/or hypertension, and the above described cutaneous manifestations. The clinical impression may be confirmed by elevated plasma 17-hydroxycorticoid levels with absence of the normal diurnal variation, increased 24-hour urinary 17-OH corticoids and 17-ketosteroid excretion, the dexamethasone suppression test, and when anterior pituitary abnormality is present, by visual field examination and radiologic examination of the sella turcica.

TREATMENT.—The treatment of Cushing's syndrome depends on the etiology, whether it be iatrogenic, secondary to adrenal tumor, or the result of ACTH secretion from the pituitary or a nonpituitary source ("the ectopic ACTH syndrome"). When the disorder is endogenous, treatment should be directed at either the pituitary (through surgery, irradiation, or isotope ablation) or at the adrenal glands by total or subtotal adrenalectomy. When the disorder is caused by an ectopic source of ACTH, treatment should be directed at the underlying disease. In instances where bilateral tumors are present and bilateral adrenalectomy is indicated, patients must be maintained on lifelong glucocorticoid and mineralocorticoid therapy. About 16% of patients with Cushing's syndrome eventually develop pituitary tumors or Addisonian hyperpigmentation, or both, following treatment by adrenalectomy (despite adequate adrenocortical replacement therapy).[9] This phenomenon is called the Nelson syndrome. Treatment with metapyrone and/or aminoglutethimide prior to adrenalectomy diminishes the incidence of complications in these patients,[37] and cyproheptadine (Periactin) appears to reduce ACTH levels and ameliorate clinical symptoms in some patients with Nelson syndrome.[36]

The Adrenogenital Syndrome

The adrenogenital syndrome is a condition in which there is excessive secretion of androgenic steroids by the adrenal cortex. It may result in adrenocortical insufficiency and salt wasting and may produce sudden death in newborns and virilization effects in patients that survive infancy (masculinization of the female [pseudohermaphroditism] and pseudoprecocious puberty in the male). The adrenogenital syndrome caused by adrenocortical hyperplasia is a genetic disorder in the biosynthesis of adrenal steroids resulting from a deficiency of one of several enzymes required for the formation of cortisol and, at times, aldosterone.

CLINICAL MANIFESTATIONS.—Virilizing adrenal tumors, although rare, are the most common type of adrenal tumor in the young. The apparent increased frequency of this disorder in females (by a 2 to 1 ratio) is probably related to the fact that clinical manifestations are more obvious in females than in males. In females, the predominant clinical manifestations are hirsutism, features of Cushing's syndrome mixed with virilism in a masculine distribution, the early appearance of pubic hair, clitoral enlargement, suppression of breast development, and a delay in menarche at the usual pubertal age. In contrast to girls with congenital adrenogenital hyperplasia, those with virilizing tumors do not develop labial fusion. Clinical features of virilization in adult females include amenorrhea; clitoral enlargement; hirsutism in a masculine distribution; acne vulgaris manifested by comedones, deep cystic and pustular lesions; deep voice; increased muscle mass; and a male habitus.[9] A similar tumor in prepubertal boys produces macrogenitosomia praecox and hirsutism without testicular maturation. In both girls and boys, muscles are well developed and there is rapid statural growth with marked advance in osseous maturation resulting in early epiphyseal closure and an inability to achieve full growth.

The *congenital adrenogenital syndrome* results in masculinization of girls in the form of pseudohermaphroditism with clitoral hypertrophy or labioscrotal fusion and the formation of a phallic urethra. Other clinical features include the premature development of pubic and axillary hair; deepening of the voice, and MSH hyperpigmentation of the skin, areolae, genitalia, palmar creases and buccal mucosa.[9] These patients are taller than normal during early childhood but are abnormally short during adolescence and adulthood because of premature closure of the epiphyses.

DIAGNOSIS.—Obvious hirsutism in young children with virilism in girls of premature sexual development in boys is strongly suggestive of congenital adrenal hyperplasia or the adrenogenital syndrome, with elevation of total neutral urinary 17-ketosteroids serving as the laboratory key to diagnosis. When 17-ketosteroid levels are extremely high, the diagnosis of a neoplasm of the adrenal cortex should be suspected. As a means of differentiating the disorders, virilizing adrenal tumors do not demonstrate suppression of plasma androgens or urinary 17-ketosteroids during a dexamethasone-suppression test. Furthermore, since tumoral secretion is not ACTH-dependent, the administration of ACTH has no effect on steroid production of patients with adrenal tumors.

TREATMENT.—The management of patients with the adrenogenital syndrome depends upon the cause and course of the disorder. Physiologic amounts of cortisone acetate administered intramuscularly and oral hydrocortisone suppress the production of adrenal androgens and improve the virilization in affected individuals, but are contraindicated in the treatment of patients with adrenocortical tumors. For patients with adrenal tumors, the treatment is surgical. Since most of these tumors are malignant in the pediatric age group, surgical removal with postoperative irradiation is frequently recommended as the treatment of choice.

Pituitary Disorders

Hyperpituitarism

The excessive secretion of growth hormone by pituitary tumors (usually an eosinophilic adenoma) produces gigantism in children whose epiphyses have not yet closed and acromegaly in adults. Although acromegaly is rare in children, transitional acromegalic features may also be seen at times in adolescents. Clinical features of excessive secretion of growth hormone include coarsening of the features with overgrowth of soft tissues, cutis verticis gyrata (coarse furrowing of the skin on the posterior aspect of the neck and vertex of the scalp); thick edematous eyelids; a large triangular-shaped nose; lantern jaw; macroglossia with, at times, a deeply furrowed tongue; a thick protruding lower lip; broad spade-like hands with short squat fingers; prominent pores; short, flat, wide rapidly growing nails, at times with absence of the lunula, longitudinal striations and splitting; hirsutism; and hyperpigmentation similar to that seen in patients with Addison's disease. The cause of hirsutism is not well understood but the hyperpigmentation appears to be related to increased secretion of MSH (melanocyte stimulating hormone).[34]

When the full clinical picture of gigantism is present, there is generally little doubt as to the diagnosis. Measurement of growth hormone levels should confirm the diagnosis. In addition, patients should be investigated for pituitary tumor and/or evidence of other endocrine abnormalities.

Hypopituitarism

Pituitary insufficiency (hypopituitarism) is a disorder or group of disorders resulting from a deficiency in secretion of one or more hormones derived from the pituitary gland. These include idiopathic hypopituitarism (panhypopituitarism, Simmond's disease), the least common variety; Sheehan's syndrome (pituitary deficiency usually arising as a result of hemorrhage or infarct); pituitary tumors; congenital abnormalities; or ablation of the pituitary gland by surgery or x-ray irradiation used for the treatment of local tumors.

The most obvious cutaneous manifestations of pituitary insufficiency are pallor and a decreased ability to tan (due to a decrease in melanin pigmentation secondary to diminished or absent secretion of a melanocyte-stimulating factor from the pituitary).[9] Other features include a smooth waxy or a myxedematous coarse dry and scaly skin (resulting from hypothyroidism). The face may be slightly puffy, pale or yellowish (secondary to carotenemia); the skin and subcutaneous tissue are thin and, when coupled with wrinkling around the eyes and mouth, may lead to an aged appearance, and gonadal hypofunction produces a gradual loss of axillary, pubic, and body hair. Other manifestations of hypopituitarism include retardation of skeletal growth and thin opaque fragile slow-growing nails (often with a loss of the lunula). In addition, brown spots may be seen beneath the nail and onycholysis or longitudinal ridging may be present.

Disorders Associated With Diabetes

Necrobiosis Lipoidica Diabeticorum

Necrobiosis lipoidica diabeticorum (NLD) is a degenerative disorder of the dermal connective tissue, often seen in patients with diabetes mellitus, characterized by atrophic plaques on the anterior surface of the lower legs. Although the etiology of this disorder is unknown, it appears to be related to an alteration of dermal collagen due to angiopathy of small vessels (possibly a diabetes-related endarteritic obliterative vascular occlusion).[38, 39]

Necrobiosis lipoidica diabeticorum precedes the onset of diabetes in 20% of patients. More than half the patients have active diabetes mellitus, and an abnormal glucose tolerance test is demonstrable in from 50% to 87% of patients with this disorder.[9] Although statistics vary, NLD occurs in 0.1 to 0.3% of diabetics. It is more frequent in children than in adults and occurs three times more often in women than in men.[40] In 90% of patients, it is localized to one or both pretibial areas; in the remaining individuals it may occur on the trunk, face, scalp, arms, palms, or soles. The disorder may occur at any age. It was noted at birth in one patient, but usually develops in the third or fourth decade of life and has a peak incidence in persons between 50 to 60 years of age.[9, 40]

A typical lesion of necrobiosis lipoidica diabeticorum begins as an erythematous papule or nodule with a sharply circumscribed border. It gradually enlarges and slowly develops into an oval yellowish-red sclerotic plaque with an irregular outline and a violaceous margin. The center of the plaque is often depressed or atrophic and shows a waxy translucent surface coursed by telangiectatic vessels (Fig 6–9). Lesions are usually asymptomatic. Trauma to the atrophic skin is poorly tolerated and ulceration, although rare in childhood, may occur in up to 30% of patients with this disorder.[41]

DIAGNOSIS.—The diagnosis of necrobiosis lipoidica diabeticorum is suggested by the presence of sharply demarcated waxy plaques with violaceous borders on the lower portion of the legs. Characteristic of the histopathology are degeneration of collagen surrounded by lymphocytes, histiocytes, and epithelioid cells, thickening of vessel walls, proliferation of vessels in the mid and lower dermis and the presence of lipid-filled giant cells.

TREATMENT.—The treatment of necrobiosis lipoidica diabeticorum is, in general, not very satisfactory. Since trauma may produce stubborn painful ulcerations, protection of the legs, elastic stockings, and bed rest may be useful. Although patients may be seen without evidence of diabetes, the presence of lesions should alert one to this possibility, and an appropriate

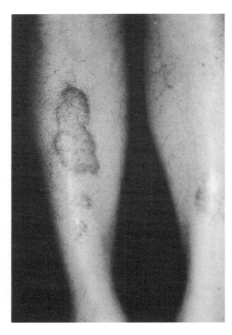

Fig 6–9.—Necrobiosis lipoidica diabeticorum. Yellowish-red oval atrophic plaques with a waxy translucent surface, telangiectatic vessels, and characteristic violaceous margins.

search for frank diabetes, latent diabetes, or a prediabetic state should be initiated.

Lesions of NLD are usually symptom free and often are only of diagnostic or cosmetic importance. Cosmetic makeup or dark hose may help hide lesions. Topical corticosteroids (alone or under occlusion) or intralesional steroids injection may improve and clear some lesions. Since patches of necrobiosis are ordinarily atrophic, caution must be exercised to prevent further atrophy or ulceration. Ulcerative lesions are best treated conservatively with compresses, topical antibiotics, or topical benzoyl peroxide in a 10% to 20% concentration.[42] Extensive ulcerations may require excision and full-thickness skin grafts. Poor healing due to vascular damage and recurrences in and around grafts, however, is not uncommon.

Diabetic Dermopathy

Diabetic dermopathy, first described in 1964 by Melin, is a characteristic dermatosis seen in 50% of patients with diabetes mallitus.[43] Seen most frequently in males, the initial lesions are round or oval, red or reddish-brown papules that slowly evolve into discrete, sharply circumscribed atrophic, hyperpigmented, or scaly patches; sometimes only depressed areas with normal skin color are seen. Lesions generally measure one centimeter or less in diameter, and although they may occur on the scalp, forearms, or trunk, they usually appear on the anterior aspect of thighs and shins of affected individuals.[43, 44]

The histologic picture of this disorder suggests a possible relationship to diabetic microangiopathy.[43, 45] Although the exact pathogenesis is still undetermined, the presence of these characteristic lesions can serve as a clue to the diagnosis of diabetes mellitus. More studies on the vascular and dermal changes, however, are required to help elucidate the true pathogenesis of this disorder.

DIAGNOSIS.—The histopathologic features of lesions consist of a combination of vascular disease and minor collagen changes. Vessel walls thickened with a PAS-positive material are seen in the upper dermis and slight collagen change and microangiopathy are seen in the dermis and subcutis.

TREATMENT.—Lesions of diabetic dermopathy are in large part uninfluenced by treatment. Individual lesions tend to disappear spontaneously after one-and-a-half to two years. The development of new lesions, however, often creates an impression that individual lesions persist for longer periods of time. Treatment should emphasize protection of the shins from trauma. Bed rest, open wet compresses, and topical antibiotics should be utilized to assist healing of inflammatory and crusted lesions.

Bullous Dermatosis in Diabetes Mellitus

Bullosis diabeticorum is a rare disorder that consists of large asymptomatic bullous lesions that develop rapidly on the distal extremities, especially the hands and feet (Fig 6–10).[46, 47] Although many of the patients have peripheral neuropathy, this complication of diabetes is not present in all. The bullae are painless, clear, and noninflammatory. They develop rapidly, without evidence of trauma, ultraviolet exposure, or vascular insufficiency and heal slowly and spontaneously.[47]

The etiology of bullosis diabeticorum is not known. Treatment consists of aseptic aspiration of incision and drainage and the use of topical antibiotics to prevent infection.

Granuloma Annulare

Granuloma annulare is a relatively common cutaneous disorder characterized clinically by papules or nodules that are grouped in a ringlike or circinate distribution. Although granuloma annulare may occur on any part of the body, it usually begins on the lateral or dorsal surfaces of the hands or feet. Females are affected twice as frequently as males. Granuloma annulare may occur at any age. Children and young adults, however, are

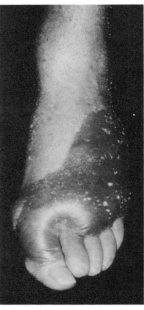

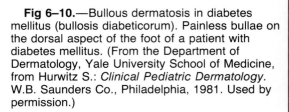

Fig 6–10.—Bullous dermatosis in diabetes mellitus (bullosis diabeticorum). Painless bullae on the dorsal aspect of the foot of a patient with diabetes mellitus. (From the Department of Dermatology, Yale University School of Medicine, from Hurwitz S.: *Clinical Pediatric Dermatology.* W.B. Saunders Co., Philadelphia, 1981. Used by permission.)

most commonly affected, with over 40% of cases appearing in children under 15 years of age.[48, 49]

The cause of granuloma annulare is unknown. Various studies have shown latent diabetes to be present in a third of patients with this disorder.[50] Although still open to controversy, this finding (demonstrated in some adults but not in children) suggests that the underlying defect may be related to diabetes and to vascular changes associated with the diabetic state.[50, 51] In some individuals granuloma annulare has been noted following trauma or insect bites. These theories, although attractive, still remain unsubstantiated and require further confirmation.[52]

Early lesions of granuloma annulare begin as smooth, flesh-colored or pale red papules that slowly undergo central involution and peripheral extension to form rings with clear centers and elevated borders of continuous papules or nodules (Fig 6–11). The rings are oval or irregular in outline and vary in size from 1 to 5 cm in diameter. Lesions may be single or multiple; multiple lesions are more common in young children than in older patients, but numerous widely disseminated lesions can occur at any age. Subcutaneous forms, most often seen on the legs, scalp, palms, and buttocks, have a similar clinical and histological appearance and often are confused with rheumatoid nodules. Rheumatoid nodules, however, are usually larger and subcutaneous rather than intradermal in location.

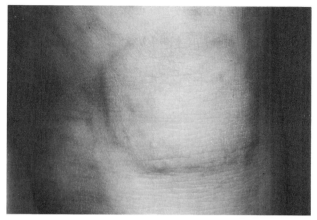

Fig 6–11.—Granuloma annulare. Flesh-colored papulonodular lesions in an annular configuration.

Lesions of granuloma annulare usually disappear spontaneously, often within several months to several years. Although 73% of lesions disappear within two years (with no residual scarring), recurrences are common and may be seen, usually at the original site, in up to 40% of patients.[48] At times, as simple a procedure as intralesional saline or a small biopsy may be followed by complete involution.

Although topical corticosteroids, corticosteroids under occlusion, and intralesional steroids are beneficial and hasten resolution of lesions, because of the potential risk of dermal atrophy associated with such therapy, reassurance of eventual spontaneous resolution may be all that is necessary for treatment of the cosmetic aspect of this disorder. Since we recognize the fact that patients with granuloma annulare (particularly adults with the generalized form of granuloma annulare) may be candidates for diabetes mellitus,[53] patients with granuloma annulare should be investigated for this possibility.

REFERENCES

1. LaFranchi S.: Hypothyroidism, congenital and acquired, in Kaplan S.A.: *Clinical Pediatric and Adolescent Endocrinology.* W.B. Saunders Co., Philadelphia, 1982, pp. 69–130.
2. Fisher D.A., Dussalt J.H., Foley T.P., Jr., et al.: Screening for congenital hypothyroidism: Results of screening one million North American infants. *J. Pediat.* 94:700–705, 1979.
3. Gardner L.I.: Historical notes on cretinism, in Gardner L.I. (ed.): *Endocrine and Genetic Diseases of Childhood and Adolescence.* W.B. Saunders Publishing Co., Philadelphia, 1975, pp. 234–238.

4. Lucky A.: Congenital hypothyroidism, in Demis J., Dobson R.L., McGuire J.: *Clinical Dermatology.* Harper & Row Publishers, Philadelphia, ed. 10. 1983, 12–32:1–7.
5. LaFranchi S.H., Murphey W.H., Foley T.P., Jr., et al.: Neonatal hypothyroidism detected by the Northwest Regional Screening Program. *Pediatrics* 63:180–191, 1979.
6. Christianson H.B.: Cutaneous manifestations of hypothyroidism including purpura and ecchymoses. *Cutis* 17:45–52, 1976.
7. Fisher D.A.: Thyroid disease, in Gellis S.S., Kagan B.M.: *Current Pediatric Therapy, 11.* W.B. Saunders Co., Philadelphia, 1984, pp. 288–293.
8. Hollingsworth D.R., Mabry C.C.: Congenital Graves disease. Four familial cases with long-term follow-up and perspective. *Am. J. Dis. Child.* 130:148–155, 1976.
9. Braverman I.M.: Endocrine and metabolic diseases, in Braverman I.M.: *Skin Signs of Systemic Disease,* ed. 2. W.B., Saunders Co., Philadelphia, 1981, pp. 619–709.
10. Cheung H.S., Nicoloff J.T., Kamiel M.B., et al.: Stimulation of fibroblast biosynthetic activity by serum of patients with pretibial myxedema. *J. Invest. Dermatol.* 71:12–17, 1978.
11. Nixon D.W., Samols E.: Acral changes associated with thyroid diseases. *J.A.M.A.* 212:1175–1181, 1970.
12. Thomas J., Collipp P.J., Sharma R.K.: Thyroid acropachy. *Am. J. Dis. Child.* 125:745–746, 1973.
13. Goette D.K.: Thyroid acropachy. *Arch. Dermatol.* 116:205–206, 1980.
14. Buckingham B.A., Costin G., Roe T., et al.: Hyperthyroidism in children: a re-evaluation of treatment. *Am. J. Dis. Child.* 135:112–117, 1981.
15. Khairi M.R.A., Dexter R.N., Burzynski N.J., et al.: Mucosal neuroma, pheochromocytoma and medullary thyroid carcinoma: multiple endocrine neoplasia type 3. (Review) *Medicine* 54:89–112, 1975.
16. Sipple J.H.: Association of pheochromocytoma with carcinoma of the thyroid gland. *Ann. J. Med.* 31:163–166, 1961.
17. Gorlin R.J., Sedano H.O., Vickers R.A., et al.: Multiple mucosal neuromas, pheochromocytoma and medullary carcinoma of the thyroid—a syndrome. *Cancer* 22:293–299, 1968.
18. Baum J.L., Adler M.E.: Pheochromocytoma, medullary thyroid carcinoma, multiple mucosal neuroma, a variant of the syndrome. *Arch. Ophthal.* 87:574–584, 1972.
19. Hurwitz S.: The Sipple syndrome. Society transactions. *Arch. Dermatol.* 110:139–140, 1974.
20. Anderson T.E., Spackman T.J., Schwartz S.S.: Roentgen findings in intestinal ganglioneuromatosis: its association with medullary thyroid carcinoma and pheochromocytoma. *Radiology* 101:93–96, 1971.
21. Steiner A.L., Goodman A.D., Powers S.R.: Study of a kindred with pheochromocytoma, medullary thyroid carcinoma, hyperparathyroidism and Cushing's disease: multiple endocrine neoplasia, type 2. *Medicine* 47:371–409, 1968.
22. Keiser H.R., Beaven M.A., Doppman J., et al.: NIH Conference. Sipple's syndrome: medullary thyroid carcinoma, pheochromocytoma and parathyroid disease. *Ann. Int. Med.* 78:561–579, 1973.
23. Brown R.S., Colle E., Tashjian A.H., Jr.: The syndrome of multiple mucosal neuromas and medullary thyroid carcinoma in childhood. Importance of rec-

ognition of the phenotype for the early detection of malignancy. *J. Pediatrics* 86:77–85, 1975.

24. Baylin S.B.: The multiple endocrine neoplasia syndromes: implications for the study of inherited tumors. *Semin. Oncol.* 5:35–45, 1978.
25. Jackson C.E., Tashjian A.H., Jr., Block M.A.: Detection of medullary thyroid cancer by calcitonin assay in families. *Ann. Int. Med.* 78:845–852, 1973.
26. Lang P.G., Jr.: The clinical spectrum of parathyroid disease. *J. Am. Acad. Dermatol.* 5:733–749, 1981.
27. Lembach R.G., Keates R.H.: Band keratopathy: its significance and treatment. *Perspect. Ophthalmol.* 1:13, 1977.
28. Smith A.G., Shuster S., Comaish J.S., et al.: Plasma immunoreactive melanocyte stimulating hormone and skin pigmentation in chronic renal failure. *Br. Med. J.* 1:658–659, 1975.
29. Wolfsdorf J.I.: Parathyroid disease, in Gellis S.S., Kagan B.M. (Editors): *Current Pediatric Therapy 11.* W.B. Saunders Co., Philadelphia, 1984, pp. 293–295.
30. Gilchrest B.A., Rowe J.W., Brown R.S., et al.: Relief of uremic pruritus with ultraviolet phototherapy. *N. Engl. J. Med.* 297:136–138, 1977.
31. Gilchrest B.A., Rowe J.W., Brown R.S., et al.: Ultraviolet phototherapy of uremic pruritus. long-term results and possible mechanism of action. *Ann. Int. Med.* 91:17–21, 1979.
32. Conley M.E., Beckwith J.B., Mancer J.F.K., et al.: Spectrum of the DiGeorge syndrome. *J. Pediatr.* 94:888–900, 1979.
33. Wara D.W.: Primary immunodeficiency disease, in Gellis S.S., Kagan B.M. (Editors): *Current Pediatric Therapy 11.* W.B. Saunders Co., Philadelphia, 1984, p. 747.
34. Nerup J.: Addison's disease—a review of some clinical, pathological and immunological features. *Dan. Med. Bull.* 21:201–217, 1974.
35. Lerner A.B., McGuire J.S.: Melanocyte-stimulating hormone and adrenocorticotrophic hormone: their relation to pigmentation. *N. Engl. J. Med.* 270:539–546, 1964.
36. DiGeorge A.M.: The endocrine system, in Vaughn V.C. III and McKay R.J.: *Nelson's Textbook of Pediatrics*, ed. 12., 1983, W.B. Saunders Co., Philadelphia, pp. 1432–1514.
37. Misbin R.L., Canary J., Willard D.: Aminoglutethimide in the treatment of Cushing's syndrome. *J. Clin. Pharmacol.* 16:645–651, 1976.
38. Bauer M.F., Hirsch P., Bullock W.D., et al.: Necrobiosis lipoidica diabeticorum. *Arch Dermatol.* 90:558–566, 1964.
39. Engel M.F., Smith J.G.: The pathogenesis of necrobiosis lipoidica, a forme fruste of diabetes mellitus. *Arch. Dermatol.* 93:272–281, 1966.
40. Muller S.A., Winkelmann R.K.: Necrobiosis lipoidica diabeticorum. A clinical and pathologic investigation of 171 cases. *Arch Dermatol.* 93:272–281, 1966.
41. Hansen T.W.: Necrobiosis lipoidica diabeticorum in Demis D.J., Dobson R.L., McGuire J. (Eds.): *Clinical Dermatology.* Harper and Row, Hagerstown, Maryland, ed. 11., 1984, 4:8, pp. 1–5.
42. Hanke C.W., Bergfeld W.F.: Treatment with benzoyl peroxide of ulcers on legs within lesions of necrobiosis lipoidica diabeticorum. *J. Dermatol. Surg. Oncol.* 4:701–704, 1978.
43. Melin H.: An atrophic circumscribed skin lesion in the lower extremities of diabetics. *Acta Med. Scand. Suppl.* 423:1–75, 1964.

44. Shelley W.B.: Diabetic dermopathy. *Consultations in Dermatology with Walter B. Shelley, 1*. W.B. Saunders Co., Philadelphia, 1972, pp. 172–175.
45. Binkley G.W.: Dermopathy in the diabetic syndrome. *Arch. Dermatol.* 92:625–634, 1965.
46. Cantwell A.R., Martz W.: Idiopathic bullae in diabetics—bullosis diabeticorum. *Arch. Dermatol.* 96:42–44, 1967.
47. Bernstein J.E., Medenica M., Soltani K., et al.: Bullous eruption of diabetes mellitus. *Arch. Dermatol.* 115:324–325, 1979.
48. Wells R.S., Smith M.A.: The natural history of granuloma annulare. *Br. J. Dermatol.* 75:199–205, 1963.
49. Muhlbauer J.E.: Granuloma annulare. *J. Am. Acad. Dermatol.* 3:217–230, 1980.
50. Romaine R., Rudner E., Altman J.: Papular granuloma annulare and diabetes mellitus: Report of cases. *Arch. Dermatol.* 98:152–154, 1968.
51. Williamson D.M., Dykes J.R.W.: Carbohydrate metabolism in granuloma annulare. *J. Invest. Dermatol.* 58:400–404, 1972.
52. Stankler L., Leslie G.: Generalized granuloma annulare. *Arch. Dermatol.* 95:509–513, 1967.
53. Huntley A.C.: The cutaneous manifestations of diabetes mellitus. *J. Am. Acad. Dermatol.* 7:427–455, 1982.

7 / Errors of Metabolism

THE INBORN DISORDERS OF METABOLISM are a group of hereditary diseases that are transmitted by mutant genes and result in various metabolic and clinical defects. Most of the severe errors of metabolism are transmitted by autosomal recessive genes requiring two heterozygous mates to produce a homozygous child manifesting the clinical disorder. The number of known inborn errors of metabolism is continually increasing and many of them once thought to result from a single enzymatic defect can now be subdivided into several distinct entities, each with different enzymatic deficiencies and varying clinical features.[1]

Phenylketonuria

Phenylketonuria (PKU, phenylpyruvic oligophrenia) is an autosomal recessive disorder characterized by mental retardation, diffuse hypopigmentation, seizures, an eczematoid dermatitis, and photosensitivity (Table 7–1). A disorder of amino acid metabolism, it is caused by a defect in phenylalanine hydroxylase, the enzyme found in liver that converts phenylalanine to tyrosine. Its frequency has been estimated to be 1 in 10,000 to 20,000 births and it affects males and females with equal frequency.

CLINICAL MANIFESTATIONS.—Ninety percent of affected infants are blond, blue eyed, and fair skinned. A peculiar musty odor, attributable to decomposition products (phenylacetic acid or phenylacetaldehyde) in the urine and sweat is characteristic and by itself often suggests the diagnosis. Infants appear to be normal at birth and develop the first manifestations of delayed intellectual development sometimes between 4 and 24 months of age. Early symptoms may include severe vomiting to such a degree that pyloromyotomy has been carried out because of a misdiagnosis of pyloric stenosis. Skeletal changes associated with this disorder include microcephaly, short stature, pes planus, and syndactyly. Eczematous dermatitis appears in 10% to 50% of patients, and affected individuals may have sclerodermatous skin lesions. While many have a typical flexural distribution of atopic dermatitis, others have an ill-defined, poorly described eczematous dermatitis that follows no specific pattern.

DIAGNOSIS.—The diagnosis of phenylketonuria depends upon the demonstration of elevated serum levels of phenylalanine (10 to 50 times that of normal) or elevated urinary levels of phenylpyruvic acid. The latter can be detected by a characteristic green or blue color that results when a few

TABLE 7–1.—ERRORS OF METABOLISM

DISORDER	INHERITANCE	DEFECT	CLINICAL FEATURES	DIAGNOSIS	TREATMENT
Phenylketonuria	Autosomal recessive (1 in 10,000 to 20,000 births)	Phenylalanine hydroxylase	90% are blond, blue-eyed and fair skinned; musty odor; eczematous dermatitis; photosensitivity; mental retardation; microcephaly; short stature	Guthrie test, Ferric chloride test, Phenistix	Low phenylalanine diet
Homocystinuria	Autosomal recessive (1 in 200,000 live births)	Cystathionine synthetase	Ectopia lentis, myopia, arachnodactyly in 50%, seizures, mental retardation, cerebrovascular accidents, sparse light or blond easily friable hair, malar flush, widepored facies, "Charlie Chaplin-like" gait and "rocker-bottom" feet	Cyanide nitroprusside test	Low methionine diet with pyridoxine (vitamin B_6)
Alkaptonuria (ochronosis)	Autosomal recessive (1 in 3 to 5 million individuals)	Homogentisic acid oxidase	Dark urine; blue to brownish-black pigment on nose, malar region, sclerae, ears, axillae, genitalia; staining of clothing (beads of ink-like perspiration); arthritis; contractures; rupture of Achilles tendon; mitral and aortic valvulitis and/or calcific aortic stenosis	Ferric ferricyanide reduction	Low protein (low phenylalanine low tyrosine) diet with added ascorbic acid
Wilson's disease (hepatolenticular degeneration)	Autosomal recessive	Abnormal ceruloplasmin metabolism	Kayser-Fleischer rings, hyperpigmentation of legs, azure lunulae, neurologic and hepatic dysfunction	Aminoaciduria, decreased or absent ceruloplasmin	Chelating agents (BAL, versenate, or D-penicillamine)

drops of urine are added to a 10% solution of ferric chloride, or the Guthrie test (a bacterial inhibition assay method widely used in the newborn period in which several drops of capillary blood easily obtained by heel stick may indicate an elevated level of phenylalanine). False positive results and the technical difficulty occasionally associated with obtaining urine from infants have led to the Phenistix tape test, which utilizes a paper strip impregnated with buffered ferric ammonia sulfate.

For dietary management to be most effective, it is imperative that it be initiated as soon as possible, the earlier the diagnosis the better. In most states in the United States, testing of the capillary blood of all newborns (the Guthrie test) is required by law. Since testing is performed early (during the first few days of life) before dietary phenylalanine intake is sufficient to cause elevated serum levels, a level above 4 to 8 mg/100 ml is considered presumptive of the diagnosis. More effective screening programs should incorporate blood testing for phenylalanine levels in the second week of life with follow-up testing of the urine for increase in phenylalanine metabolites (phenylpyruvic acid and o-OH-phenylacetic acid) at 1 to 2 months of age.

TREATMENT.—Dietary management consists of a diet low in phenylalanine content. Appropriate diets should be started at as early an age as possible. This can be initiated by the use of Lofenalac (Mead-Johnson), a hydrolysate formula from which most of the phenylalanine has been removed. When kept on appropriate restriction of phenylalanine, the patient becomes free of seizures, the electroencephalogram reverts to normal, the eczema clears, and the skin and hair regain their normal color. The effect of treatment on intellectual function depends upon the age at which therapy is initiated. With initiation of appropriate therapy prior to 6 weeks to 2 months of age, normal mental development can usually be achieved. With delay in therapy beyond this period, the beneficial effect is lessened. When initiated after 2½ years of age, little benefit can be achieved. However, the diagnosis of PKU must be firmly established before treatment is initiated since phenylalanine restriction in infants without phenylpyruvic oligophrenia frequently results in dire results.

Present evidence indicates that the final intelligence quotient is significantly higher if the average phenylalanine levels are kept in a range of 5 to 15 mg/ml. Since overtreatment with resulting phenylalanine deficiency is now a well-recognized hazard, blood phenylalanine levels should be determined at regular intervals—once or twice a week for the first months, perhaps every other week until six months of age, and, as the child's growth rate slows, monitoring at monthly intervals until the diet is discontinued.

As yet there is no agreement as to how long the low phenylalanine diet should be continued. In recent years many physicians have discontinued the diet when the patient reached 4 to 6 years of age. There is some evidence that after this age, the intellectual level is maintained, presumably since the brain has completed the critical growth phase during which it is sensitive to damage by elevated levels of phenylalanine and its metabolites. Long-term studies, however, are required in order to determine whether or not differences in intelligence quotients and behavior exist between groups whose treatment was terminated after the first four years of life and those who are continued on low phenylalanine diets.[2]

Homocystinuria

Homocystinuria is an autosomal recessive disorder of methionine metabolism associated with an absence or deficiency of cystathionine synthetase, the hepatic enzyme that catalyzes the formation of cystathionine from homocystine and serine. Estimated to have an incidence of 1 in 20,000 births, with no sexual predilection, it is characterized by ectopia lentis, arachnodactyly, chest and spinal deformities (as seen in the Marfan syndrome), seizures, developmental retardation, cerebrovascular accidents, and increased urinary excretion of homocystine (Table 7–1). The hallmark feature of this disorder is subluxation of the ocular lenses.

CLINICAL FEATURES.—The typical appearance of affected individuals usually develops during the first or second year of life. It consists of sparse, light or blond, easily friable hair; malar flush; a coarse, wide-pore appearance of the facial skin; and erythematous blotches on the skin of the face and extremities suggestive of livedo reticularis. The skin has been described as thin, and children may become quite flushed with exertion. Patients usually are tall and thin, resembling individuals with the Marfan syndrome. Bowed extremities are common and arachnodactyly is said to occur in about 50% of cases.[1] In addition, platyspondyly is characteristically seen on x-ray and kyphoscoliosis, pectus carinatum and genu valgum are common. Some patients have rocker-bottom feet, and most have a shuffling, toe-out "Charlie Chaplin-like" gait.

Central nervous system involvement is manifested by developmental retardation which becomes evident within months to years after birth and although average intelligence has been reported in patients with homocystinuria, mental retardation may be severe by adolescence. Disturbances of gait are common, many electroencephalographic abnormalities may be noted, and severe focal or generalized seizures may occur.

Other abnormalities include hepatomegaly, hyperinsulinemia with deranged carbohydrate metabolism, and inguinal hernia. Focal neurologic signs may develop as the result of cerebrovascular accidents and thromboembolism may occur at any age presenting a persisting mortal threat. Coronary occlusion, renal artery involvement with an associated hypertension, peripheral arterial occlusions, and pulmonary, intracranial, vena cava and portal vein thrombosis are also seen in individuals with this disorder.[1]

DIAGNOSIS.—Homocystinuria and the Marfan syndrome have several features in common. Mental retardation, generalized osteoporosis, and arterial and venous thromboses, however, are features of homocystinuria not found in patients with the Marfan syndrome. Glaucoma is a frequent complication in patients with homocystinuria as well as in patients with the Marfan syndrome. Most homocystinuric patients are myopic, and ectopia lentis is seen in 90% of patients. A curious difference between homocystinuria and the Marfan syndrome is the fact that the dislocation of the lens is generally congenital and upward in the Marfan syndrome, but acquired, downward, and progressive in patients with homocystinuria.

The presence of homocystinuria is suggested by the clinical features and may be confirmed by a urinary cyanide-nitroprusside test and by amino acid chromatography of the serum and urine. Unfortunately, not all neonates with homocystinuria will have an increased blood methionine level and can be missed by neonatal screening. The cyanide-nitroprusside test, when positive, consists of a beet-red color indicating the presence of a compound containing a sulfhydryl group. A positive test result should be followed by a quantitative analysis of the amino acids of the urine. The presence of homocystine in the urine establishes the diagnosis.

TREATMENT.—The treatment of homocystinuria consists of a low methionine diet with cystine as a supplement and some patients respond to pyridoxine phosphate (vitamin B_6), a cofactor for cystathionine synthetase in dosages of 50 to 1000 mg/day with prevention or at least amelioration of clinical complications (dislocation of the ocular lenses, mental retardation, and skeletal changes).[3, 4] Dietary management, to achieve maximum effect, should be instituted early.

Alkaptonuria (Ochronosis)

Alkaptonuria (ochronosis) is an inborn error of tyrosine metabolism in which homogentisic acid, an intermediate product in the metabolism of phenylalanine and tyrosine, accumulates in the tissues and is excreted in the urine because of a lack of homogentisic acid oxidase, an enzyme normally found in the liver and kidney. A rare autosomal recessive disorder with an incidence of 1 in 200,000 live births, the disorder is characterized by homogentisic aciduria, dark urine, blue to bluish-brown or black-brown cartilagenous pigmentary changes and to some extent dermal deposition of pigment (ochronosis), degenerative joint disease, and vascular abnormalities (Table 7–1).

CLINICAL MANIFESTATIONS.—Although alkaptonuria can be detected in infancy by the presence of dark brown stains on urine-moistened diapers, the disorder is usually inapparent until adulthood. Homogentisic acid has an affinity for connective tissue and is polymerized to a blue to brownish-black cutaneous pigmentation which becomes most apparent on the nose, the molar region of the face, the ears, axillae, genitals, sclerae, eyelashes, and nail beds. The ears, besides appearing blue to blue-brown in color, also become tender and stiff from staining of the underlying cartilage.[5, 6] Dusky pigmentation of the hands is associated with underlying discoloration of the tendons; the fingernails may appear blue to gray, and subcutaneous leg calcifications have been described. Perspiration, especially in the axillary, inguinal, and malar regions, may contain appreciable amounts of pigment that appear as beads of ink on the skin, with staining of the clothes as a presenting complaint.

SYSTEMIC MANIFESTATIONS.—Dark urine, a classic finding of this disorder, may not occur in every alkaptonuric patient. Oxidation of homogentisic acid in the urine to a melanin-like pigment is responsible for the brown-black color change; addition of alkali to the urine will hasten this phenomenon.

Spondylitis and osteoarthritis of the major weight-bearing joints, arthritic complications of alkaptonuria, are believed to be a direct result of the deposition of the black pigment in cartilage.[7, 8] Most debilitating is the progressive arthritis which begins in the fourth decade. Calcified intervertebral discs are common. The spine, knees, shoulders, and hips are the most commonly affected joints. Other complications include synovial effusions, contractures, calcification of the large joints and, at times, rupture of the Achilles tendon.

Degenerative cardiovascular disease may be seen as myocardial infarction, often leading to death in these patients. Valvular changes secondary to pigment deposition and subsequent calcification may result in mitral and aortic valvulitis and/or calcific aortic stenosis.[9, 10]

DIAGNOSIS.—The diagnosis of alkaptonuria is made when freshly passed urine darkens on alkalinization. Other causes of black or dark urine include porphyria, myoglobinuria, melanoma, and hemoglobinuria. These pigments can be distinguished by specific chemical tests, thus differentiating the disorders. Other pigmentary disorders such as argyria, hemochromotosis, Addison's disease, pellagra, and porphyria can be differentiated from alkaptonuria by their clinical manifestations, distribution of pigment, and in some cases cutaneous punch biopsy. Differentiation of ochronotic pigment from melanin is difficult but may be differentiated by the fact that it reduces ferric ferriccyanide but not acid silver nitrate. Atabrine and chloroquine may produce a similar bluish pigmentation, but the clinical history and characteristic involvement of the nails, skin, and oral mucosa by these antimalarial agents helps distinguish these disorders.

TREATMENT.—The treatment of ochronosis (alkaptonuria) is best achieved by a low protein diet with dietary control of phenylalanine and tyrosine intake. Long-term application of this diet, however, is frequently impractical. Since vitamin C prevents the homogentisic acid inhibition of lysyl hydroxylase and appears to reduce the binding of homogentisic acid to tendon and cartilage, early institution of ascorbic acid therapy appears to be helpful in the management of this disorder.

Hepatolenticular Degeneration (Wilson's Disease)

Hepatolenticular degeneration (Wilson's disease) is a chronic progressive familial disorder characterized by a triad of basal ganglia degeneration with progressive central nervous system degeneration, cirrhosis of the liver, and a pathognomonic pigmentation of the corneal margins (the Kayser-Fleischer ring) (Table 7–1). Inherited as an autosomal recessive trait resulting in excessive tissue accumulation of copper, two types of this disturbance are described: (1) abnormalities in metabolism and progressive failure of tubular transfer mechanisms for amino acids, glucose, uric acid, calcium, and phosphate; and (2) the ability to synthesize ceruloplasmin resulting in an increase of copper in tissues, especially the liver and brain.

CLINICAL FEATURES.—Hepatolenticular degeneration manifests itself in the first three decades of life and usually begins during adolescence. Although initial signs of this disorder are frequently neurologic (tremors, dysarthria, ataxia, incoordination, or personality changes), signs of liver insufficiency (jaundice, ascites, hepatomegaly, hematemesis, and spider angiomas) are frequently the first clinical features of this condition.[11]

Kayser-Fleischer rings are seen as golden brown or greenish brown pigmentation localized near the limbus of the cornea. Best visualized with side lighting, this discoloration is produced by the deposition of copper in Descemet's membrane at the periphery of the cornea. Blue or azure lunulae of the nails have been reported in individuals with this disorder, but also have been observed in a normal individual and in a person who had ingested phenolphthalein.[12] On the anterior aspects of the lower legs, hyperpigmentation may be seen due to increased melanin deposition with no increase in copper or iron on biopsy specimens of the skin.[13]

TREATMENT.—Hepatolenticular degeneration is a progressive disease and becomes inevitably fatal with death resulting from a complicating infection or liver failure. Treatment depends upon removal of accumulated copper depositions in the body. Chelating agents such as BAL (2–3 dimercaptopropanol), versenate, or a penicillamine are helpful, with D-penicillamine as the most effective agent for this disorder. However, penicillamine can produce allergic or toxic reactions, fever, cutaneous rashes, leukopenia, thrombocytopenia, and elastosis perforans serpiginosa.

Menkes' Kinky Hair Syndrome

Menkes' kinky hair syndrome (trichopoliodystrophy) is a rare, X-linked recessive neurodegenerative disorder that affects infant males and is characterized by coarse facies, pili torti, temperature instability, seizures, psychomotor retardation, arterial intimal changes, low or absent plasma copper and ceruplasmin, growth failure, increased susceptibility to infection, and death, generally by age three to four years.[14–16] Originally thought to be a disorder of copper deficiency, the disorder now appears to be a copper storage disease with the observed defects resulting from inappropriate systemic copper distribution[17] (Table 7–2).

CLINICAL FEATURES.—Clinical features often include premature birth, hypothermia, and relatively normal development until two to six months of age, when drowsiness and lethargy are noted, intractable seizures begin, and growth and development cease.

The face takes on a characteristic appearance with pallid skin, pudgy tissues, horizontal tangled eyebrows and a cupid's bow-like upper lip. Usually the hair is fine, dull, sparse, and poorly pigmented in infancy, stands on end, and looks and feels like steel wool (Fig 7–1). Additional features include a seborrheic rash, which may be coincidental, and, at times, superficial fissuring;[18] tortous cerebral and other medium-sized arteries; osteoporosis; frequent subdural hematomas; and widening of the metaphyses with spurring and frequent fractures, at times simulating the radiologic findings characteristic of patients with the battered child syndrome. Although pili torti is generally a prominent feature of this disorder, other less frequently reported hair abnormalities include monilethrix and trichorrhexis nodosa.

DIAGNOSIS.—The combination of clinical features, bone abnormalities, and low plasma copper and ceruplasmin levels establishes the correct diagnosis in patients with this disorder. Radiographic examination of the skull may disclose scattered wormian bones, especially in the posterior sagittal and lambdoidal sutures. Long bone x-rays show metaphyseal spurs and subperiostial calcifications along the shafts, particularly of the femora. In some

TABLE 7–2. MENKES' KINKY HAIR SYNDROME
(TRICHOPOLIODYSTROPHY)

1. X-linked recessive (affects infant males)
2. A disorder of copper storage and distribution
3. Coarse facies, premature birth, hypothermia, seborrheic rash, dull sparse poorly pigmented hair, pili torti, monilethrix and trichorrhexis nodosa
4. Low plasma copper and ceruplasmin levels
5. Treatment unsatisfactory to date

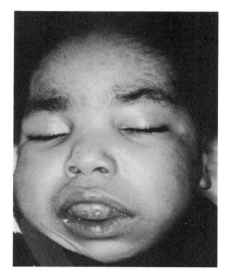

Fig 7–1.—"Steel wool"-like hair, psychomotor retardation and coarse features in a child with Menkes' kinky hair syndrome. (From the Department of Dermatology, Yale University School of Medicine.)

cases anterior flaring of the ribs has also been recorded.[1] In suspected cases of pregnant women, prenatal diagnosis by copper incorporation studies on cultured cells have allowed the diagnosis of an infant in utero.[19]

TREATMENT.—Since the demonstration of a defect in intestinal absorption and utilization of copper, parenteral copper and ceruplasmin therapy have been attempted with results varying from a temporary arrest to clinical worsening of the disorder. Although treatment has raised plasma copper and ceruplasmin levels to normal, possible irreversible damage prior to diagnosis (presumably in utero) cautions against undue optimism for the value of intravenous copper therapy for patients with this disorder.

The Lesch-Nyhan Syndrome

The Lesch-Nyhan syndrome, an inherited disorder of purine metabolism affecting males, is characterized by mental retardation, choreoathetoid movement, self-mutilation and gout-like manifestations of hyperuricemia.[20] A sex-linked (X-linked) disorder, the Lesch-Nyhan syndrome is caused by a deficiency of hypoxanthineguanine phosphoribosyl transferase (HG-PRTase) which leads to an overproduction of uric acid and the clinical features associated with this disorder (Table 7–3).

CLINICAL MANIFESTATIONS.—Patients appear normal at birth and may develop normally for a period of six to eight months, the first recognizable sign of the disease often manifesting as a result of orange uric acid crystals (resembling grains of sand) in the diaper, as renal stones, or as hematuria during the early months of life.

TABLE 7–3.—LESCH-NYHAN SYNDROME

1 X-linked
2. Hypoxanthine-guanine phosphoribosyl transferase (HG-PRTase) deficiency
3. Hyperuricemia, mental retardation, spastic cerebral palsy, choreoathetosis, and aggressive self-mutilating behavior
4. Orange uric acid crystals (resembling grains of sand) in diaper often first sign
5. Diagnosis: increased levels of uric acid in blood and urine
6. Allopurinol (100–300 mg/day) helpful

The onset of cerebral manifestations may be subtle, with difficulty in sitting or standing without help, involuntary movements, dystonia, spasticity, and increased deep tendon reflexes. Although mental retardation may vary in degree, it usually is severe and abnormal behavior remains a striking characteristic of the disease. The main clinical feature of this disorder is a loss of tissue about the mouth or fingers which occurs as a result of the child's habit of compulsive self-destructive biting of this area. In time, without adequate restraint, all of the lower lip that is accessible to the teeth may be chewed away. The face, fingers, and wrists may also be mutilated, and since young children frequently bite others (such as parents or nurses) particular caution should be exercised when handling children with this disorder.[20, 21]

DIAGNOSIS.—Diagnosis of the Lesch-Nyhan syndrome can be established by the clinical presentation and laboratory demonstration of increased levels of uric acid in the blood and urine. Heterozygous females may be detected by the presence of two populations of fibroblasts in tissue culture of fibroblasts grown from a skin biopsy, with only one cell-line showing the key enzyme.

TREATMENT.—The management of this disorder includes the use of allopurinol (in dosages of 100 to 300 mg daily in divided doses) in an effort to control uric acid levels, tophaceous deposits, nephropathy and gouty arthritis. Physical restraints (hand bandages and elbow splints) may be used to help control the self-mutilating behavior of patients. Lip biting may require extraction of deciduous teeth, but permanent teeth should be spared, since lip biting usually diminishes with age.

Biotin Deficiency

Biotin, part of the vitamin B complex, is required for the function of three carboxylase enzymes: (1) 3-methyl crotonyl-C_OA carboxylase, essential for the catabolism of leucine; (2) propionyl-C_OA carboxylase, essential for the catabolism of isoleucine, threonine, valine, and methionine; and (3) pyruvic acid carboxylase, required for the gluconeogenesis and regulation of carbohydrate metabolism.[22]

Biotin deficiency may be induced by a biotin deficient diet containing large quantities of raw egg white which contains avidin, a protein which binds to biotin, thus preventing its absorption in the intestine. The resulting biotin deficiency is manifested by anorexia, lassitude, a pale tongue, grayish pallor of the skin, atrophy of the lingual papillae, anemia, muscle pains, dryness of the skin and a scaly dermatitis (Fig 7–2), all of which disappear following biotin administration or by cooking, boiling, or steaming of egg white which causes avidin to lose its biotin-binding capacity. Another dietary form of biotin deficiency can also occur in patients receiving biotin-deficient parenteral therapy.[23, 24]

Besides nutritionally-induced biotin deficiency, there are two metabolic forms of biotin-responsive carboxylase deficiency disorders: an acute neonatal form and a juvenile form. The neonatal form of biotin-responsive multiple carboxylase deficiency appears in the first few weeks of life with a metabolic acidosis, ketosis, and an erythematous rash. A result of deficient holocarboxylase synthetase activity, patients with this form of the disorder do not survive without the benefit of early diagnosis and treatment[25–28] (Table 7–4).

The juvenile form of the disorder, a condition that develops two or three months after birth, appears to be the result of impaired biotin absorption and/or transport. It is characterized by seizures, intermittent acidosis, recurrent infections, dermatitis (often periorificial), sparse hair (alopecia), keratoconjunctivitis, ataxia, hypotonia, and glossitis.

DIAGNOSIS.—The diagnosis of biotin deficiency can be established by a decreased concentration of plasma biotin and an increase in the urinary

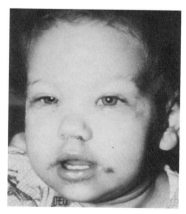

Fig 7–2.—Scaly periorificial dermatitis in a child with biotin-responsive carboxylase deficiency. (Courtesy of Dr. Mary Williams, San Francisco, California.)[26]

TABLE 7–4.—BIOTIN DEFICIENCY

1. Dietary (biotin deficient diet or ingestion of raw eggs)
2. Biotin-deficient parenteral therapy
3. Metabolic forms
   a. Neonatal (multiple carboxylase deficiency)
      1. Metabolic acidosis, ketosis and erythematous rash
      2. Patients do not survive without early treatment
   b. Juvenile form (impaired biotin absorption and/or transport)
      1. Ataxia, hypotonia, seizures, intermittent acidosis, recurrent infections
      2. Periorificial dermatitis and alopecia
4. Diagnosis confirmed by low plasma biotin and an increase in urinary metabolites
5. Avoidance of raw eggs (for avidin-type) and IV or oral biotin supplementation

metabolites 3-hydroxyisoraleric acid, 3-methylcrotonyl-glycine, 3-hydroxypropionic acid, methylcitric acid, and lactic acid.

TREATMENT.—The neonatal form of biotin deficiency is fatal but biotin deficiency associated with the ingestion of raw eggs and the juvenile form of the disorder can be treated by intravenous multivitamins containing 60 micrograms of biotin, or by the oral administration of 10 mg of biotin daily.[26, 28]

Disorders of Tyrosine Metabolism

Although the relationship of tyrosine to the synthesis of melanin has been well known since the early and mid-twentieth century, the effect of dietary tyrosine on the skin was not cited in the dermatologic literature until ophthalmologic and cutaneous involvement became recognized as clinical features of tyrosinemia.[29] Clinical disorders of tyrosine metabolism include: (1) neonatal tyrosinemia, (2) tyrosinemia I, and (3) tyrosinemia II (the Richner-Hanhart syndrome) (Table 7–5). Of these, only the Richner-Hanhart syndrome exhibits cutaneous manifestations.

Neonatal tyrosinemia.—Infants (particularly those that have birth weights below 2500 grams) exposed to high protein diets may develop a syndrome of tyrosinemia, lethargy, and motor impairment termed neonatal tyrosinemia. A relative deficiency of p-hydroxyphenyl-pyruvate oxidase in premature infants has been hypothesized as the basis of this disorder. Data on the levels of this enzyme and tyrosine aminotransferase, however, are lacking since neonatal tyrosinemia is a self-limiting disorder. Investigative studies would require liver biopsies which would create a potential risk to this group of otherwise healthy infants. Affected infants can be treated by a low protein diet with, perhaps, ascorbic acid supplementation. Although

TABLE 7–5.—Disorders of Tyrosine Metabolism

1. Neonatal tyrosinemia
   a. A relative deficiency of p-hydroxyphenyl-pyruvate oxidase in prematures
   b. Tyrosinemia, lethargy, and motor impairment
   c. May be treated by a low protein diet with ascorbic acid supplementation
2. Tyrosinosis (tyrosinemia I)
   a. Autosomal recessive inheritance
   b. A deficiency in fumarylacetoacetate (FAA) hydrolase
   c. Failure to thrive, vomiting, diarrhea, cabbage-like odor, hepatomegaly, and often death in first year of life
   d. A milder form with chronic liver disease, renal tubular dysfunction (with deToni-Fanconi syndrome), vitamin D-resistant rickets, pancreatic islet cell hyperplasia, and (in ⅓ of cases) hepatomas
   e. Treatment: a low tyrosine, low phenylalanine and low methionine diet
3. Tyrosinemia II (Richner-Hanhart syndrome)
   a. Autosomal recessive
   b. Tyrosinemia, keratitis, palmar and plantar hyperkeratosis with erosions, and, at times, mental retardation
   c. Diagnosis confirmed by increased levels of tyrosine in blood and urine and increased urinary tyrosine metabolites
   d. Treatment: low tyrosine, low phenylalanine diet (Mead Johnson 3200 AB)

the urinary excretion of tyrosine and p-hydroxyphenylpyruvic acid may be aided by the administration of ascorbic acid, the efficacy of vitamin C supplementation for patients with this disorder remains questionable.

Tyrosinosis (tyrosinemia I).—Tyrosinosis (tyrosinemia I) is an autosomal recessive disorder characterized by failure to thrive, vomiting, diarrhea, and hepatomegaly. A deficiency in fumarylacetoacetate (FAA) hydrolase, resulting in an increase in succinylacetone (a metabolite that interferes with cell growth and inhibits delta-amino levulinic acid dehydratase), appears to be associated with the cause of this disorder.[29–31] The acute form of this disorder is caused by a severe enzyme deficiency and is associated with liver failure, a cabbage-like odor, and often death during the first year of life. In a milder chronic form of the disease, patients are seen to have chronic liver disease with cirrhosis, renal tubular dysfunction with the deToni-Fanconi syndrome, vitamin D-resistant rickets, acute intermittent porphyria-like symptoms, pancreatic islet cell hyperplasia, hypoglycemia; in over one-third of patients, hepatomas may be present.[29]

The treatment of tyrosinemia I consists of a low tyrosine, low phenylalanine, and low methionine diet. Supplemental dietary cysteine has also been recommended, but its value remains questionable.[29]

Tyrosinemia II (Richner-Hanhart syndrome).—The Richner-Hanhart syndrome (tyrosinemia II, oculocutaneous tyrosinosis) is an autosomal recessive disorder that affects both sexes equally and is manifested by tyrosinemia, bilateral keratitis, palmar and plantar hyperkeratosis and erosions, and, at times, mental retardation. A result of a deficiency of hepatic tyrosine aminotransferase, the disease is characterized by ocular, neurologic and cutaneous features. Ophthalmic abnormalities often present as the first sign of this condition. Usually appearing during the first few months of life, they consist of photophobia, increased lacrimation, redness and inflammation of the eyes, dendritic ulcers, bilateral keratitis often leading to corneal opacities and thick corneal and conjunctival plaques with increased vascularity.

Cutaneous changes appear shortly after the ocular lesions and, limited to the palms and soles (especially the distal phalanges, thenar and hypothenar eminences), they are manifested by painful erosions and blisters (Fig 7–3), often with crusting and hyperkeratosis. The keratoses may vary from crusting and hyperkeratotic lesions 1 to 2 mm in diameter, sometimes in a linear configuration, to diffuse hyperkeratosis of the palms and soles. With pain a common feature, young children frequently prefer crawling rather than walking during the first few years of life.[29, 31–33]

Neurologic features vary from mild to moderate degrees of mental retardation. Since they can be prevented or modified by appropriate therapy, early diagnosis and treatment of this disorder is suggested.

DIAGNOSIS.—The diagnosis of tyrosinemia II is established by the clinical features and increased levels of tyrosine in the blood and urine of affected patients. Other laboratory abnormalities include elevated levels of urinary tyrosine metabolites (p-hydroxyphenylacetic acid, p-hydroxyphenylpyruvic acid, and N-acetyl tyrosine).

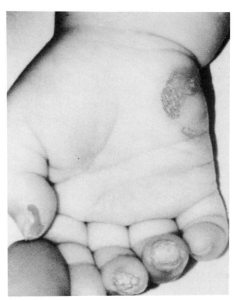

Fig 7–3.—Erosions on the palm and fingertips in a child with tyrosinemia II (Richner-Hanhart syndrome, oculocutaneous tyrosinosis). (Courtesy of Dr. Lowell A. Goldsmith, Rochester, New York.)[29]

TREATMENT.—The lowering of plasma tyrosine levels can be initiated with a low-tyrosine, low-phenylalanine diet commercially available as Mead Johnson 3200 AB. With appropriate therapy, the ophthalmic and cutaneous manifestations clear over a period of a few days to weeks.[34-36] However, dietary management must not be terminated since discontinuation of therapy results in recurrence or exacerbations of the disorder.

The Hyperlipidemias

The hyperlipidemias (hyperlipoproteinemias) represent a group of metabolic diseases characterized by persistent elevation of plasma cholesterol, triglycerides, or both. Since plasma lipids circulate in the form of high molecular weight complexes bound to protein, the term hyperlipidemia also indicates an elevation of lipoproteins, hence justification for introduction of the term hyperlipoproteinemia for this group of disorders.

Plasma lipoproteins differ significantly in electrostatic charges, thus permitting their separation by electrophoretic techniques into four major fractions (chylomicrons and beta-, prebeta-, and alpha-lipoproteins). By means of ultracentrifugation, it is also possible to separate the plasma lipoproteins into four major groups (chylomicrons and very low density, low density, and high density lipoproteins), which correlate well with those separated by electrophoresis. These recently introduced techniques allow classification of the familial hyperlipidemias into five groups, designated as hyperlipoproteinemias I through V, each with its own specific clinicopathologic, prognostic, and therapeutic features[37-39] (Table 7–6).

Clinical Manifestations of Xanthomas

Xanthomas are lipid-containing papules, nodules, or tumors that may be found anywhere on the skin and mucous membranes. Although the mechanism of their formation is not completely understood, it appears that serum lipids infiltrate the tissues where they are phagocytized by macrophages (histiocytes) and deposited, particularly in areas subjected to stress and pressure. Although they may suggest the presence of hyperlipidemia and can provide clues to the underlying disorder, when seen alone they are not diagnostic. Complete clinical and biochemical evaluations are required before the true nature of the underlying disorder can be determined.[40]

Depending on their gross appearance, anatomic location, and mode of development, several forms of xanthomas have been categorized: *plane, eruptive* or *papuloeruptive, tendinous,* or *tuberous.* Recognition of these lesions is important inasmuch as they present easily visible cutaneous clues to underlying metabolic abnormalities and frequently assist in diagnosis of specific metabolic disease entities.

TABLE 7-6.—THE HYPERLIPOPROTEINEMIAS

TYPE	CLINICAL FEATURES	BIOCHEMICAL FEATURES	INHERITANCE
I Bürger-Grütz	Common in infancy and early teens Episodic abdominal pain Eruptive xanthomas Lipemic plasma Lipemia retinalis	Exogenous fat-induced hyperlipemia	Autosomal recessive
II Familial hypercholesterolemia	Onset in childhood or adulthood Crops of eruptive xanthomas, tendinous and tuberous xanthomas Xanthelasma Atherosclerosis and coronary disease	High cholesterol levels	Autosomal dominant
III Broad beta disease	Onset in adulthood (uncommon in childhood) Plane xanthomas in palmar creases A high incidence of cardiovascular disease	Endogenous hyperlipemia Abnormal glucose tolerance Increased cholesterol, betalipoproteins, and triglycerides	Autosomal recessive
IV Familial hyperbetalipoproteinemia	Unusual before age 20 Eruptive tuberous xanthomas on elbows, knees, heels, and wrists Obesity Hepatosplenomegaly Abdominal pain Lipemia retinalis Premature cardiovascular disease	Endogenous carbohydrate-induced hyperlipidemia Laboratory findings similar to those in type III	Autosomal recessive
V Familial hyperchylomicronemia with hyperbetalipoproteinemia	Combination of types I and IV Rare in childhood Eruptive, tuberous, and palmar xanthomas Obesity Hepatosplenomegaly Lipemia retinalis	Exogenous and endogenous Increase in both chylomicrons and prebetalipoproteins	? Recessive inheritance

(From Hurwitz S.: *Clinical Pediatric Dermatology.* W. B. Saunders Co., Philadelphia, 1981)

    1.—*Plane xanthomas.*—Soft, flat, macular or slightly elevated yellow to orange or brownish-yellow intracutaneous plaques, plane xanthomas are generally seen on the face, sides of the neck, upper trunk, elbows, and knees, but may occur anywhere on the body and have a marked predilection for surgical or acne scars and the palmar creases. The most frequently seen xanthomas are those that occur on or near the eyelids during middle age. Termed *xanthelasmas* or *xanthoma palpebrarum*, they rarely occur in children or adolescents. When present, however, they require studies for diabetes mellitus, Hand-Schüller-Christian disease, myeloma, and hepatic or liver disorders; a search for xanthomas elsewhere on the body; and an investigation of plasma lipids for evidence of familial hyperlipidemia. Although approximately two-thirds of individuals with xanthelasma may have normal lipid levels, these cutaneous lesions may be the first clues to the presence of hyperlipoproteinemia type II disease. If the physician is to prevent the vascular consequences of type II disease, early detection is helpful. Lesions that develop in palmar creases and flexural surfaces of the fingers, termed *xanthoma striatum planum*, generally portend the presence of hepatic disease or familial hyperlipidemia (types II and III).

2.—*Papulo-eruptive xanthomas.*—Small red to yellow papular lesions that have an erythematous base, these lipoidal lesions appear in crops and consist of multiple small red to yellow-orange raised solid papules, sometimes surrounded by an erythematous halo at the base of the lesion. Although they may involve the trunk and oral mucosa, they have a predilection for sites subjected to pressure or trauma, particularly the extensor surfaces of the arms, legs, and buttocks (Fig 7–4). Papuloeruptive xanthomas are almost always associated with hypertriglyceridemia and are generally seen in patients with uncontrolled diabetes mellitus, in mild diabetics who are asymptomatic yet have high triglyceride levels, or in patients with hyperlipoproteinemia types I, III, IV, and V.

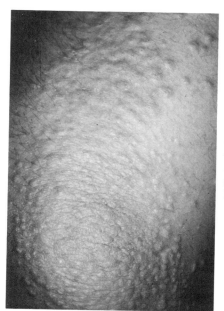

Fig 7–4.—Eruptive xanthomas on the knee of a 13-year-old child with type III lipoproteinemia. (From Hurwitz S.: *Clinical Pediatric Dermatology.* W.B. Saunders Co., Philadelphia, 1981. Used by permission.)

3.—*Tendon xanthomas.*—Multiple skin-colored or yellowish, smooth, freely movable subcutaneous nodules and tumors, these xanthomas have a predilection for the extensor tendons of the elbows, knees, heels, hands, and feet. These nontender, firm nodules measure 1 cm or more in diameter and are best seen or palpated on the Achilles tendon and the tendons on the dorsal aspect of the hands.

4.—*Tuberous xanthomas.*—Large, firm, nodular or tumorous, sessile or pedunculated, flesh-colored or yellowish, tuberous xanthomas are lipid deposits that occur on extensor surfaces subject to stress or trauma, particularly the elbows, knees, hands, and buttocks. Located in the dermis and subcutaneous layers, they can enlarge to 5 cm or more in diameter and are not attached to underlying structures. Generally associated with increased serum triglycerides (either on an acquired or familial basis), tuberous xanthomas are most frequently seen in association with types II, III, and IV lipoproteinemia.

5.—*Tendinous xanthomas.*—Firm, subcutaneous papules or nodules, tendinous xanthomas have a predilection for the extensor tendons of the fingers, patellae, and elbows. They frequently occur in association with xanthelasma, tuberous lesions, and coronary atherosclerosis. Although they may occur in patients with hypertriglyceridemia, they generally indicate the presence of hypercholesterolemia and appear almost exclusively in familial lipoproteinemia types II and III.

Classification of the Hyperlipoproteinemias

The classification of the hyperlipidemic disorders is based upon the classification by Fredrickson and Lees. Based upon electrophoretic and ultracentrifugal analyses of serum lipoproteins, they are designated as type I, hyperchylomicronemia; type II, increased betalipoprotein; type III, increased beta- and prebetalipoprotein; type IV, increased prebetalipoprotein; and type V, combined hyperchylomicronemia and hyperprebetalipoproteinemia (of these, types I and II are the most commonly seen in childhood)[39] (Table 7–6).

Type I hyperlipoproteinemia (Bürger-Grütz Disease).—A rare autosomal recessive disorder, type I hyperlipoproteinemia is characterized by an elevation of fasting serum triglycerides carried in the form of chylomicrons. The defect in type I disease, expressed as soon as the infant takes fat, probably lies in the faulty removal of normal chylomicrons from the serum because of a deficiency of lipoprotein lipase activity. Hyperlipemia is usually discovered accidentally because of lactescence (manifested by a creamy or chocolate appearance of whole blood), or because of the appearance of xanthomas, bouts of abdominal pain, or hepatic and splenic enlargements. Occasionally the disease may be noted for the first time during examination of a patient presenting with severe abdominal pain and signs of peritoneal irritation.

Episodic abdominal pain, seen in approximately one-half of affected children, is very common and frequently manifested by clinical signs of acute abdominal distress. General malaise and anorexia are common, and abdominal spasms, rigidity, rebound tenderness, leukocytosis, and fever may be present. Sometimes, particularly in patients under the age of 6, the pain is caused by lipid accumulations in the liver and spleen. In others it may be due to splenic infarct or pancreatitis associated with this disorder.

About two-thirds of children with type I disease are seen with xanthomas which, in almost all cases, are of the eruptive type. They may appear at any site, including the mucous membranes, and are most commonly seen on the buttocks, thighs, arms, forearms, chest, back, and face. Xanthelasmas and tendinous xanthomas account for less than 2% of the lesions seen in such patients. Eruptive xanthomas usually occur suddenly when the hyperlipemia is severe, and resolve rapidly when the chylomicrons decrease after institution of a low fat diet.

Type II hyperlipoproteinemia (familial hypercholesterolemia).—Best understood and most important from a pediatric point of view, type II hyperlipoproteinemia is an autosomal dominant disorder characterized by cutaneous xanthomas, increased concentrations of plasma cholesterol, and a high incidence of coronary artery disease.

Seen in approximately 1 in 250 to 500 persons in the general population, there are two groups of patients with type II disease. In patients homozygous for this disorder, plasma cholesterol levels are extremely high (often reaching 700 to 1000 mg/100 ml). Cutaneous xanthomas usually develop during childhood, often in the first years of life, and affected individuals frequently die of ischemia heart disease in their twenties and thirties. In a second group, affected persons are presumably heterozygous for this disorder. They develop tendon xanthomas (usually after age 30), and even though serum cholesterol levels are markedly elevated, patients have a normal longevity without a significant increase in atherosclerosis and coronary heart disease.

Although the exact defect in type II disease is not completely understood, it appears to be related to a derangement of cholesterol metabolism. Recent studies suggest deficiency of hydroxymethylglutaryl coenzyme A reductase (HMG-CoA reductase) with an associated defect in fibroblast cell receptors that bind betalipoproteins, with a resulting elevation of plasma betalipoprotein and cholesterol.[41]

Cutaneous xanthomas reportedly occur in 40% to 50% of patients with type II disease. These include tendinous xanthomas in 40% to 50% of cases, xanthelasmas in 23%, and tuberous lesions in 10% to 15% of affected individuals. Large pendulous tuberous xanthomas may occur in children with this disorder; eruptive xanthomas, however, are unusual.

Arcus cornea (also termed *arcus lipoides* or *arcus juvenilis*), consisting of lipid deposits of cholesterol, triglycerides, and phospholipids around the edge of the cornea, is commonly seen in association with this disease. The significance of arcus cornea depends upon the age of the patient. When seen in childhood, it is almost always a sign of hyperlipoproteinemia.

Type III hyperlipoproteinemia (familial hyperbeta- and prebetalipoproteinemia).—Often referred to as "broad beta disease," type III hyperlipoproteinemia is an autosomal recessive disorder characterized by xanthomas, a high incidence of cardiovascular disease, frequent abnormal tolerance to glucose, and an increase in serum levels of both cholesterol and triglycerides. The precise nature of type III disease is unknown, but it appears to be associated with a disturbance in the clearance of remnant lipoproteins, with accumulations of both cholesterol and triglycerides. It is uncommon in childhood and nearly always first diagnosed in adulthood (usually around middle age) (Fig 7–4).

Electrophoresis of plasma proteins shows a broad beta band. Seventy-five percent to 80% of patients with this disorder have xanthomas. They may include the full range of xanthomatous lesions from eruptive xanthomas to tendinous nodules. Soft planar xanthomas (striatum palmare) in the palmar creases are a common feature of familial type III hyperlipoproteinemia. However, since they may also be seen in individuals with the type II disorder and in patients with liver disease, they are not an exclusive feature of type III hyperlipoproteinemia. Atherosclerotic vascular complications are common in patients with type III disease. Although both coronary and peripheral artery diseases may occur, the latter are more common in patients with type III as compared to type II forms of this disorder.

Type IV disease (familial hyperbetalipoproteinemia).—The most common form of familial hyperlipoproteinemia, type IV, is an endogenous carbohydrate-induced disorder (in contrast to type I, which is fat-induced). Characterized by obesity and elevation of serum prebetalipoproteins, type IV disease may be familial or acquired. The familial type appears to be inherited as an autosomal dominant disease. Usually not seen before the age of 20, type IV hyperlipoproteinemia may appear in children with renal disease or in diabetics who have become ketotic. The cutaneous lesions seen with this disorder are eruptive, tuberous, and palmar in distribution. Cardiovascular disease is extremely common and hepatosplenomegaly, abdominal pain, and lipemia retinalis may occur.[39]

Type V disease (familial hyperchylomicronemia with hyperprebetalipoproteinemia).—A combination of type I and type IV disease, type V is a complex abnormality of both endogenous and exogenous origin characterized by increased concentrations of both chylomicrons and prebetalipoproteins. Although the exact mode of inheritance is still unclear, it appears to be a recessive disorder. Patients are usually obese, and their lipemia is often discovered in late adolescence or early adulthood because of the eruptive xanthomas, hepatosplenomegaly, and acute abdominal crises similar to those seen in individuals with type I disease. Although type V hyperlipoproteinemia may have its onset in adolescence, it has rarely been reported in childhood.[42]

Tangier Disease

Tangier disease (familial high density lipoprotein deficiency) is a unique, rare heritable disorder characterized by hypocholesterolemia, an almost complete absence of plasma high density lipoprotein (HDL), and storage of cholesterol esters in many tissues of the body. Seen in children as well as adults, it derives its name from the Chesapeake Bay Island home of the first two patients described with this disorder.

The biochemical defect of Tangier disease is uncertain but appears to be related to a defect in the synthesis of high density lipoprotein associated with a double dose of a rare mutant gene. The clinical manifestations include hypocholesterolemia (50 to 125 mg per 100 ml) and low phospholipid levels in association with normal or slightly elevated triglycerides (150 to 250 mg per 100 ml) and enlarged tonsils with distinctive alternating bands of red, orange, or yellowish-white striations overlying the normal red mucosa. Lipid deposits may be accompanied by a persistent maculopapular eruption over the trunk and abdomen, hepatosplenomegaly, lymph node enlargement, infiltration of the cornea in adults, and alterations in the intestinal and rectal mucosa. Several patients have had recurrent peripheral neuropathy.

The prognosis in Tangier disease is unknown. Children may have no detectable abnormality except in the tonsils and plasma. Adults, however, have shown more extensive cholesterol ester deposition in the rectal mucosa, skin, and cornea.[39]

The Mucopolysaccharidoses

The mucopolysaccharidoses are inherited disorders of mucopolysaccharide metabolism characterized by widespread accumulation of mucopolysaccharide (the major component in the ground substance of connective tissue) in tissues and cultured skin fibroblasts, with excessive excretion in the urine.[43] First described by Hunter in 1917 (and labeled "gargoylism" in 1936), these disorders can now be divided into at least six somewhat related clinical entities on the basis of their clinical features, their mode of

TABLE 7-7.—THE MUCOPOLYSACCHARIDOSES

SYNDROMES	CLINICAL FEATURES	BIOCHEMICAL FEATURES	INHERITANCE
Hurler (MPS I-H)	Severe retardation Corneal clouding Hepatosplenomegaly Chondrodystrophy Dwarfism Grave manifestations and early demise	Chondroitin sulfate B, haparan monosulfate Excessive urinary excretion of dermatan sulfate and heparan sulfate	Autosomal recessive
Scheie (MPS I-S) (formerly MPS V)	Corneal clouding Severe osteochondrodystrophy Aortic incompetence Retinitis pigmentosa	Keratosulfate Excessive urinary excretion of dermatan sulfate and heparan sulfate	Autosomal recessive
Hunter (MPS II)	Less severe than Hurler's Longer survival Lack of corneal involvement Cutaneous markers over scapula, posterior axilla, or thigh Atypical retinitis pigmentosa Aggressive behavior	Chondroitin sulfate B heparan monosulfate	X-linked recessive
Sanfilippo (MPS III)	Severe neurologic involvement Mild somatic changes	Heparitin monosulfate Excessive urinary excretion of heparan sulfate	Autosomal recessive
Morquio (MPS IV)	Normal intelligence Striking dwarfism Corneal opacity Severe osteoporosis and atlanto-axial dislocation	Chondroitin sulfate B Marked urinary excretion of keratin sulfate and chondroitin sulfate	Autosomal recessive
Maroteaux-Lamy (MPS VI)	Normal intelligence Dwarfism Severe corneal and bony lesions	Chondroitin sulfate B Increased urinary excretion of dermatan sulfate	Autosomal recessive

(From Hurwitz S.: *Clinical Pediatric Dermatology*. W.B. Saunders Co., Philadelphia, 1981.)

inheritance, and the nature of the accumulated mucopolysaccharide[43–45] (Table 7–7).

Although the precise biochemical defect is still not well understood, current evidence suggests a deficiency of beta-galactosidase, leading to abnormal accumulation of mucopolysaccharides in cells of the connective tissue and many organs. The usual distinguishing features of the various syndromes of mucopolysaccharidosis (MPS) are based on the presence or degree of somatic and skeletal involvement, mental retardation, corneal clouding, cardiopulmonary changes, hepatosplenomegaly, and hearing loss, and on the mode of inheritance and the nature of their accumulated poly-saccharides (Table 7–7). The Hunter syndrome (MPS II) is an X-linked recessive disorder; all others are autosomal recessive. They can be differ-entiated from the mucolipidoses, a group of disorders characterized by an accumulation of sphingolipids or glycolipids in the visceral and mesenchy-mal cells, which exhibit clinical and skeletal signs of the mucopolysacchar-idoses but differ from them by the normal urinary excretion of uronic acid containing acid mucopolysaccharides (with the exception of mucosulfati-dosis), and by the presence of clinical features usually seen in the sphin-golipidoses (Niemann-Pick disease and Gaucher disease).[46]

The cutaneous changes of all six forms of mucopolysaccharidosis consist of pale, coarse, and dry skin with hirsutism, especially over the back and extremities, and thickened, roughened, taut inelastic skin, especially over the fingers.

Hurler syndrome.—The most common of the mucopolysaccharidoses, Hurler syndrome (mucopolysaccharidosis I-H, MPS 1 in McKusick's origi-nal classification), an autosomal recessive disease with a deficiency of alpha-L-iduronidase and dermatan sulfate in the connective tissues and central nervous syndrome, is the classic prototype of this group of disorders. Seen in approximately 1 out of 100,000 births, it appears in the first year of life and is particularly grave, with demise occurring in almost all cases before age 10. Death, when it occurs, is usually associated with cardiac failure or respiratory infection.

Cardinal features of the Hurler syndrome include coarsening of facial features; macrocephaly with frontal bulging; premature closure of the su-tures, with hyperostosis frequently leading to a scaphocephalic skull; flat-tened nasal bridge with a saddle-shaped appearance; hypertelorism; pro-tuberant tongue; short neck; protuberant abdomen due to hepatic and splenic enlargement; deformity of the chest; shortness of the spine; laxity of the abdominal wall with inguinal and umbilical hernias; broad hands with stubby fingers; a claw hand due to stiffening of the phalangeal joints; limitation of extensibility of the joints; severe, progressive mental retarda-tion; and marked retardation of growth (Figs 7–5, 7–6). Although the ma-jority of infants are normal or above normal in length during the first year of life, growth rate decreases by two years of age. By age three almost all patients are below the third percentile for stature. Clouding of the cornea develops in all patients with Hurler syndrome. On inspection this feature is most apparent if light is shone on the cornea from the side (slit lamp examination confirms the finding).[46, 47]

Diagnosis is based upon the clinical picture and identification of exces-sive mucopolysaccharides in the urine by the toluidine blue test and the

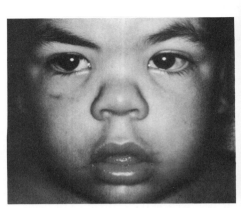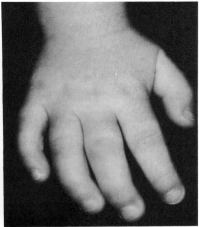

Fig 7–5 (left).—Coarse facial features in a child with Hunter syndrome (Mucopolysaccharidosis II). (From Hurwitz S.: *Clinical Pediatric Dermatology.* W.B. Saunders Co., Philadelphia, 1981. Used by permission.)

Fig 7–6 (right).—Mucopolysaccharidosis II (Hunter's syndrome). Broad stubby fingers with stiffening and limiting of extension of the phalangeal joints result in a claw hand-appearance in patients with the Hurler and Hunter syndromes (MPS I and II).

gross albumin turbidity test. Routine histopathologic examination of the skin shows vacuolization of the cytoplasm in some of the epidermal cells (due to mucopolysaccharide), with displacement of the nucleus to one side, and occasional solitary swollen cells at all levels of the epidermis. Large vacuolated mononuclear cells ("gargoyle cells") are present beneath the basement membrane as well as in the periappendageal and perivascular areas.

There is no effective definitive treatment of mucopolysaccaridosis. Although initial reports of beneficial effects from plasma infusions were promising, subsequent studies indicate no clinical or biochemical results from this technique.[48, 49] Prenatal diagnosis of the mucopolysaccharidoses is now possible through the study of cultured amniotic fluid cells and the amniotic fluid itself. The clinical course of patients is usually progressively downhill, with death in those with the fully expressed syndrome from either respiratory infection or cardiac failure, generally before the age of 10.[43]

Scheie syndrome.—Originally considered a distinctive form of mucopolysaccharidosis, the Scheie syndrome (mucopolysaccharidosis I-S, formerly MPS V) now appears to represent a variant of the Hurler syndrome

(MPS 1-H). It is characterized by stiff joints, coarse facies, corneal cloud-ing, excessive body hair, retinitis pigmentosa, aortic regurgitation, few other somatic effects, and normal intellect. Patients with Scheie syndrome excrete excessive amounts of dermatan sulfate and heparan sulfate. The Hurler and Scheie syndromes, despite their striking clinical differences, are similar by fibroblast culture. They both are corrected by the Hurler factor and both show deficiency of the same enzyme, alpha-L-iduroni-dase.[50]

Hunter syndrome.—The Hunter syndrome (mucopolysaccharidosis II, MPS II) is distinguished from the Hurler syndrome by an X-linked reces-sive inheritance, longer survival, lack of corneal clouding, characteristic cutaneous markers, and a different pattern of mucopolysaccharide excretion (chrondroitin sulfate B and heparitin sulfate). The clinical picture in all respects is generally less severe than that seen in the Hurler syndrome. Mental retardation progresses at a slower rate, humping of the lumbar area (gibbus) does not occur, and progressive deafness is a frequent feature. Hearing loss is present in about 50% of patients with Hunter syndrome, and children are often brought to a physician at about three years of age because of lack of speech. Although deafness also occurs in the Hurler syndrome (MPS I), severe mental retardation and death at an early age make it an inconspicuous feature of this disorder.

Distinctive cutaneous changes are highly characteristic of MPS II (Hunter syndrome) and probably represent a marker of this disorder. These pathognomonic lesions consist of firm flesh-colored to ivory-white papules and nodules that often coalesce to form ridges or a reticular pattern in symmetrical areas between the angles of the scapulae and posterior ax-illary lines (Fig 7–7), the pectoral ridges, the nape of the neck, and/or the lateral aspects of the upper arms and thighs. They appear before age 10 and can spontaneously disappear. Although a reliable marker when pres-ent, the majority of cases reported with this syndrome fail to mention this finding, so the precise incidence of this cutaneous feature is unknown.[51]

Sanfilippo syndrome.—The Sanfilippo syndrome (MPS III) is an autoso-mal recessive disorder characterized by aggressive behavior, severe mental retardation, coarse hair, coarse immobile facies, and relatively less severe somatic changes than those seen in MPS I and MPS II. Thickening of the skin and subcutaneous tissues produces coarse features, with prominent eyebrows, thickened nares, thick lips, and a lack of expressive facial move-ment.[52, 53] The hair is coarse and loss of extension of the interphalangeal joints of the hands develops, but not to a degree that causes the typical claw hand deformities seen in patients with Hurler and Hunter syndromes. When the diagnosis is indeterminate, examination of urinary mucopolysac-

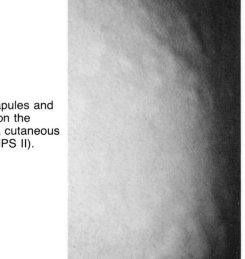

Fig 7–7.—Flesh-colored papules and nodules in a reticular pattern on the shoulder and scapular area (a cutaneous marker of Hunter syndrome MPS II).

charides reveals excessive excretion of heparan sulfate (the only mucopolysaccharide excreted in excessive amounts in this disorder.[43]

Morquio syndrome.—The Morquio syndrome (MPS IV) is an autosomal recessive disorder characterized by normal intelligence, striking dwarfism (usually not apparent until the child reaches two or three years of age), and distinctive skeletal findings with marked osteoporosis of all bones. Usually the joints are not stiff. A barrel chest with pigeon breast (pectus carinatum) deformity, relatively short trunk and neck, an appearance of disproportionately long extremities, and looseness of some joints are characteristic features. Marked excretion of keratan sulfate and chrondroitin sulfate A (about two or three times greater than normal) in the urine is a characteristic feature during childhood in patients with the Morquio syndrome. These findings, however, slowly decrease, reaching normal levels during adulthood.[46]

Maroteaux-Lamy syndrome.—Mucopolysaccharidosis VI (Maroteaux-Lamy syndrome) is an autosomal recessive disorder characterized by dwarfism, coarse facies, clouding of the corneas (frequently with severe impairment of vision), severe osseous changes, flexion contractures of the hands, normal intellect, and increased urinary excretion of dermatan sulfate. No estimates as to its incidence exist (owing in part to the fact that this syndrome has only recently been delineated). Most authorities, however, consider this disorder extremely rare.[54]

The Mucolipidoses

The mucolipidoses are a group of disorders that exhibit clinical skeletal signs of the mucopolysaccharidoses and clinical features seen in patients with sphingolipidoses. This group includes three disorders specifically termed mucolipidosis I, II, and III, gangliosidosis, juvenile sulfatidosis, fucosidosis, mannosidosis, and perhaps, lipogranulomatosis.

Mucolipidosis I.—Mucolipidosis I is an autosomal recessive disorder characterized by mild Hurler-like clinical manifestations, moderate progressive mental retardation, skeletal changes of dysostosis multiplex, normal urinary mucopolysaccharide excretion, and coarse refringent inclusions in cultured fibroblasts similar to but without the clear perinuclear halo of those seen in mucolipidosis II. Previously called lipomucopolysaccharidosis, mucolipidosis I (ML I) is a lysosomal storage disease that results from a deficiency of acid neuraminadase with accumulation of sialic acid-rich macromolecular compounds.[55] This disorder should be differentiated from the cherry red spot-myoclonus syndrome which also demonstrates a deficiency of acid neuraminidase.[56]

The cherry red spot-myoclonus syndrome, characterized by bilateral macular cherry red spots, progressive myoclonus beginning in adolescence without mental retardation, and progressive visual deterioration, differs from ML I in that hepatosplenomegaly, dysostosis multiplex, coarse facies, and dwarfism are not observed. The cherry red spot-myoclonus syndrome occurs in two forms: one with a partial secondary betagalactosidase deficiency and mental deterioration, and a second with normal levels of beta galactosidase and no mental deterioration.[56]

Mucolipidosis I should be included in the differential diagnosis of disorders that display a Hurler's syndrome-like phenotype in infancy. The measurement of urinary levels of bound sialic acid represents a simple screening procedure. Confirmation of the diagnosis can be accomplished by the demonstration of isolated acid neuraminidase deficiency in cultures of skin fibroblasts.

Mucolipidosis II.—Mucolipidosis II (ML II, I-cell disease) is an autosomal recessive Hurler-like disorder characterized by small orbits and prominent eyes, puffy and swollen eyelids, a pattern of tortuous veins around the orbits, fullness of the lower part of the face, full rounded cheeks that appear flushed because of many fine telangiectases, a prominent maxilla (which produces a fishmouth appearance), gingival hypertrophy, a severe type of dysostosis multiplex, short neck, thick and rigid skin (particularly on the ears and neck), stiffness of all joints with considerable reduction in range of motion, and death, usually due to severe respiratory infection and cardiac failure at about four years of age.

Mucolipidosis II can be distinguished from the Hurler syndrome by the presence of hypertrophic gums, vacuolated lymphocytes in the peripheral blood, striking inclusions ("I-cell disease" refers to these) in fibroblast cultures from cutaneous biopsy, normal urinary mucopolysaccharide excretion, and a 10- to 100-fold increase in the specific activity of several plasma acid hydrolases.[57, 58] Prenatal diagnosis of this disorder can be confirmed by enzyme assays of amniotic fluid.[59]

Mucolipidosis III.—Mucolipidosis III (pseudo–Hurler polydystrophy) is an autosomal recessive disorder characterized by mental retardation, early restriction of joint mobility, and normal mucopolysacchariduria. Children with this disorder usually present at or about the age of three years, with stiffness of the joints as the main complaint. The facies is variable, but most patients have coarse facies, short stature, fine ground-glass corneal clouding, and a moderate degree of mental retardation with an I.Q. of 65 to 85. Aortic valve disease is present in most patients with this disorder.

GM₁ gangliosidosis.—GM_1 gangliosidosis, caused by generalized accumulation of GM_1 ganglioside due to a beta galactosidase deficiency, is characterized by coarse facies with depressed nasal bridge, full cheeks and puffy eyelids, corneal clouding, cherry red macules, kyphoscoliosis, roentgenographic changes of dysostosis multiplex, hepatosplenomegaly, marked psychomotor retardation, progressive cerebral deterioration, and death usually before the age of 2. Features resembling the mucopolysaccharidoses include bone changes, hepatosplenomegaly, and corneal clouding. Those suggesting a sphingolipidosis include large head, cherry red spot of the macula, and progressive neurologic deterioration.

Juvenile sulfatidosis.—Juvenile sulfatidosis with mucopolysacchariduria (also called the Austin type of leukodystrophy) is a very rare Hurler-like disorder characterized by mild Hurler-like features, slowly progressive neurologic deterioration that begins in the second year of life, and death, generally in the early teens.

"Stiff Skin" Syndrome

A unique combination of skin and joint defects, presumably a form of focal mucopolysaccharidosis, termed the *stiff skin syndrome* has been reported in four patients.[60] This disorder is characterized by localized areas of stony-hard skin, mild hirsutism, limited mobility of various joints, and normal urinary mucopolysaccharide excretion. In one patient the areas of skin with less severe involvement had a cobblestone appearance suggestive of that occurring in patients with the Hunter type of mucopolysaccharidosis.

Although the exact nature of this disorder is unknown, the presence of abnormal amounts of hyaluronidase-digestible acid mucopolysaccharide in the dermis, as well as an increase in cytoplasmic metachromatic material in cultured fibroblasts, suggests a focal abnormality of mucopolysaccharide metabolism. The presence of this constellation of findings in a mother and her two children suggests a heritable disorder of the autosomal dominant type. The fact that the siblings were the progeny of a consanguineous marriage between cousins, however, cannot exclude an autosomal recessive pattern of inheritance.

REFERENCES

1. Freiberger H.F., Pinnel S.R.: Heritable disorders of connective tissue, in Moschella S.L. (ed.), *Dermatology Update. Reviews for Physicians*, 1979 edition, Elsevier, New York, 1979, pp. 221–253.
2. Holtzman N.A., Welcher D.W., Mellitis E.D.: Termination of restricted diet in children with phenylketonuria: randomized controlled study. *N. Engl. J. Med.* 293:1121–1124, 1975.
3. Schimke R.N.: Low-methionine diet of homocystinuria. *Ann. Intern. Med.* 70:642–643, 1969.
4. Carson N.A.J., Carré I.J.: Treatment of homocystinuria with pyridoxine. *Arch. Dis. Child.* 44:387–392, 1969.
5. Layman C.W.: Ochronosis. *Arch. Dermatol. Syph.* 67:553–560, 1953.
6. Wyre D.: Alkaptonuria with extensive ochronosis. *Arch. Dermatol.* 115:561–563, 1979.
7. O'Brien W.M., Banfield W.G., Sokoloff L.: Studies on the pathogenesis of ochronotic arthropathy. *Arthritis Rheum.* 4:137–152, 1961.
8. Kutty W., Igbal Q., Teh E.: Ochronotic arthropathy. *Arch. Pathol.* 98:55–57, 1974.
9. Gould E., Redd C., DePalma D., et al.: Cardiac manifestations of ochronosis. *J. Thorac. Cardiovasc. Surg.* 72:788–791, 1976.
10. Levine H., Parisi A., Holdsworth D., Cohn L.: Aortic valve replacement for ochronosis of the aortic valve. *Chest* 74:466–467, 1978.
11. Dobyns W.V., Goldstein N.P., Gordon H.: Clinical spectrum of Wilson's disease (hepatolenticular degeneration). *Mayo Clin. Proc.* 54:35–42, 1979.
12. Leff I.L.: Azure lunulae. *Arch. Dermatol.* 80:224–226, 1959.
13. Leu M.L., Strickland G.T., Wang G.C., et al.: Skin pigmentation in Wilson's disease. *J.A.M.A.* 211:1542–1543, 1970.
14. Menkes J.H., Alter M., Steigleder G.K., et al.: A sex-linked recessive disorder with retardation of growth, peculiar hair, and focal cerebral and cerebellar degeneration. *Pediatrics* 29:764–779, 1962.
15. Danks D.M., Campbell P.E., Stevens B.J., et al.: Menkes' kinky hair syndrome: an inherited defect in copper absorption with widespread effects. *Pediatrics* 50:188–201, 1972.
16. Bucknall W.E., Haslam R.H.A., Holtzman N.A.: Kinky hair syndrome: response to copper therapy. *Pediatrics* 52:653–657, 1973.
17. Hart D.B.: Menkes' syndrome: an updated review. *J. Am. Acad. Dermatol.* 9:145–152, 1983.
18. Ricci M.A., Tunnessen W.W., Jr., Pergolezzi J.J., et al.: Menkes' kinky hair syndrome. *Cutis.* 30:55–58, 1982.
19. Horn N.: Copper incorporation studies on cultured cells for prenatal diagnosis of Menkes' disease. *Lancet* 1:1156–1158, 1976.

20. Lesch M., Nyhan W.L.: A familial disorder of uric acid metabolism and central nervous system function. *Amer. J. Med.* 36:561–570, 1964.
21. Nyhan W.L.: Clinical features of the Lesch-Nyhan syndrome. *Arch. Int. Med.* 130:214–220, 1972.
22. Sweetman L., Surh L., Baker H., et al.: Clinical and metabolic abnormalities in a boy with dietary deficiency of biotin. *Pediatrics* 68:553–558, 1981.
23. Mock D.M., Delorimer A.A., Liebman W.B., et al.: Biotin deficiency: an unusual complication of parenteral alimentation. *N. Engl. J. Med.* 304:820–823, 1981.
24. McClain C.J., Baker H., Onstad G.R.: Biotin deficiency in an adult during home parenteral nutrition. *J.A.M.A.* 247:3116–3117, 1982.
25. Packman S., Sweetman L., Baker H., et al.: The neonatal form of biotin–responsive multiple carboxylase deficiency. *J. Pediatr.* 99:418–420, 1981.
26. Williams M.L., Packman S., Cowan M.J.: Alopecia and periorificial dermatitis in biotin-responsive multiple carboxylase deficiency. *J. Am. Acad. Dermatol.* 9:97–103, 1983.
27. Thoene J., Baker H., Yoshino M., et al.: Biotin-responsive carboxylase deficiency associated with subnormal plasma and urinary biotin. *N. Engl. J. Med.* 304:817–820, 1981.
28. Lee E.B.: Metabolic diseases and the skin, in *Symposium on Pediatric Dermatology (Part II). Ped. Clinics N. Amer.* W.B. Saunders Co., 1983, pp. 597–608.
29. Goldsmith L.A.: Tyrosinemia II: Lessons in molecular pathophysiology. *Pediatric Dermatology* 1:25–34, 1983.
30. Lindblad B., Lindstedt S., Steen G.: On the enzyme defects in hereditary tyrosinemia. *Proc. Natl. Acad. Sci. USA* 74:4641–4645, 1977.
31. Strife C.F., Zuroweste E.L., Emmett E.A., et al.: Tyrosinemia with acute intermittent porphyria. aminolevulinic acid dehydratase deficiency related to urinary aminolevulinic acid levels. *J. Pediatr.* 90:400–404, 1977.
32. Goldsmith L.A., Kang E., Bienfang D.C., et al.: Tyrosinemia with plantar and palmar keratosis and keratitis. *J. Pediatr.* 83:798–805, 1973.
33. Hunziker N.: Richner-Hanhart syndrome and tyrosinemia type II. *Dermatologica* 160:180–189, 1980.
34. Goldsmith L.A., Reed J.: Tyrosine-induced eye and skin lesions: a treatable genetic disease. *J.A.M.A.* 236:382–384, 1976.
35. Zaleski W.A., Hill A., Kushniruk W.: Skin lesions in tyrosinosis: response to dietary treatment. *Br. J. Dermatol.* 88:335–340, 1973.
36. Ney D., Bay C., Schneider J.A., et al.: Dietary management of oculocutaneous tyrosinemia in an 11-year-old child. *Am. J. Dis. Child.* 137:995–1000, 1983.
37. Fleischmajer R., Dowlati Y., Reeves J.R.T.: Familial hyperlipidemias—diagnosis and treatment. *Arch. Dermatol.* 110:43–50, 1974.
38. Fredrickson D.S., Levy R.J., Lees R.S.: Fat transport in lipoproteins: an integrated approach to mechanisms and disorders. *N. Engl. J. Med.* 276:32–44; 94–103; 148–156; 215–225; 273–281, 1967.
39. Polano M.K., Baes H., Hulsmans A.M., et al.: Xanthomata in primary hyperlipoproteinemia—a classification based on the lipoprotein pattern of the blood. *Arch. Dermatol.* 100:387–400, 1969.
40. Lloyd J.K.: Hyperlipoproteinemia in childhood. *Aust. Paediatr. J.* 8:264–272, 1972.
41. Goldstein J.L., Brown M.S.: Familial hypercholesterolemia: A genetic regulatory defect in cholesterol metabolism. *Am. J. Med.* 58:147–150, 1975.

42. Yeshuron D., Chung H., Gotto A.M., Jr., et al.: Primary type V hyperlipoproteinemia in childhood. *J.A.M.A.* 236:2518–2520, 1977.

43. McKusick V.A., Kaplan D., Wise D., et al.: Genetic mucopolysaccharidoses. *Medicine* 44:445–483, 1965.

44. Hunter C.: A rare disease in two brothers. *Proc. Roy. Soc. Med.* 10:104–116, 1917.

45. Gerich J.E.: Hunter's syndrome. Beta-galactosidase deficiency in the skin. *N. Engl. J. Med.* 280:799–802, 1969.

46. Gorlin R.J., Pindborg J.J., Cohen M.M., Jr.: *Syndromes of the Head and Neck, ed. 2.* McGraw-Hill, New York, 1976.

47. McKusick V.A.: Heritable Disorders of Connective Tissue, ed. 4. C.V. Mosby Company, St. Louis, 1972.

48. DiFerrante N., Nichols B.L., Connelly P.V., et al.: Induced degradation of glycosaminoglycans in Hurler's and Hunter's syndromes by plasma infusion. *Proc. Natl. Acad. Sci., U.S.A.,* 68:303–307, 1971.

49. Dekaban A.S., Holden K.R., Constantopoulos G.: Effects of fresh plasma or whole blood transfusions on patients with various types of mucopolysaccharidosis. *Pediatrics* 50:688–692, 1972.

50. Hopwood J.J., Muller V., Smithson A., et al.: A fluorometric assay using 4-methylumbelliferyl alpha-L-iduronide for the estimation of alpha-L-iduronidase activity and the detection of Hurler and Scheie syndromes. *Clin. Chem. Acta* 92:257–265, 1979.

51. Prystkowsky S.D., Maumanee I.H., Freeman R.G., et al.: A cutaneous marker in the Hunter syndrome. A report of four cases. *Arch. Dermatol.* 113:602–605, 1977.

52. Leroy J.C., Crocker A.C.: Clinical definition of Hurler-Hunter phenotypes: review of 50 patients. *Am. J. Dis. Child.* 112:518–530, 1966.

53. Danks D.M., Campbell P.E., Cartwright E., et al.: Sanfilippo syndrome: clinical, biochemical, radiologic, hematologic, and pathologic features of nine cases. *Aust. Paediatr. J.* 8:174–186, 1972.

54. Spranger I.W., Koch F., McKusick V.A., et al.: Mucopolysaccharidosis VI (Maroteaux-Lamy disease). *Helv. Paediatr. Acta* 25:337–362, 1970.

55. Kelly T.E., Bartoshesky L., Harris V.J., et al.: Mucolipidosis I (acid neuraminidase deficiency). Three cases and delineation of the variability of the phenotype. *Am. J. Dis. Child.* 135:703–708, 1981.

56. Rapin I., Goldfischer S., Katzman R., et al.: The cherry red spot-myoclonus syndrome. *Ann. Neurol.* 3:234–242, 1978.

57. Terashima Y., Katsuya T., Isomura S., et al.: I-cell disease, report of three cases. *Am. J. Dis. Child.* 129:1083–1090, 1975.

58. Gellis S., Feingold M.: Picture of the Months, I-cell disease (mucolipidosis II). *Am. J. Dis. Child.* 131:1137–1138, 1977.

59. Aula P., Rapola J., Antio S., et al.: Prenatal diagnosis and fetal pathology of I-cell disease (mucolipidosis II). *J. Pediatr.* 87:221–226, 1975.

60. Esterly N.B., McKusick V.A.: The stiff skin syndrome. *Pediatrics* 47:360–369, 1971.

8 / Neurocutaneous Disorders

THE NEUROCUTANEOUS DISORDERS consist of a group of conditions with cutaneous, nervous system, and internal manifestations. Since the skin and nervous system share a common embryologic origin, it is not surprising that there are a number of hereditary neurologic conditions associated with unique cutaneous markers. Of these, neurofibromatosis, tuberous sclerosis, incontinentia pigmenti, hypomelanosis of Ito (incontinentia pigmenti achromians), nevus achromicus, the Vogt-Koyanagi-Harada, Alezzandrini, multiple lentigines, basal cell nevus and epidermal nevus syndromes have striking cutaneous markers.

Neurofibromatosis

Neurofibromatosis (von Recklinghausen disease) is an autosomal dominant disorder characterized by cutaneous pigmentation (café au lait spots); neurofibromas of the skin, peripheral and central nervous systems; varied manifestations in bone, soft tissue, muscle and endocrine system; and hamartomas of the iris termed Lisch nodules. Estimated to occur approximately once in 2500 to 3000 births, with no significant difference in respect to sex, race, or color, hereditary factors are responsible for about 50% of cases; the other 50% probably represent new mutations[1-5] (Table 8–1).

CLINICAL MANIFESTATIONS.—Neurofibromatosis is a heterogeneous disorder in which at least three (and perhaps as many as seven) variants exist. Type 1, the central variety of von Recklinghausen's neurofibromatosis, is characterized by bilateral acoustic neuromas and an absence of significant numbers of café au lait spots and neurofibromas; type 2, a peripheral variety in which there are many neurofibromas and café au lait spots but minimal central nervous system involvement; and type 3, a relatively uncommon mixed variety, with a combination of central and peripheral involvement.[6] Riccardi currently describes four other variants.[7] The cutaneous characteristics of type 4 (variant neurofibromatosis) are intermediate between those of type 1 and type 2 neurofibromatosis. Type 5 (segmental neurofibromatosis) is characterized by involvement of only one body segment and unlike the other types of neurofibromatosis which are autosomal dominant in nature, segmental neurofibromatosis is considered the result of a postzygotic mutation and is not heritable. Type 6 disease is characterized by the presence of café au lait spots and an absence of cutaneous neurofibromas, and patients with type 7 disease (late-onset neurofibroma-

TABLE 8–1.—NEUROFIBROMATOSIS

1. Autosomal dominant
   a. 1 in 2,500 to 3,000 births
   b. 50% represent new mutations
2. Cutaneous and ophthalmic manifestations
   a. Café au lait spots
   b. Axillary freckling (Crowe's sign)
   c. Neurofibromas
   d. Blue-red and pseudoatrophic macules
   e. Lisch nodules (94% of patients over 6 years)
3. Systemic manifestations
   a. Neurologic, osseous, endocrine
   b. 7% are at risk for severe disease and another 5% are
   at risk for moderate disease

tosis) have no café au lait spots and develop their cutaneous neuromas during adulthood.[7]

Café au lait spots.—The café au lait spots associated with neurofibromatosis are considered a hallmark of the disease. Although usually present at birth, they may make their appearance during the first few months or even up to one year of age and often continue to increase in size and number during the first decade, especially the first two years of life (most patients with neurofibromatosis demonstrate their café au lait spots by the age of nine).[4] Generally seen as sharply defined oval pale-brown patches averaging 2 to 5 cm in length, giant café au lait spots as large as 15 cm in diameter may also be noted.

Crowe and associates have postulated that the existence of six or more café au lait spots greater than 1.5 cm in diameter probably indicates the presence of neurofibromatosis[2, 8] (Fig 8–1). Although 10% to 20% of normal individuals have one or more café au lait spots, these characteristic macules are seen in 95% of patients with neurofibromatosis and 78% of patients with von Recklinghausen disease demonstrate six or more such lesions.[2, 8] The "six spot" criterion, while not a hard and fast rule, is valuable, particularly in young children and adolescents before the cutaneous neurofibromas make their appearance. In children 5 years of age or under, however, smaller lesions are also significant in the diagnosis of this disorder. In this age group, five or more café au lait spots 0.5 centimeter or greater is suggestive of the diagnosis of neurofibromatosis.[9]

Another form of café au lait pigmentation, termed axillary "freckling" (Crowe's sign), also serves as a valuable diagnostic aid in the early recognition of neurofibromatosis (Fig 8–2). Seen in 20% to 50% of the patients with the disease, axillary freckling appears as multiple 1 to 4 mm café au lait spots in the axillary vault. Lack of sun exposure in this area prevents confusion with true freckles. Since such axillary pigmentation is not seen

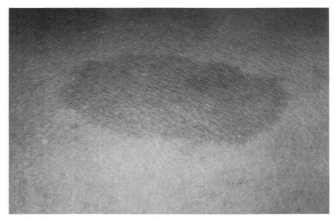

Fig 8–1.—Café au lait spot. Six café au lait spots larger than 1.5 cm in diameter suggests a diagnosis of neurofibromatosis (von Recklinghausen disease) in older children and adults. In children five years of age or less, 5 or more café au lait spots 0.5 cm or greater probably indicate the presence of this systemic disorder.

in any other condition, it is highly pathognomonic of von Recklinghausen disease.[10]

Microscopic examination of café au lait spots reveals increased pigment in the basal layer of the epidermis in patients with neurofibromatosis. Giant pigment granules measuring up to 5 cm in diameter in both melanocytes and basal cells (frequently not found in the café au lait spots of normal individuals) have been observed in the melanocytes and keratinocytes of the epidermis, particularly in the cafe au lait spots of patients with neurofibromatosis.[11–13] Giant pigment granules, however, are not specific for the café au lait spots of neurofibromatosis since they are occasionally found in café au lait spots of persons without neurofibromatosis,[14] may be absent in the café au lait spots of adult patients with neurofibromatosis,[15] are absent in the café au lait spots of children with this disorder,[11, 16] and also have been noted in patients with the multiple lentigines syndrome, in the melanocytic macules of Albright's syndrome, nevus spilus, and normal human epidermis.[17] The presence of giant pigment granules is not a specific finding in patients with neurofibromatosis, and the absence of giant pigment granules in café au lait spots in children does not necessarily rule out the presence of neurofibromatosis.[12, 16, 17] In addition, the café au lait spots in patients with neurofibromatosis contain more dopa-positive melanocytes per square centimeter than the surrounding normal skin. In individuals without neurofibromatosis, there are fewer dopa-positive melano-

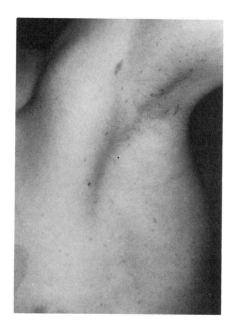

Fig 8–2.—Axillary freckling (Crowe's sign). Multiple 1 to 4 mm café au lait spots in the axillary vault is pathognomonic for neurofibromatosis.

cytes per square centimeter in the café au lait spots than in the normal surrounding skin.[15]

Café au lait spots also occur in the Albright syndrome (polyostotic fibrous dysplasia with sexual precocity in girls). In the Albright syndrome, the pigmented lesions are dark brown and frequently have a jagged, irregular border (resembling the coast of Maine). This is in contrast to the smooth outline (resembling the coast of California) and light brown color of the spots seen in von Recklinghausen disease. In Albright's disease the café au lait spots are large, few in number, follow a dermatomal distribution, are more commonly seen over the neck and buttocks, often are located on the same side as the bone lesions, and generally stop at the midline.[17]

Other cutaneous pigmentary changes have been noted in patients with neurofibromatosis but lack the diagnostic significance attributed to axillary freckling and multiple café au lait spots. These include minute, freckle-like café au lait spots distributed in other regions of the body, areas of leukoderma, and diffuse graying or bronzing of the skin suggestive of the color seen in patients with argyria.[1]

Neurofibromas.—Von Recklinghausen disease is also characterized by dermal fibromas and dermal or subcutaneous neurofibromas of Schwann cell origin derived from peripheral nerve sheaths. Solitary neurofibromas without other cutaneous findings are not diagnostic of neurofibromatosis and may be seen in individuals without evidence of this disorder. Whereas neurofibromas occurring as solitary lesions without cafe au lait spots or family history of neurofibromatosis may arise in adulthood, the cutaneous tumors of neurofibromatosis generally appear in late childhood or adolescence—their appearance is frequently associated with puberty. They vary in number from a few to many hundreds, with a progressive increase in size and number as the patient becomes older. Neurofibromas may occur anywhere on the body, with no specific site of predilection other than the fact that they usually avoid the palms and soles. They may appear as superficial tumors varying in size from 1 to 2 mm to several centimeters in diameter or as discrete beaded, nodular, elongated masses seen along the course of nerves, usually the trigeminal or upper cervical nerves (plexiform neuromas). Plexiform neuromas usually involve the limbs, are often associated with hypertrophy of the underlying soft tissues and bones and are not necessarily confined to patients with neurofibromatosis.

Although generally flesh-colored, neurofibromas tend to have a distinctive violaceous hue when small. As they enlarge they become pink, blue, or pigmented. Small tumors may be deep-seated, sessile, or dome-shaped; as they become larger they become globular, pear-shaped, pedunculated, or pendulous (Fig 8–3). With moderate digital pressure the smaller lesions may be invaginated into an underlying dermal defect, an almost pathognomonic maneuver termed "buttonholing".

Although a benign course for neurofibromas is usual, some of the tumors may undergo malignant change. Neurofibrosarcomas, also referred to as

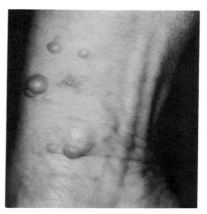

Fig 8–3.—Neurofibromas. Flesh-colored globular and dome-shaped nodules in a patient with neurofibromatosis (von Recklinghausen disease). With moderate digital pressure the smaller lesions may be invaginated into an underlying dermal defect, an almost pathognomonic maneuver termed "buttonholing."

malignant Schwannomas, may develop in patients with neurofibromatosis, but this is not common.[17] Because of a tendency to report unusual cases, the literature reflects a high incidence of malignant transformation, with a range between 2% and 16%. A more accurate figure for this complication appears to be 2% to 3%. Although fibrosarcomatous malignant degeneration has occurred in early childhood, it is rare before the age of forty. Malignant degeneration may be heralded by rapid enlargement of pain. Malignant growth, however, once it develops is often slow, with few metastases. The prognosis, however, for neurofibrosarcomas is poor. Extensive spread along the involved nerve requires aggressive surgical treatment, and local recurrences are common.

Blue-red macules and pseudoatrophic macules.—Blue-red macules and pseudoatrophic macules have also been described as characteristic lesions of neurofibromatosis. They arise before or after puberty, become slightly elevated and domeshaped, and new lesions may continue to appear. The blue-red lesions may have small blood vessels leading to the conglomerate appearance of telangiectasia and a reddish or bluish discoloration (due to stasis of blood) on exposure to cold.[18]

Lisch nodules.—Yellowish-brown pigmented neurofibromas on the iris (Lisch nodules) have recently been described in individuals with the classic form of neurofibromatosis.[4, 5] Seen in 94% of children over 6 years of age and 97% of postpubertal patients, these lesions are not symptomatic and increase in number with age. They are not found in normal persons or in patients with the central, acoustic or segmental forms of neurofibromatosis.[5] Since 6% of patients with neurofibromatosis who are five years of age or less, and 3% of postpubertal patients do not have Lisch nodules, their absence does not discount the diagnosis.[3]

Systemic manifestations.—In almost all patients, neurofibromatosis may be diagnosed in the first year of life, and some form of systemic problem or compromise generally develops before the age of 20.[3] There is marked variability, however, in the overall severity and progression of classical neurofibromatosis. It can cause serious problems, and even death in the newborn,[19] or may produce only a mild or insignificant problem throughout the life of the affected individual.

The severity of cutaneous involvement is not indicative of the extent of disease in other organs. Neurological manifestations have been reported in as high as 40% of patients and may involve any part of the central nervous system. The acoustic nerve (VIII) and optic nerve (II) are the most commonly involved of the cranial nerves. Deafness is common in neurofibromatosis and gliomas of the optic nerve, with exophthalmos, decreased visual acuity, or restricted ocular movements are occasionally seen as complications of this disorder.

Neurologic disease occurs in more than half the cases of neurofibromatosis and includes retardation, seizure disorders, and tumors. Seizures are said to occur in 8% to 13% of patients (of these about half are associated with intracranial tumors). Mental retardation, seen in 10% to 20% of patients, may vary from a mild learning disability to severe retardation.[20] The degree of mental deficiency, although occasionally severe, is usually mild to moderate and not progressive.

As many as 50% of patients with neurofibromatosis may have osseous defects associated with this disorder. All bony changes may be explained by the development of neurofibromas lying within or in close proximity to involved bone. Of these, spinal deformity, particularly scoliosis or kyphosis, is the most common and may be seen in over 10% of patients.

The autonomic nervous system may also be affected and the gastrointestinal tract is involved in about 10% of patients with neurofibromatosis. Intestinal neurofibromas with bleeding of the overlying mucosa have been reported. Complications, therefore, include vague abdominal discomfort, melena, hematemesis, bowel obstruction and even intestinal perforation.[21] Endocrine disorders associated with neurofibromatosis include acromegaly, menstrual abnormalities, delayed or incomplete sexual development, gynecomastia, hyper- and hypothyroidism, infertility, Addison's disease, hyperparathyroidism, and diabetes. In children the most common endocrine abnormality that occurs is sexual precocity. Between 5% and 20% of patients with pheochromocytoma also have neurofibromatosis; only 1 of every 223 patients with neurofibromatosis, however, is found to have a pheochromocytoma.[2]

DIAGNOSIS.—The diagnosis of neurofibromatosis depends upon the number and size of café au lait spots (the earliest manifestation of this disorder), axillary freckling when present, Lisch nodules, and cutaneous neurofibromas. In individuals with inconclusive cutaneous changes, giant pigment granules or an increased number of melanocytes in the café au lait macules compared to the surrounding skin, although not diagnostic, may help establish the diagnosis. If, at any age, Lisch nodules, neurofibromas, and café au lait spots are present, the diagnosis of neurofibromatosis is established. If there are at least six café au lait spots larger than 1.5 cm in size, the diagnosis of neurofibromatosis is likely, but not definitively established. If axillary freckling is also present, the condition is even more likely. A careful search of the skin for neurofibromas, ocular examination (by an ophthalmologist using a slit-lamp microscope) for Lisch nodules, and determination of whether other family members are known to have or are suspected of having neurofibromatosis is helpful.

If the diagnosis of neurofibromatosis is in doubt, or at least not confirmed, this point should be made clear and, when warranted, referrals should be made for appropriate evaluation. If the diagnosis is certain or likely and the child's family history is negative, both parents should be examined for cutaneous lesions and slit-lamp ocular examinatin should be performed in an effort to establish the presence or absence of Lisch nodules.

TREATMENT.—Since many patients have minor or incomplete forms of this disorder, reassurance for parents of children affected with neurofibromatosis is often helpful. Treatment consists of surgical excision of tumors that are disfiguring, interfere with function, or are subject to irritation, trauma, or infection. Periodic complete physical examinations are necessary, with particular attention to possible hypertension, skeletal deformities, endocrine disorders, gastrointestinal complications, and involvement of cranial nerves II and VIII. Although malignant degeneration of cutaneous tumors before age 50 is rare, complete surgical excision with histopathologic examination is mandatory if cutaneous neurofibromas become painful or show signs of rapid enlargement.

Genetic counseling is another important aspect of treatment, since there is a 50% chance of transmitting neurofibromatosis with each pregnancy. About 7% of all patients with neurofibromatosis are at risk for severe disease, and at least another 5% are at risk for moderate disease. In addition, an affected adult has about a 40% chance of having a mildly affected child and a 12.5% chance of having a moderately to severely affected child. In most affected families, 75% of patients afflicted with the disorder will have minimal to mild disease; of these, there is a 25% lifetime risk of moderate to severe involvement.[22] Patients with a combination of juvenile xanthogranuloma and neurofibromatosis may have a predisposition to leukemia. Patients with this combination, accordingly, should be watched for this possibility (see Chapter 12).

Tuberous Sclerosis

Tuberous sclerosis is a relatively uncommon disease of irregular but dominant autosomal inheritance occurring with an incidence of about 5 to 7 per 100,000 individuals. Of these, 50% to 70% of cases appear to arise from new mutations. It is classified as a neurocutaneous syndrome in which the brain, eyes, skin, heart, kidneys, lungs, and bones may be affected. The full entity classically is defined by a triad of seizures, mental deficiency, and a variety of pathognomonic skin lesions (Table 8–2). The latter include adenoma sebaceum, shagreen patches, periungual and gingival fibromas, and hypopigmented macules. Although café au lait spots have an increased incidence (26%) in this disorder, they are not a diagnostic sign of tuberous sclerosis.[23]

TABLE 8–2.—TUBEROUS SCLEROSIS

1. Autosomal dominant
   a. 5 to 7 per 100,000 individuals
   b. 50% to 70% represent new mutations
2. Cutaneous manifestations
   a. Hypopigmented macules (in 70%–90% of cases)
   b. Adenoma sebaceum (angiofibromas)
   c. Shagreen patches
   d. Periungual and gingival fibromas
   e. Tooth pits?
3. Systemic manifestations
   (CNS involvement, cardiac rhabdomyomas, retinal gliomas, renal hamartomas, cystic lesions in lungs, osseous lesions)

Primarily a defect in the organization of connective tissue in which hyperplasia of ectodermal and mesodermal tissue leads to a variety of hamartomas in the nervous system, skin, heart, kidneys, and other organs, the exact pathogenesis of tuberous sclerosis is unclear. The development of lesions, however, appears to depend upon a faulty differentiation of embryonic cells. Whether this is the fault of an abnormality in cell competence or in embryologic organizers is unclear.[24]

CLINICAL MANIFESTATIONS.—Adenoma sebaceum, present in 80% to 90% of cases, is the most common skin manifestation associated with this disorder. The term *adenoma sebaceum* is a misnomer; these lesions represent angiofibromas, hamartomas composed of fibrous and vascular tissue. The lesions usually appear as 1 to 4 mm dome-shaped nodules with a smooth surface. They range from pink to red in color and often are accompanied by fine telangiectasia. Lesions of adenoma sebaceum are usually located in a bilaterally symmetrical distribution in the nasolabial folds, nose, cheeks, and chin and sometimes on the forehead and scalp (Fig 8–4). They are rarely found on the upper lip except for the central area immediately below the nose. The lesions, rarely present in birth, usually appear sometime between the second and fifth birthdays, often not until puberty. Since only 13% of children with tuberous sclerosis develop the facial lesions of adenoma sebaceum during the first year of life, this is not the best early marker of this condition.

Fibromas also develop around and under the nails of the fingers and toes (periungal and subungual fibromas) and on the gums (gingival fibromas). The periungual and subungual fibromas, seen in about 50% of patients, appear at puberty as firm, flesh-colored growths. Because of their late appearance, they too are of little value in the early diagnosis of this disorder.

Shagreen patches are seen in 21% to 83% of patients with tuberous sclerosis. They develop during early childhood, usually between the patient's

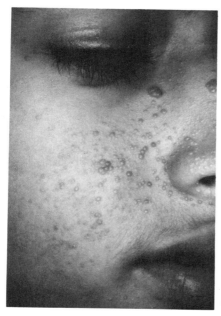
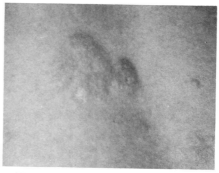

Fig 8–4 (left).—Adenoma sebaceum. Small discrete reddish-pink dome-shaped angiofibromas on the nose and cheek of an 11-year-old male with tuberous sclerosis.

Fig 8–5 (right).—Shagreen patches. Slightly elevated flesh colored plaques of connective tissue with an orange-peel (peau d'orange) surface on the lumbosacral area of a 13-year-old girl with tuberous sclerosis.

second and fifth birthdays. They generally develop on the trunk (most frequently the lumbosacral area) and appear as flesh-colored to yellowish or yellowish-orange slightly elevated plaques of dermal connective tissue (Fig 8–5). Seen as single or multiple lesions measuring 2 to 10 cm or more in diameter, they frequently have an orange-peel or pigskin appearance resembling shagreen leather.

White macules, seen in 70% to 90% of patients with tuberous sclerosis, are a particularly valuable early marker of this disorder. Although delayed appearance of hypopigmented macules in patients with tuberous sclerosis has been reported,[25] reports of their late appearance is questionable since these hypopigmented lesions can frequently be overlooked during infancy unless careful examination (including the use of a Wood's lamp in a completely darkened room) has been undertaken. Hypopigmented macules, therefore, generally appear at birth or shortly thereafter, may enlarge as the infant grows, and persist throughout life, but otherwise do not change in size or shape (Fig 8–6). In addition to the characteristic hypopigmented macules, there is also an increased incidence of tuberous sclerosis in patients with poliosis and partial albinism, and individuals with tuberous sclerosis also have an increased number of café au lait spots.[23, 26, 27] Although

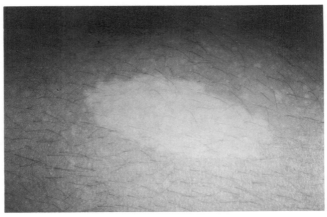

Fig 8–6.—Lance-ovate ash leaf-shaped hypopigmented macule on the leg of an 11-year-old boy with tuberous sclerosis.

the etiologies of hyperpigmentation and hypopigmentation are unknown, since melanocytes are derived from the neural crest and in many ways function as nerve cells, it is not surprising that these changes are found in patients with disorders involving the central nervous system.

A striking feature of the white spots of tuberous sclerosis is the marked variability in size and shape of lesions. They range in size from 0.4 to 7 cm or more, with the majority of lesions measuring between 1 and 3 cm in diameter. They usually are oval or semioval in appearance and have highly irregular margins. Although ash-leaf-shaped lance-ovate hypopigmented macules have been described as the characteristic lesions of tuberous sclerosis,[28] in our series only 18% of the white spots of tuberous sclerosis were found to be truly ash-leaf in shape.[23]

The white spots of tuberous sclerosis have often been termed "vitiliginous" by nondermatologists, but these partially depigmented lesions are unrelated to vitiligo and can be differentiated by many characteristics. Vitiligo represents an acquired form of hypopigmentation characterized by sharply demarcated "ivory-white" macules surrounded by hyperpigmented skin. The completely depigmented ivory-white macules of vitiligo may appear on any part of the body. They frequently have a bilateral or symmetrical distribution, with involvement of the skin of the face and neck, of the backs of hands and forearms, over bony prominences, and in body folds and periorificial areas. They often change in size and shape, frequently spread, and occasionally may show partial to complete repigmentation. Conversely, the leukoderma of tuberous sclerosis is usually present at birth and is located over the abdomen, back, and anterior and lateral surfaces of the arms and legs. The white spots of tuberous sclerosis are dull-white, with incomplete depigmentation (in comparison to the ivory-white color of vitiligo), do not alter in shape or size with age, and appear to be related to a defect of melanosome melanization. The basic cause of this pigmentary disturbance remains obscure.

The difference between hypopigmented lesions of tuberous sclerosis and vitiligo can be further demonstrated by the use of electron microscopy. Whereas the completely depigmented lesions of vitiligo reveal an absence or decrease in the number of melanocytes, the partially depigmented macules of tuberous sclerosis have a normal number of melanocytes with a decrease in the size, synthesis, and melanization of melanosomes.[28]

Another peculiar form of speckled leukoderma in tuberous sclerosis may be seen as small 1 to 3 mm hypopigmented lesions (white freckles) in a confetti-like pattern over the pretibial area in some patients with tuberous sclerosis. Although occasionally seen in normal individuals, they too can help in the diagnosis of patients with this disorder.[23] There also appears to be an increased incidence of tuberous sclerosis in patients with partial albinism,[26, 27] and the presence of one or more tufts of white hair in an infant with seizures is suggestive of a diagnosis of tuberous sclerosis.[29]

In view of the high frequency of white macules present at birth in patients with tuberous sclerosis, all infants and children, particularly those with seizure disorders, should be screened for the characteristic but easily overlooked dull-white macules that are now recognized as the earliest cutaneous markers of tuberous sclerosis. In individuals with light pigmentation, however, these macules can be extremely faint and illumination of the skin with a Wood's light in a darkened room may be required to detect hypopigmented lesions that contrast poorly with the surrounding normal skin.

Tooth pits (seen as punctate, round or oval, 1 to 2 mm randomly arranged enamel defects), particularly in the permanent teeth, may represent another marker of tuberous sclerosis. Recent studies suggest that when tooth pits are seen in numbers of five or more, they may prove to be pathognomonic of this disorder.[30]

The systemic lesions of tuberous sclerosis may produce severe symptoms and possibly death. Central nervous system involvement may lead to convulsions and mental retardation. Seizures, seen in 80% of patients with tuberous sclerosis, may begin as infantile spasms, in which sudden repetitive myoclonic contractions of most of the body musculature are combined with flexion, extension, opisthotonos, and tremors.[31, 32] By two to three years of age, focal or generalized seizures and mental retardation may become evident. Extensive CNS involvement leads to hypsarrhythmia (salaam seizures), with electroencephalographic findings of multifocal high voltage spikes and slow chaotic waves. Later in life the seizure pattern may change to a petit mal variety and in less severe cases, generalized or focal motor seizures may develop.[22, 32]

Retardation may be mild or severe and appears in 62% of affected individuals. Sclerotic calcification in the brain is visible as "tubers" by x-ray in approximately 50% to 75% of individuals. In young children, when skull x-rays are not diagnostic, computerized axial tomographic (CAT) scan findings of small calcifications, ventricular dilatation, or both, are frequently helpful in the diagnosis of this disorder.[20, 33, 34] Sixty per cent of patients with tuberous sclerosis have renal hamartomas which cause enlarged cystic kidneys resembling those of polycystic kidney disease. Rhabdomyomas in the heart may be associated with congestive heart failure, murmurs, cyanosis, or sudden death. The eyes may have characteristic retinal lesions (gliomas) referred to as phakomas. Fundoscopy may show multiple, raised, mulberry-like lesions on or adjacent to the optic nerve head or flat, disclike lesions in the periphery of the retina. Ophthalmologic examination may reveal flat, partially transparent, noncalcified tumors, nodular calcified tumors, or a tumor containing features of both.[35] Cystic lesions in the lungs may rupture and produce spontaneous pneumothorax, often with a radiographic "honeycombed" appearance. About 85% of patients with tuberous sclerosis have osseous manifestations with the bones, particularly those of the hands and feet, demonstrating cysts and periosteal thickenings.[26]

DIAGNOSIS.—Although formes frustes of tuberous sclerosis are common, the appearance of characteristic skin lesions in children with epilepsy, mental retardation, or both should establish a diagnosis of tuberous sclerosis. The diagnosis is readily apparent when the classic triad of adenoma sebaceum, epilepsy, and mental retardation is present. In the absence of all features of the syndrome, however, diagnosis depends upon the cutaneous manifestations, family history (with examination of family members), ophthalmologic examination, bone survey for cortical thickening and phalangeal cysts, skull x-rays, computerized axial tomography (CAT scans),[36] intravenous pyelography or ultrasonic examination of the kidney for renal hamartomas, and chest x-ray for honeycombing of the lungs.

MANAGEMENT.—Seizure disorders associated with tuberous sclerosis often respond to anticonvulsant therapy. Death, when it occurs, may result from status epilepticus, pulmonary or renal insufficiency, or cardiac failure. Adenoma sebaceum requires no treatment except for cosmetic reasons. Best results are seen following cryosurgery, electrodesiccation and curettage, dermabrasion or argon laser beam therapy. Although surgery may be required for relief of symptoms from internal tumors of tuberous sclerosis, surgical removal is often unsatisfactory. Genetic counseling against childbearing is recommended for individuals (even those with mild forms of tuberous sclerosis), since their children may be more severely affected than they are. However, 50% to 70% of patients with tuberous sclerosis may be mutations and, unless there is evidence of tuberous sclerosis in other members of the family, genetic counseling is not completely effective in the prevention of new cases. Recognition of cutaneous markers, however, may help screen previously unrecognized or mildly affected individuals with *formes frustes* of the disorder.

Since genetic counseling is an integral part of treatment of patients and families of patients with tuberous sclerosis, the incidence of family cases is frequently underestimated because of the variability of expression and incomplete examination of parents. It has been suggested that all family members at risk for tuberous sclerosis have skin examination, funduscopic examination through a dilated pupil, cranial computerized tomography, and excretory urogram. A recent review of apparently unaffected parents, however, suggests modification of this protocol to include skull, hand and foot roentgenograms and ultrasound examination instead of the excretory urogram.[36]

Although it has been stated that "most patients with tuberous sclerosis die before age 25, with death usually caused by malignant CNS neoplasm or status epilepticus,"[37] that "30% of affected children die before age 5," that 5% to 15% die before adulthood,"[22] and that "only 5% live beyond the age of 30,"[38] many patients with mild or abortive forms of the disorder go unrecognized and probably go on to live out a normal life span. These high morbidity figures are overly pessimistic and require further evaluation.

Incontinentia Pigmenti

Incontinentia pigmenti (Bloch-Sulzberger syndrome) is a hereditary disorder that affects the skin, central nervous system, eyes, and skeletal system.[38] Although the genetics of this disorder have not been delineated, the familial tendency with almost exclusive involvement in females (97%) suggests that transmission is X-linked dominant, prenatally lethal to hemizygous males.[39] Females with the abnormal gene on one of their two X chromosomes are heterozygous for this condition and are not severely affected. Males with the abnormal gene on their single X chromosome are hemizygous and generally so severely affected that they frequently die in utero. This explains the predominance of female patients with this disorder.[39, 40] The fact that males with incontinentia pigmenti are no more severely affected than their female counterparts suggests that the disease in living male patients may be the result of spontaneous mutation.[39]

CLINICAL MANIFESTATIONS.—Incontinentia pigmenti generally appears at birth or shortly thereafter (90% of patients have cutaneous lesions within the first two weeks of life and 96% have their onset before the age of 6

TABLE 8–3.—INCONTINENTIA PIGMENTI

1. X-linked dominant, prenatally lethal to males
   (97% are females, living males probably represent mutations)
2. Four cutaneous phases
   (inflammatory vesicles or bullae, verrucous lesions, whorled
   hyperpigmentation, and hypopigmentated patches)
3. Eosinophilia in over 70% of patients (often until 20th week of life)
4. Systemic manifestations in 79% (20% at birth)
   (dental 68%, ocular 35%, CNS 30%, cardiac occasionally and
   skeletal 13%)

weeks). Although the cutaneous lesions have three or perhaps four distinct phases, their sequence is irregular and overlapping of stages is common (Table 8–3).

Phase 1.—The first phase of incontinentia pigmenti begins with inflammatory vesicles or bullae that develop in crops over the trunk and extremities, often persisting for weeks to months (Fig 8–7). An interesting and unexplained feature of this phase of the disorder is the high degree of eosinophilia (from 18% to 50%) which is present in 75% of patients during the first two weeks with mean blood eosinophilia exceeding 5% until the 20th week of life. Biopsy of a small blister during this vesicular stage reveals an inflammatory dermatitis with epidermal vesicles filled with eosinophils.

Phase 2.—The vesicular stage is followed by an intermediate phase characterized by irregular linear warty or verrucous lesions on one or more extremities, usually the backs of the hands and feet. This stage, seen in 70% of patients with incontinentia pigmenti, resolves spontaneously, usually within several months.

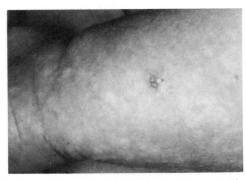

Fig 8–7.—Vesicular and verrucous lesions on the arm of a 5-day-old infant with incontinentia pigmenti. (Courtesy of Dr. Haskell Rosenbaum, Waterbury, Connecticut.)

Phase 3.—During or shortly following this intermediate verrucous stage, a highly characteristic pigmentary state begins. The pigmentation that is the hallmark of the disease, seen in almost 100% of patients, is characterized by bands of slate-brown or blue-gray splattered Chinese-figure-like patches arranged in swirl-like formations on the extremities and trunk (Fig 8–8). This stage increases in intensity until the patient's second year of life. It persists for many years and gradually fades and, in many cases, completely disappears in adolescence or early adulthood. It is from this pigmentary stage that the disease derives its name (because histologically melanin appears to drop down from the melanocytes into the dermis).

Although the pigmentary changes were originally considered to be a postinflammatory phenomenon secondary to the vesiculo-bullous or verrucous stages, the pigment fails to follow the pattern, shape, or location of the bullous and verrucous lesions. Recent electron microscopic studies, however, conclude that all three stages are related to each other and that the pigmentary incontinence can be explained as a phagocytic phenomenon.[41]

Phase 4.—A fourth phase consisting of depigmented lesions has also recently been reported in individuals with incontinentia pigmenti.[42] Seen as

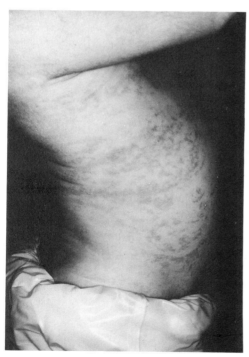

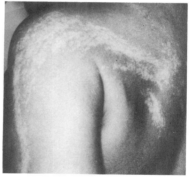

Fig 8–8 (left).—Chinese figure-like hyperpigmentation on the trunk of a 2-year-old girl with incontinentia pigmenti.
   Fig 8–9 (right).—Hypomelanosis of Ito (incontinentia pigmenti achromians). Patterned macular, linear, or swirls of hypopigmentation (approximately 50% of patients with hypomelanosis of Ito have internal manifestations).

isolated streaked hypopigmented lesions, or in conjunction with other manifestations, they have been noted on the arms, thighs, trunk, and particularly the calves of children as well as adults. The histologic features, incidence, and pathogenesis of these hypopigmented lesions are poorly defined. Their presence, however, may serve as a clue to the hereditary pattern and may play a role in the genetic counseling of families of individuals with this disorder.

SYSTEMIC MANIFESTATIONS.—Systemic manifestations are seen in a high percentage of patients with incontinentia pigmenti. Almost 80% of patients have one or more abnormalities of the hair, eyes, central nervous system, and/or structural development. Thirty percent of patients have central nervous system involvement. Of these, 3.3% have seizures, and although many individuals are bright or have normal intellect, 16% have low mentality and 13% have spastic abnormalities. Ophthalmic changes are present in 35% of patients; 18% have strabismus; and an equal number demonstrate more serious eye involvement (cataracts, optic atrophy, or retinal damage). Alopecia is seen in 38% of patients; nail dystrophy is present in 7% of individuals; and 68% of patients have dental anomalies (delayed dentition, partial anodontia, pegged or conical teeth).[39] Occasionally, cardiac anomalies and skeletal malformations (such as microcephaly, syndactyly, supernumerary ribs, hemiatrophy, or shortening of the arms or legs) may occur. In a four-generation study of a family with incontinentia pigmenti, several members also had wooly nevus syndrome and six of the seven had alopecia, agenesis or hypoplasia of eyebrows and eyelashes.[43]

DIAGNOSIS.—The combination of bullae and linear nodular or warty lesions in a female infant is pathognomonic of this disorder; the pigmentation in older children is a hallmark of the disease. Because of the risk of involvement of other children and a potential for ocular, dental, osseous, and neurological changes, it is important that pediatricians, usually the first to see the patient, be familiar with this entity and be able to diagnose and counsel patients seen with this disorder.

Histopathologic examination of vesicular lesions in the first stage of incontinentia pigmenti reveal a dermal infiltrate composed of lymphocytes, polymorphonuclear leukocytes, and numerous eosinophils and mononuclear cells in the vesicles as well as the epidermis and dermis. Features of the second stage consist of acanthosis, irregular papillomatosis, and hyperkeratosis. The basal cells show vacuolization and a decrease in their melanin content. The dermis shows a mild chronic inflammatory infiltrate intermingled with melanophages. The third stage is characterized by extensive deposits of melanin within melanophages located in the upper dermis. The epidermis also shows thinning in this stage and in some cases the amount of melanin in the basal layer is diminished and the cells of the basal layer show vacuolization and degeneration.

TREATMENT.—No special therapy is required for the skin lesions of incontinentia pigmenti. Genetic counseling for carrier females is advisable, however, since almost 80% of affected children have associated congenital defects (cataracts, microcephaly, spastic paralysis, strabismus, alopecia, delayed or impaired dentition, epilepsy, or mental retardation).

Hypomelanosis of Ito (Incontinentia Pigmenti Achromians)

Incontinentia pigmenti achromians (hypomelanosis of Ito) is a peculiar condition of hypopigmentation first described by Ito in 1952.[44] The name was first coined because hypopigmentation of the skin appeared in a linear swirled pattern that resembled a negative image of the hyperpigmentation seen in patients with incontinentia pigmenti (Fig 8–9).[45] Histologic examination of the hypopigmented areas reveals a decrease in melanin granules in the basal area with a complete absence of melanin in some areas. With the dopa reaction, the hypopigmented areas have been shown to contain fewer and smaller melanocytes than normal and sparse, short dendrites.[46] Since there is no histologic evidence of pigment incontinence and the disorder appears to be distinct from and unrelated to incontinentia pigmenti, these two disorders should not be confused with one another (Table 8–4). The more appropriate term of this disease appears to be *hypomelanosis of Ito*.

Although multiple cases of hypomelanosis of Ito have been described in several families, it may represent an autosomal dominant disorder, but its genetic pattern remains unclear.[47, 48] The disorder is often seen at birth or early in infancy or childhood, and persists for many years. In a few patients the lesions may be patchy and confined to relatively limited areas of the body (see nevus achromicus); in most patients, however, the hypopigmented areas are more extensive, often bilateral, and appear to be more pronounced on the ventral surface of the trunk and the flexor surfaces of the limbs.

Approximately 50% of patients with hypomelanosis of Ito have internal manifestations. These include central nervous system dysfunction (seizure disorders and delayed development), ocular disturbances (strabismus, heterochromia iridis, microphthalmia, and nystagmus), muculoskeletal anom-

TABLE 8–4.—HYPOMELANOSIS OF ITO
(INCONTINENTIA PIGMENTI ACHROMIANS)

1. Genetic pattern unclear (perhaps autosomal dominant)
2. Hypopigmentation often in a linear swirled pattern
3. 50% have systemic manifestations (CNS dysfunction, ocular disturbances, musculoskeletal anomalies, hair, nail and dental anomalies)

alies (macrocephaly, scoliosis, asymmetry of the limbs, weakness, hypotonicity, asymmetry of the head, dwarfism, small stature, delayed fontanelle closure, spina bifida occulta, genu valgum, luxatio coxae, polydactyly, lordosis, and bifid thumbs), hair anomalies (diffuse alopecia, generalized hirsutism, facial hypertrichosis, coarse, curly or slow growing hair), cleft lip and palate, malformed auricles, hypertelorism, skin anomalies (decreased sweat response, decreased capillary resistance, incontinentia pigmenti, morphea, and ichthyosis), dental anomalies (anodontia and dental dysplasia), transverse ridging of the nails, hepatomegaly, diaphragmatic hernia, and diastasis recti.[45, 47–51]

The report of familial cases of incontinentia pigmenti achromians and incontinentia pigmenti and the fact that one mother and child had skin lesions of incontinentia pigmenti before the onset of incontinentia pigmenti achromians suggests a possible relationship between the two disorders.[50]

DIAGNOSIS.—Since hypopigmented lesions appear infrequently in early infancy and young children, the appearance of such lesions, particularly in the absence of previous inflammatory skin disease, should alert the physician to possible association with systemic disease. The distinguishing features of incontinentia pigmenti achromians include: (1) depigmented areas that are not preceded by inflammatory lesions; (2) the presence in males as well as females; (3) absence of histologic findings of incontinentia pigmenti and (4) a possible autosomal dominant transmission. Association of incontinentia pigmenti achromians (hypomelanosis of Ito) with nevus depigmentosus suggests that individuals with nevus depigmentosus (nevus achromians) also be investigated for possible systemic abnormalities.

TREATMENT.—All patients with systemitized hypopigmented lesions, and patients with nevus achromicus, should be investigated for anomolies, and a careful developmental evaluation should be attained. If scoliosis or asymmetry is present, since the likelihood of seizures with this combination is high, an electroencephalogram and neurologic assessment are indicated.[50, 51]

Nevus Achromicus

Nevus achromicus is a congenital disorder characterized by single macular lesions, band, or bizarre streaks of hypopigmentation that lack the characteristic swirling pattern seen in patients with incontinentia pigmenti achromians (hypomelanosis of Ito).[52] Although many authorities consider nevus achromicus (nevus depigmentosus) to be a distinct nosologic entity, others are less restrictive in their classification and consider nevus achromicus to be a variant of hypomelanosis of Ito.[6, 54, 55] Affected areas may be quite small or may cover large segments of the body, and, present at birth, they grow only with the growth of the individual. This disorder may be seen in association with hemihypertrophy and severe mental retardation, and if considered a form of hypomelanosis of Ito, the myriad of systemic manifestations may be seen in patients with incontinentia pigmenti achromians.[53]

Probably seen more frequently than the literature indicates, the hypopigmented areas are usually confined to one side of the body, but may be bilateral or systematized, and are most often located on the trunk. They are generally irregular in shape, frequently occur in long bands or streaks, and show varying degrees of melanin deficiency and a reduced number of functional melanocytes.

The Waardenburg Syndrome

The Waardenburg (also termed Klein-Waardenburg) syndrome is a rare autosomal dominant disorder characterized by congenital neural deafness, lateral displacement of the medial canthi and lacrimal puncta of the eyelids (dystopia cantharum), broad nasal root, partial albinism, white forelock, and heterochromia irides.[56] There are now two types of this disorder. In the first, only 20% have decreased hearing; in the second type, up to 60% have hearing loss. Patients with the latter disorder do not have the characteristic dystopia cantharum that was once thought to be a hallmark of the Waardenburg syndrome.[57] Other features include excessive and occasionally confluent eyebrows, hypoplasia of the ala nasi, mild mandibular prognathism, impaired speech with or without cleft lip or cleft palate, and a variety of skeletal deformities.

Measurements of the interocular distance can help determine the presence or absence of dystopia cantharum, a highly diagnostic feature of this disorder, which is seen in 69% of patients with the Waardenburg syndrome. If the inner canthal distance divided by the interpupillary distance is greater than 0.6, this lateral displacement of the inner canthi may help confirm the diagnosis.[58]

Vogt-Koyanagi-Harada Syndrome

The Vogt-Koyanagi-Harada syndrome (Vogt-Koyanagi syndrome) is a rare, possibly autoimmune disorder characterized by bilateral uveitis, alopecia, vitiligo, poliosis (which may be limited to the eyebrows and eyelashes or may also involve the scalp and body hair), dysacousia (a condition in which certain sounds produce discomfort), and deafness. Usually seen in adults in the third and fourth decades of life, the disorder also occurs in children and adolescents. The Vogt-Koyanagi and the Vogt-Koyanagi-Harada syndromes appear to be one and the same, except that meningeal irritation or encephalitic symptoms are described in association with the latter condition. In this variant a prodromal febrile episode, with ence-phalitic or meningeal symptoms, lymphocytosis, and increased pressure of the cerebrospinal fluid, is followed by bilateral uveitis (often with choroidi-tis and optic neuritis). One explanation for this association may be that a virus that infects the leptomeninges can also infect cutaneous melanocytes, destroying the latter (if this process is rapid, the meninges may also be-come inflamed, thus producing the symptoms of meningitis).[59]

Although the etiology of the Vogt-Koyanagi-Harada syndrome remains unknown, it has been hypothesized tht this disorder is associated with an abnormal host response to an infective agent, possibly a virus, with an allergic sensitization to uveal melanocyte antigens and destruction of mel-anin in the hair and skin.[59, 60] The condition has been associated with the HLA antigen BW22J, a variant of BW22, observed in the Japanese[61] and the HLA-D antigen of Japanese origin (LD–Wa).[62]

CLINICAL COURSE.—All patients with the Vogt-Koyanagi-Harada syn-drome have a self-limiting bilateral uveitis. As the uveitis subsides, the following features develop: poliosis (in 80% to 90%); temporary auditory impairment; vitiligo, usually symmetrical (in 50% to 60%); and alopecia (in 50% of affected individuals). The hearing usually returns to normal, but the pigmentary changes, which generally appear about three weeks to three months after the onset of the uveitis, tend to be permanent. The uveitis generally takes a year or more to clear, and although most cases show some recovery of visual acuity, only partial recovery may occur at times, and some individuals may be left with a residual visual defect.

The Alezzandrini Syndrome

The Alezzandrini syndrome is a rare disorder of unknown origin pri-marily seen in adolescents and young adults. Possibly related to the Vogt-Koyanagi-Harada syndrome, it is characterized by unilateral degen-erative retinitis with visual impairment, which is followed, at times, after an interval of months or years, by bilateral deafness and unilateral vitiligo and poliosis, which appear on the same side of the face.

Multiple Lentigines Syndrome (Leopard Syndrome)

In 1969 Gorlin and his associates published a review of an autosomal dominant disorder with high penetrance and variable expressivity charac-terized by striking cutaneous pigmentation.[63] The various aspects of this syndrome are best remembered by the term "leopard syndrome," a mne-monic device derived from an acronym that encompasses many of the pro-tean manifestations of this disorder; lentigines, electrocardiographic con-duction defects, ocular hypertelorism, pulmonary stenosis, abnormalities of genitalia, retardation of growth, and deafness[64] (Table 8–5).

TABLE 8–5.—Multiple
Lentigenes Syndrome
(Leopard syndrome)

1. Lentigines
2. Electrocardiographic conduction defects
3. Ocular hypertelorism
4. Pulmonary stenosis
5. Abnormalities of genitalia
6. Retardation of growth
7. Deafness

CLINICAL MANIFESTATIONS.—The cutaneous marker heralding this syndrome consists of hundreds of small, light tan, dark brown, or black pinpoint lentigines ranging from 1 to 5 mm to several cm in size which are usually congenital in nature. They may also be present soon after birth and generally become obvious between the ages of two and five years. With time they increase in number, depth of color, and size, and there is marked increase in number at the time of puberty. Light and electron microscopy confirm them to be lentigines with characteristic acanthosis, increase in melanocytes, and melanin deposition. The cutaneous lesions tend to be concentrated on the neck and upper trunk, but may also appear on the irides of the eyes and on the skin of the face and scalp, arms, palms, soles, and genitalia, only sparing the oral mucosa. Occasionally formes frustes of this disorder occur in which the characteristic lentigines are absent.[65]

Skeletal aberrations may include retardation of growth (below the 25th percentile), hypertelorism, pectus deformities (carinatum or excavatum), dorsal kyphosis, winged scapulae, and prognathism. Cardiac abnormalities, commonly seen in this disorder, may consist of valvular pulmonary stenosis, subaortic stenosis, or cardiac conduction defects. Endocrine disorders include gonadal hypoplasia, hypospadias, undescended testicles, hypoplastic ovaries, and delayed puberty. Congenital neurosensory hearing loss, abnormal electroencephalograms, and slowed peripheral nerve conduction may complete the findings in this disorder.

The NAME (LAMB) Syndrome

In 1973, Rees reported the case of an 18-year-old male with brown macules, an embolic stroke, and a left atrial endotheliomyxoma;[66] in 1980, Atherton described a 10-year-old boy with generalized brown macules, multiple blue nevi, multiple congenital pigmented nevi, multiple myxoid tumors of the skin, and bilateral atrial myxomas;[67] and in 1984, Rhodes, et al. described a 13-year-old girl with a congenital nevocellular nevus, black macules of the face and vulva, brown macules of the lips and perioral skin, multiple blue nevi, thyroid nodules, and an atrial myxoma.[68] Two eponyms have been proposed to describe these cardiocutaneous disorders, the NAME syndrome (Nevi, Atrial myxoma, Myxoid neurofibromas, and Ephilides), coined by Atherton and the LAMB syndrome (Lentigines, Atrial myxoma, Mucocutaneous myxomas, and Blue nevi) to distinguish this syndrome from the multiple lentigines (Leopard) syndrome. The black and brown macules of the face and vulva in Rhodes' cases consisted of lentiginous proliferations of large, intensely dopa-reactive melanocytes. These cases emphasize the necessity for cardiac evaluation for a potentially fatal (but surgically treatable) atrial myxoma in individuals with multiple melanocytic and myxomatous tumors of the skin and mucosa.[68]

The Basal Cell Nevus Syndrome

The basal cell nevus syndrome (nevoid basal cell carcinoma syndrome, Gorlin syndrome) is an autosomal dominant disorder with low penetration characterized by childhood onset of multiple basal cell epitheliomas associated with other abnormalities such as odontogenic jaw cysts, bifid ribs, other anomalies of the vertebrae, neurologic, ophthalmic and musculoskeletal anomalies, and intracranial calcification[69–72] (Table 8–6). The most obvious cutaneous feature of the syndrome is the appearance of multiple basal cell epitheliomas early in life.

CLINICAL MANIFESTATIONS.—The skin lesions of the basal cell nevus syndrome may appear as early as the second year of life, frequently develop at puberty, and generally occur between puberty and 35 years of age. They involve, in decreasing order of frequency, the face, neck, back, thorax, abdomen, and upper extremities.[72] Lesions appear as flesh-colored to pale brown dome-shaped papules that measure 1 mm to 1 cm in diameter and erupt in crops periodically throughout the lifetime of affected in-

TABLE 8–6.—THE BASAL CELL NEVUS SYNDROME

1. Autosomal dominant with low penetration
2. Basal cell epitheliomas (usually between puberty and age 35)
3. Palmar or plantar pits (usually in second decade or later)
4. Osseous malformations: jaw cysts, defective dentition, frontal and temporoparietal bossing, prognathism, splayed or bifid ribs, spina bifida, scoliosis, shortened 4th metacarpals
5. Neurologic abnormalities: mental retardation, EEG abnormalities, seizures, calcification of dura and falx cerebri, medulloblastomas early in life
6. Ophthalmic abnormalities (in ⅓ of cases): hypertelorism, dystopia canthorum, strabismus, congenital blindness due to corneal opacities, cataracts, glaucoma, and colobomas of retina and iris
7. Associated endocrine features: ovarian fibromas and calcifications, hypogonadism in males, cryptorchism or testicular agenesis, adenocortical adenomas, pseudohypoparathyroidism

dividuals. Secondary changes such as ulceration, crusting, and bleeding rarely occur before puberty, but if left untreated, these lesions can become extremely destructive. Unlike ordinary basal cell carcinomas, the basal cell nevi do not appear to be induced by prolonged exposure to sunlight.[73]

In addition to nevoid basal cell carcinomas, affected individuals have other cutaneous stigmata. These include small milia on the face, numerous comedonal lesions, large epidermal cysts of the limbs, lipomas, fibromas, café au lait pigmentation, multiple pigmented nevi, and ectopic calcium deposits in the skin. Shallow 2 to 3 mm palmar and plantar pits, a characteristic feature of the syndrome, are seen in 60% of affected individuals. These defective areas of keratinization usually first appear during the second decade of life or later. Palmar and plantar pits also frequently have an underlying area of erythema, which on casual observation appear as multiple small red spots on the palms and soles.

Neurologic abnormalities include mental retardation, electroencephalographic abnormalities, agenesis of the corpus collosum, a peculiar calcification of the dura and falx cerebri, seizures, congenital communicating hydrocephalus, nerve deafness, and, in some patients, medulloblastomas, which generally appear during the first two years of life.[69]

Ophthalmic abnormalities, documented in approximately one-third of patients with this disorder, include hypertelorism and lateral displacement of the medial canthi (dystopia canthorum), strabismus, congenital blindness due to corneal opacities, cataracts, glaucoma, and colobomas of the retina and iris. Associated endocrine findings include ovarian fibromas and calcifications, pseudohypoparathyroidism, hypogonadism in males, cryptorchism or testicular agenesis, and adrenal cortical adenomas.

Musculoskeletal anomalies, present in 60% to 75% of patients, consist of frontal and temporoparietal bossing, prognathism, mandibular and maxillary bone cysts, splayed or bifid ribs, kyphoscoliosis, cervical or upper thoracic vertebral fusion, spina bifida, a marfanoid build, pectus excavatum and carinatum, and shortened fourth metacarpals (seen in 10% of affected individuals).

DIAGNOSIS.—Diagnosis of the basal cell nevus syndrome is generally made by finding multiple basal cell carcinomas of the skin in children or young adults who also have characteristic, irregular, pink- to skin-colored pits of the palms and soles. The basal cell epitheliomas are indistinguishable on histopathologic examination from ordinary basal cell carcinomata. Roentgenologic examinations may reveal jaw cysts, osteomas, calcification of the falx cerebri, pelvic calcification, and bifid ribs.

TREATMENT.—The relatively benign course of these lesions suggests a nonradical therapeutic approach such as simple surgical excision or electrodesiccation and curettage. Radiotherapy, particularly in childhood, is not recommended in the management of this disorder.

Epidermal Nevus Syndrome

The epidermal nevus syndrome has been delineated as a congenitally acquired syndrome consisting of deformities of the skin, the skeletal system, the central nervous system, and the cardiovascular system (Table 8–7). Associated anomalies include cutaneous disorders (epidermal nevi, areas of hypopigmentation, other nevi, and café au lait spots), kyphoscoliosis, vertebral defects, hemihypertrophy, short limbs, phocomelia, angiomas of the skin, patent ductus arteriosus, coarctation and hypoplasia of the aorta, ocular abnormalities, and central nervous system involvement, with brain tumor, hydrocephaly, mental retardation, neural deafness, cranial nerve palsies, motor paralyses and convulsive disorders.[73–75] Local invasion of the face resulted in one death and four eye enucleations, and four patients developed hypotension and/or bradycardia during anesthesia.[76] Although there have been several cases of benign and malignant tumors reported in association with the epidermal nevus syndrome, it is not established whether the association is real or a matter of chance. Although it appears that most cases of epidermal nevus syndrome occur sporadically, accumulated data suggest that, in some cases, an autosomal dominant transmission may be present.[73]

DIAGNOSIS.—The nature of the verrucous lesions ranges from large unilateral hypertrophic deformities of the epidermis (nevus unius lateris) to whorled, brush stroke-like scaly lesions involving variable areas of the skin surface (ichthyosis hystrix) or large orange velvety changes of the scalp such as are seen in nevus sebaceus of Jadassohn[75, 78, 79] (Fig 8–10). It now appears that the linear nevus sebaceus syndrome and epidermal nevus syndrome are probably the same entity, the only difference being that of topography. Biopsies from patients with lesions in the sebaceous gland area (scalp, face, and ears) show sebaceous gland hyperplasia; those with lesions on the arms, legs, and trunk (where a sebaceous component is not prominent) show histopathologic features of epidermal nevi (nevus unius lateris).[78, 79]

The predominant histologic features of epidermal nevi consist of hyper-

TABLE 8–7.—EPIDERMAL NEVUS SYNDROME

1. Epidermal nevi (nevus unius lateris, bilateral epidermal nevi, ichthyosis hystrix)
2. Skeletal abnormalities: kyphoscoliosis, vertebral defects, hemihypertrophy, short limbs, phocomelia
3. CNS involvement: brain tumor, hydrocephaly, mental retardation, neural deafness, cranial palsies, motor paralyses, seizures
4. Cardiovascular: patent ductus, coarctation and hypoplasia of aorta

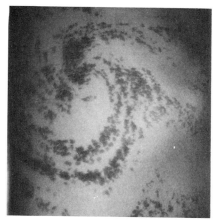

Fig 8–10.—Nevus unius lateris (a systematized epidermal nevus in a whorled pattern on the left side of the chest in an 8-year-old boy). Localized and systematized linear nevi may be associated with skeletal deformities and central nervous system disease.

keratosis, papillomatosis, and acanthosis. Nevus cells are absent, but in some cases, an increase in melanin pigment in the basal layer may be present. Hyperkeratosis, vacuolization (ballooning) of the cells, and microvesicles, as seen in epidermolytic hyperkeratosis, may be seen in some lesions, particularly in the ichthyosis hystrix form of the disorder. In some patients, both histologic patterns may be noted in a single lesion or in lesions from different areas of the same patient.

TREATMENT.—Patients with large epidermal nevi require a careful family history and thorough physical evaluation, with particular emphasis on the affected individual's developmental pattern and musculoskeletal, nervous, ocular, and cardiovascular systems. Periodic electroencephalograms and radiologic examination of the long bones, pelvis, and vertebral column are also advisable.

REFERENCES

1. Butterworth T.: Neurocutaneous Syndromes—von Recklinghausen's disease, in *Clinical Genodermatology*. Williams and Wilkins Co., Baltimore, Md., 1962, pp. 101–105.
2. Crowe F.W., Schull W.J., Neel J.V.: *A Clinical, Pathologic Genetic Study of Multiple Neurofibromatosis*. Charles C Thomas, Springfield, Illinois, 1956.
3. Riccardi V.M.: The multiple forms of neurofibromatosis. *Pediatrics in Review* 3:293–298, 1982.
4. Riccardi V.M.: The pathophysiology of neurofibromatosis. *J. Am. Acad. Dermatol* 3:157–166, 1980.
5. Riccardi V.M.: von Recklinghausen neurofibromatosis. *N. Engl. J. Med.* 305:1617–1627, 1981.
6. Braverman I.M.: Neurocutaneous disorders, in Braverman I.M.: *Skin Signs of Systemic Disease*, ed. 2. W.B. Saunders Co., Philadelphia, 1981, pp. 777–808.

7. Riccardi V.M., interview, in *Skin & Allergy News*, New York, March 1984.

8. Crowe F.W., Schull W.J.: Diagnostic importance of the café au lait spot in neurofibromatosis. *Arch Int. Med.* 91:758–766, 1963.

9. Whitehouse D.: Diagnostic value of the café au lait spot in children. *Arch. Dis. Child.* 41:316–319, 1966.

10. Crowe F.W.: Axillary freckling as a diagnostic aid in neurofibromatosis. *Ann. Int. Med.* 61:1142–1143, 1962.

11. Benedict P.H., Szabo, G., Fitzpatrick T.B., et al.: Melanotic macules in Albright's syndrome and in neurofibromatosis. *J.A.M.A.* 25:618–626, 1968.

12. Jimbo K., Szabo G., Fitzpatrick T.B.: Ultrastructural giant pigment granules (macromelanosomes) in cutaneous pigmented macules of neurofibromatosis. *J. Invest. Dermatol.* 61:300–309, 1973.

13. Morris T.J., Johnson W.G., Silvers D.N.: Giant pigment granules in biopsy specimens for café au lait spots in neurofibromatosis. *Arch. Dermatol.* 118:385–388, 1982.

14. Eady R.A.J., Cowen T.C.: Summaries of papers: nevus spilus: a light and electron microscopical study. *Br. J. Dermatol.* 93, Suppl. 11:16, 1975.

15. Johnson B.L., Charneco D.R.: Café au lait spots in neurofibromatosis and in normal individuals. *Arch. Dermatol.* 102:442–446, 1970.

16. Silvers D.N., Greenwood R.S., Helwig E.B.: Café au lait spots without giant pigment granules. *Arch. Dermatol.* 110:87–88, 1974.

17. Lever W.F., Schaumburg-Lever G.: Tumors of Neural Tissue, Neurofibromatosis. in *Histopathology of the Skin*, ed. 6. J.P. Lippincott Co., Philadelphia, 1983, pp. 667–674.

18. Westerhof W., Konrad K.: Blue-red macules and pseudoatrophic macules. Additional cutaneous signs of neurofibromatosis. *Arch. Dermatol.* 118:557–581, 1982.

19. Apter N., Chemke J., Hurwitz N., et al.: Neonatal neurofibromatosis: unusual manifestations with malignant clinical course. *Clin. Genet.* 7:388–393, 1975.

20. Callen J.P.: The skin, the eye, and systemic disease. *Cutis* 24:501–511, 1979.

21. Kleitsch W.P., Kehne J.H., Gutch C.F.: Gastrointestinal hemorrhage due to neurofibromatosis. *J.A.M.A.* 147:1434–1436, 1951.

22. Shelley E.D., Bellur S.N., Koya D.R.: Neurocutaneous disorders, in Callen J.P. (Ed.): *Cutaneous Aspects of Internal Disease*. Year Book Medical Publishers, Inc. Chicago, 1981, pp. 593–625.

23. Hurwitz S., Braverman I.M.: White spots in tuberous sclerosis. *J. Pediatr.* 77:587–594, 1970.

24. Moolton S.E.: The hamartial nature of the tuberous sclerosis complex, and its bearing on the tumor problem. *Ann. Int. Med.* 69:589–623, 1942.

25. Oppenheimer E.Y., Rosman N.P.: Delayed appearance of hypopigmented macules in tuberous sclerosis. *Neurology* 29:570, 1979.

26. Nickel W.R., Reed W.B.: Tuberous sclerosis. *Arch. Dermatol.* 85:209–216, 1962.

27. Hurwitz S.: Society Transactions. Discussion on tuberous sclerosis. *Arch. Dermatol.* 104:336–337, 1971.

28. Fitzpatrick T.B., Szabo G., Hori Y., et al.: White leaf-shaped macules. Earliest visible sign of tuberous sclerosis. *Arch. Dermatol.* 98:1–6, 1968.

29. McWilliam R.P., Stephenson J.B.P.: Depigmented hairs, the earliest sign of tuberous sclerosis. *Arch. Dis. Child.* 53:961–963, 1978.

30. Hoff M., von Gransven M.F., Jongeblood W.L., et al.: Enamel defects asso-

ciated with tuberous sclerosis. *Oral Surg., Oral Med., Oral Path.* 40:261–269, 1975.

31. Roth J.C., Epstein C.J.: Infantile spasms and hypopigmented macules—early manifestations of tuberous sclerosis. *Arch. Neurol.* 25:547–551, 1971.

32. Papiglione G., Moynahan E.J.: The tuberous sclerosis syndrome: clinical and EEG studies in 100 children. *J. Neurol. Neurosurg. Psychiatry* 39:666–673, 1975.

33. Martin G.I., Kaiserman D., Liegler D., et al.: Computer-assisted cranial tomography in early diagnosis of tuberous sclerosis. *J.A.M.A.* 235:2323–2324, 1976.

34. Gomez M.R., Mellinger J.F., Reese D.F.: The use of computer transaxial tomography in the diagnosis of tuberous sclerosis. *Mayo Clin. Proc.* 50:553–556, 1975.

35. Nyboer J.H., Robertson D.M., Gomez M.R.: Retinal lesions in tuberous sclerosis. *Arch. Ophthalmol.* 94:1277–1280, 1976.

36. Cassidy S.B., Pagan R.A., Pepin M., et al.: Family studies in tuberous sclerosis: evaluation of apparently unaffected parents. *J.A.M.A.* 249:1302–1304, 1983.

37. Reed W.B., Nickel W.R., Campion G.: Internal manifestations of tuberous sclerosis. *Arch. Dermatol.* 87:715–728, 1963.

38. Butterworth T., Wilson McC., Jr.: Dermatologic aspects of tuberous sclerosis. *Arch Derm. Syph.* 43:1–41, 1941.

39. Carney R.G.: Incontinentia pigmenti: a world statistical analysis. *Arch. Dermatol.* 112:535–542, 1976.

40. Gordon H., Gordon W.: Incontinentia pigmenti: clinical and genetic studies of two familial cases. *Dermatologica* 140:150–168, 1961.

41. Schamburg-Lever G., Lever W.F.: Electron microscopy of incontinentia pigmenti. *J. Invest. Dermatol.* 61:151–158, 1973.

42. Wiley H.E. III, Frias J.L.: Depigmented lesions in incontinentia pigmenti: a useful sign. *Am. J. Dis. Child.* 128:546–547, 1974.

43. Wiklund D.A., Weston W.L.: Incontinentia pigmenti. a four-generation study. *Arch. Dermatol.* 116:701–703, 1980.

44. Ito M.: Studies on melanin 1. Incontinentia pigmenti achromians: a singular case of nevus depigmentosus systematicus bilateralis. *Tohoku J. Exper. Med.* 55 (Supl. 1):57–59, 1952.

45. Hamado T., Saito T., et al.: Incontinentia pigmenti (Ito). *Arch. Dermatol.* 96:673–676, 1967.

46. Nordlund J.J., Klaus S.N., Gino J.: Hypomelanosis of Ito. *Acta Derm. Venereal.* (Stockholm) 57:261–264, 1977.

47. Schwartz M.F., Esterly N.B., Fretzin D.F.: Hypomelanosis of Ito (incontinentia pigmenti achromians): a neurocutaneous syndrome. *J. Pediatr.* 90:236–240, 1977.

48. Rubin N.G.: Incontinentia pigmenti achromians. *Arch. Dermatol.* 105:424–425, 1972.

49. Jelinek J.E., Bart R.S., Schiff G.M.: Hypomelanosis of Ito ("Incontinentia Pigmenti Achromians"). *Arch. Dermatol.* 117:596–601, 1973.

50. Takematsu H., Sato S., Igarashi M., et al.: Incontinentia pigmenti achromians (Ito). *Arch. Dermatol.* 119:391–395, 1983.

51. Cram D.L., Fukuyama K.: Unilateral systematized hypochromic nevus. *Arch. Dermatol.* 109:416, 1974.

52. Coupe R.L.: Unilateral systematized achromic nevus. *Dermatologica* 134:19–35, 1967.
53. Solomon L.M., Esterly N.B.: Pigmentary abnormalities, nevus achromicus. in *Neonatal Dermatology.* W.B. Saunders Publishing Co., Philadelphia, 1973, p. 106.
54. Hurwitz S.: Disorders of hypopigmentation, in *Clinical Pediatric Dermatology.* W.B. Saunders Co., Philadelphia, 1981, pp. 343–353.
55. Jimbo W.K., Fitzpatrick T.B., Szabo G., et al.: Congenital circumscribed hypomelanosis: a characteristic based on electron microscopic study of tuberous sclerosis, nevus depigmentosus and piebaldism. *J. Invest. Dermatol.* 64:50–62, 1975.
56. Waardenburg P.J.: A new syndrome combining developmental anomalies of the eyelids, eyebrows and nose root with pigmentary defects of the iris and head hair with congenital deafness. *Am. J. Hum. Genet.* 3:195–253, 1951.
57. Gorlin R.J.: Speaking on hereditary syndromes, Second International Congress of Pediatric Dermatology, Chicago, Illinois, August 23–26, 1979.
58. Reed W.B., Stone V.M., Boder E., et al.: Pigmentary disorders in association with congenital deafness. *Arch. Dermatol.* 95:176–186, 1967.
59. Nordlund J.J., Albert D., Forget B., et al.: Halo nevi and the Vogt-Koyanagi-Harada syndrome—manifestations of vitiligo. *Arch. Dermatol.* 116:690–692, 1982.
60. Hammer H.: Lymphocyte transformation test in sympathetic ophthalmitis and the Vogt-Koyanagi-Harada syndrome. *Br. J. Ophthalmol.* 55:850–852, 1971.
61. Tagawa Y., Sugiura S., Yakura H., et al.: HLA and Vogt-Koyanagi-Harada syndrome. *N. Engl. J. Med.* 295:173, 1976.
62. Yakura H., Wakisaka A., Aizawa M., et al.: HLA-D antigen of Japanese origin (LD-Wa) and its association with Vogt-Koyanagi-Harada syndrome. *Tissue Antigens* 8:35–42, 1976.
63. Gorlin R.J., Anderson R.C., Blaw M.: Multiple lentigines syndrome. *Am. J. Dis. Child.* 117:652–662, 1969.
64. Gorlin R.J., Anderson R.C., Moller J.H.: Leopard (multiple lentigines) syndrome revisited. *Laryngoscope* 81:1674–1681, 1971.
65. Nordlund J.J., Lerner A.B., Braverman I.M., et al.: The multiple lentigines syndrome. *Arch. Dermatol.* 107:259–261, 1973.
66. Rees J.R., Ross F.M.G., Keen G.: Lentiginosis and left atrial myxoma. *Br. Heart J.* 35:874–876, 1973.
67. Atherton D.J., Pitcher D.W., Wells R.S., et al.: A syndrome of various pigmented lesions, myxoid neurofibroma and atrial myxoma: The NAME syndrome. *Br. J. Dermatol.* 103:421–429, 1980.
68. Rhodes A.R., Silverman R.A., Harrist T.J., et al.: Mucocutaneous lentigines, cardiomucocutaneous myxomas, and multiple blue nevi: The "LAMB" syndrome. *J. Am. Acad. Dermatol.* 10:72–82, 1984.
69. Howell, J.B., Caro M.R.: Basal-cell nevus: its relationship to multiple cutaneous cancers and associated anomalies of development. *Arch. Dermatol.* 79:67–80, 1959.
70. Gorlin R.J., Goltz R.W.: Multiple nevoid basal-cell epithelioma, jaw cysts, and bifid rib syndrome. *N. Engl. J. Med.* 262:908–912, 1960.
71. Gorlin R.J., Yunis J.J., Tuna N.: Multiple nevoid basal cell carcinoma, odontogenic, keratinocyte and skeletal anomalies: a syndrome. *Acta Derm. Venereol.* 43:39–55, 1963.

72. Gorlin R.J., Pindborg J.J., Cohen M.M., Jr.: Multiple nevoid basal cell carcinoma syndrome, in *Syndromes of the Head and Neck*, ed. 2. McGraw-Hill Book Co., New York, 1976, pp. 520–526.
73. Solomon L.M., Esterly N.B.: Epidermal and other congenital organoid nevi. in *Current Problems in Pediatrics*, Vol. VI, No. 1. Year Book Medical Publishers, Chicago, 1975, pp. 3–56.
74. Solomon L.M., Fretzin D.F., Dewald R.L.: The epidermal nevus syndrome. *Arch. Dermatol.* 97:273–285, 1968.
75. Solomon L.M.: Epidermal nevus syndrome. *Mod. Probl. Paediatr.* 17:27–30, 1975.
76. Southwick G.J., Schwartz R.A.: The basal cell nevus syndrome: disasters occurring among a series of 36 patients. *Cancer* 44:2294–2305, 1979.
77. Diamond R.L., Amon R.B.: Epidermal nevus and rhabdomyosarcoma. *Arch. Dermatol.* 112:1424–1426, 1976.
78. Lovejoy F.H., Jr., Boyle W.E.: Linear nevus sebaceous syndrome: report of two cases and review of the literature. *Pediatrics* 52:382–387, 1973.
79. Holden K.R., DeKaban A.S.: Neurologic involvement in nevus unius lateris and nevus linearis sebaceus. *Neurology* 22:879–887, 1972.

9 / The Skin and the Gastrointestinal Tract

THERE ARE MANY DISORDERS that affect both the skin and gastrointestinal tract. Many of these (hereditary hemorrhagic telangiectasia, scleroderma, Henoch-Schönlein purpura) are included in other sections of this text. This chapter will cover acrodermatitis enteropathica, dermatitis herpetiformis, epidermolysis bullosa, Peutz-Jeghers syndrome, dyskeratosis congenita, pyoderma gangrenosum, Gardner's and Oldfield's syndromes, and familial Mediterranean fever.

Acrodermatitis Enteropathica

Acrodermatitis enteropathica is a hereditary disorder that appears in early infancy and is characterized by acral and periorificial vesicobullous, pustular, and eczematoid skin lesions; alopecia; nail dystrophy; diarrhea; glossitis; stomatitis; and frequent secondary infection due to bacterial or candidal organisms (Table 9–1). Although the clinical characteristics of this disease were originally described by Danbolt and Closs in 1930, it was not until 1942 that they defined the disorder as a specific entity and, because of the acral distribution of skin lesions and associated gastrointestinal abnormalities, designated it by its present name.[1]

The inheritance pattern of acrodermatitis enteropathica is believed to be autosomal recessive with nearly equal incidence in male and female patients. Involvement in siblings, but not in parents, and a history of familial occurrence in 65% of patients conforms to this suggested mode of transmission.[1, 2]

The etiology of acrodermatitis enteropathica remained controversial until 1973 when Moynahan first demonstrated low serum zinc levels and a rapid response to the administration of zinc sulfate in patients with this disorder.[3] Although many questions regarding the precise pathogenesis remain unanswered, the basic defect appears to be related to a gastrointestinal malabsorption of zinc.[4] Three hypotheses have been proposed to explain reduced absorption of zinc in acrodermatitis enteropathica, but so far none has been satisfactorily documented. Moynahan has suggested that the malabsorption is caused by the formation of an unabsorbable peptide-zinc complex in the intestinal lumen. Others, however, suggest that the malabsorption is caused by the lack of zinc-binding ligands in the small intestine[5, 6]

TABLE 9–1.—ACRODERMATITIS ENTEROPATHICA

1. An autosomal recessive gastrointestinal malabsorption of zinc
2. Periorifical dermatitis, diarrhea, and alopecia (the characteristic triad); photophobia; drooling; red hair; growth retardation; irritability; frequent impetiginization and *Candida albicans* infection
3. Dx: low serum zinc levels (50 micrograms/100 ml or lower)
4. Rx: zinc gluconate or sulfate (5 mg/kg/day—usually 100 to 200 mg/day)

(the absorption of zinc in the intestine is thought to be assisted by a ligand that binds zinc and facilitates the transport of the trace element across the mucosa), or by trapping of zinc in the wall of the intestinal tract[7] (it appears that the zinc-binding ligand absent from the child's intestine is supplied by the mother's breast milk). In addition to the classic inherited disease which requires lifelong zinc supplementation, syndromes of zinc deficiency mimicking acrodermatitis enteropathica are now being seen in individuals receiving long-term parenteral nutrition with inadequate zinc supplementation,[8–11] patients who have had intestinal bypass procedures,[12, 13] premature infants fed exclusively human milk,[14–16] as a complication of regional enteritis,[17] in chronic alcoholics with poor nutrition, and in individuals on zinc deficient vegetarian diets.[18] Essential fatty acid deficiencies can also produce a similar picture.[19] Zinc deficiency in infants and children receiving parenteral nutrition without zinc supplements is a particularly acute problem in premature infants who have lower body stores of zinc than full-term infants.[20]

CLINICAL MANIFESTATIONS.—The triad of dermatitis, diarrhea, and alopecia classically appears at the time of weaning from breast to cow's milk. Although some patients are never diagnosed until adulthood, it appears that these individuals actually had their disease in a mild form during childhood. The onset of symptoms, therefore, usually begins early in life, generally between the age of one or two weeks to 20 months, with an average age of onset at nine months.

Typically, infants with acrodermatitis enteropathica are listless, anoretic, and apathetic. Tissue wasting is present with an associated failure to thrive. During periods of exacerbation, frothy, bulky, foul-smelling diarrhea stools, typical of those in patients with celiac syndrome, are seen. Other findings include conjunctivitis, photophobia, stomatitis, perléche, recurring monilial or bacterial infection, and alopecia of the scalp, eyelashes or eyebrows, or both. Children suffering from this disorder exhibit a uniform appearance, mainly because of the alopecia and periorificial lesions.

The syndrome usually begins with small moist erythematous lesions localized around the body orifices (mouth, nose, ears, eyes, and perineum) and symmetrically located on the buttocks and extensor surface of major joints (the acral aspect of this disorder) (Fig 9–1). The cutaneous lesions are similar to those of severe moniliasis or pustular psoriasis, depending upon the areas that are affected.

Drooling and change of hair color to red are additional findings seen during the active phase of the disease.[21] Other features include growth retardation in 80% and mental changes in the form of schizoid features, with frequent crying, irritability, and restlessness during periods of exacerbation in 40% of patients.[2, 22]

The basic cutaneous lesion of acrodermatitis enteropathica is a vesiculobullous eruption that arises from an erythematous base. The blisters quickly collapse, begin to dry and crust, and sharply marginated lichenified or psoriasiform plaques develop at these sites. On the face, the eroded and crusted peribuccal plaques may appear impetiginized, and secondary infection with *Candida albicans* is common. When the fingers and toes are involved, there is marked erythema and swelling of the paronychial tissues, often with subsequent nail deformity. If unrecognized or untreated, acrodermatitis enteropathica follows an intermittent but relentlessly progressive course and, as a consequence of general disability, infection, or both, frequently ends in fatality.[2]

Recent investigations of the monocyte system suggest suppression of cellular chemotaxis of monocytes and neutrophils in patients with acrodermatitis enteropathica. Since patients with this disorder suffer from frequent and persistent bacterial and monilial infection, it has been theorized that a zinc-dependent defect in chemotaxis may contribute to this susceptibility.

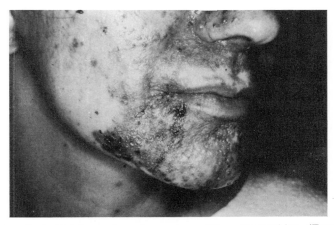

Fig 9–1.—Periorificial eruption of acrodermatitis enteropathica. (From Braverman I.M.: *Skin Signs of Systemic Disease*. W.B. Saunders Co., Philadelphia, 1970. Used by permission.)

These findings suggest an important role for zinc in neutrophil and monocyte chemotaxis and a correctable immune defect in patients with this disorder.[23]

DIAGNOSIS.—The diagnosis of acrodermatitis enteropathica is based on the clinical features of a dermatitis localized around the body orifices, buttocks, and extensor surfaces of the major joints, scalp, fingers, and toes; diarrhea; alopecia; and low serum zinc levels. Skin biopsy is not diagnostic and shows a variable picture dependent upon the age and clinical appearance of the lesions. There may be hyperkeratosis, parakeratosis, intraepidermal pustules, spongiosis, acanthosis with downward projection of the rete pegs, and a mild polymorphic infiltrate in the upper region of the dermis. A decrease in zinc levels in plasma, red blood cells, hair, and urine may be considered diagnostic (serum zinc levels of 70–110 micrograms/100 ml are considered normal, and levels of 50 micrograms/100 ml or lower appear to be diagnostic of this disorder).[24] Blood zinc determinations should always be done prior to treatment in order to determine that the patient actually has acrodermatitis enteropathica. However, there may be sources of error caused by zinc contamination of glass tubes and rubber stoppers. Blood samples should be collected in acid-washed sterile plastic tubes with the use of acid-washed plastic syringes.

TREATMENT.—Diiodohydroxyquin is no longer considered the treatment of choice for this disorder. Zinc gluconate or sulfate, without diiodohydroxyquin or breast milk, is highly effective in dosages of 5 mg/kg/day given two or three times a day. With adequate therapy (100 to 200 mg per day in most patients) improvement in temperament and a decrease in irritability usually can be noted within one or two days, the appetite improves in a few days, and diarrhea and skin lesions begin to respond within two or three days after the initiation of therapy. Hair growth begins after two or three weeks of therapy and an increase in the growth of the infant generally occurs within approximately two months. Available in tablets containing up to 15 mg of elemental zinc (the amount of elemental zinc is usually listed on the product label as the zinc equivalent), zinc sulfate or gluconate may be given in fruit juice, is well tolerated by patients, and provides a safe and inexpensive form of therapy for this formerly severe disorder of infancy and childhood.[25–57] After complete improvement, the amount of zinc can be tapered to the lowest effective dosage.

Dermatitis Herpetiformis

Dermatitis herpetiformis (Duhring's disease) is a chronic recurrent cutaneous disease of unknown cause characterized by an intensely pruritic papulovesicular and, at times, bullous eruption that responds dramatically to orally administered doses of sulfones or sulfapyridine. Although the disorder may affect individuals of all ages, it generally occurs during the second to fourth decades of life. It is uncommon in infancy and childhood, and affects males more frequently than females. Blacks are rarely afflicted.

The cause of dermatitis herpetiformis (DH) remains unknown. It seems to be related to deposition of IgA at the dermal-epidermal junction of the skin. In some individuals, immunologic processes may be associated with the pathogenesis of both dermatitis herpetiformis and adult celiac disease. Helping substantiate this hypothesis is the fact that 60% to 70% of patients with dermatitis herpetiformis have small bowel abnormalities indistinguishable from those seen in celiac-type gluten-sensitive enteropathy.[28, 29] As a corollary to this theory, it has been suggested that antigluten immunoglobulins formed in the gut are released into the circulation and ultimately lodge in the skin to produce the cutaneous lesions of dermatitis herpetiformis. Circulating antigluten antibodies reported in sera of patients with dermatitis herpetiformis,[30] and IgA circulating immune complexes found in the sera of some patients with DH following wheat ingestion[31] help substantiate this hypothesis.

Although the cutaneous abnormality may not be caused by the same agents as that of gluten-sensitive enteropathy, there appears to be a strong genetic link and an unusually high frequency of HLA-B8 and HLA-DRW3 antigens in patients with both of these disorders.[32, 33] Relatives of patients with dermatitis herpetiformis have been shown to have a high prevalence of villous atrophy assumed to be caused by celiac sprue.[34] To further support this concept, patients with dermatitis herpetiformis whose rashes are controlled by strict gluten-free diet are shown to have an exacerbation of their disorders when challenged by dietary gluten.[35] Although all patients cannot be controlled by gluten-free diet alone, a large proportion can obtain cutaneous and intestinal improvement on a strict gluten-free diet[36] and a gluten-free diet frequently permits reduction in the level of sulfone therapy.[37]

CLINICAL MANIFESTATIONS.—Dermatitis herpetiformis in childhood usually occurs in children over 8 years of age, persists into adulthood, and is fundamentally the same disease as seen in adults.[38] The disorder is characterized by an extremely pruritic, symmetrically grouped papulovesicular eruption that affects the extensor surfaces: the elbows, knees, sacrum, buttocks, and shoulders (Table 9–2). In association with the onset of intense pruritus or burning, erythematous and, at times, urticarial lesions may develop. Characteristic of this disorder are minute clear, relatively tense vesicles that measure from 0.3 to 4.0 mm in diameter. These vesicles rupture easily, either spontaneously or when scratched, and frequently erythematous lesions, small grouped papules and vesicles, superficial hyperpig-

TABLE 9–2.—Dermatitis Herpetiformis

1. An immunologic process related to celiac-type gluten-sensitive enteropathy?
2. Pruritic symmetrically grouped papulovesicular lesions on extensor surfaces
3. Diagnosis:
   a. Subepidermal microabscesses (with polymorphonuclear leukocytes and eosinophils) in dermal papillae
   b. IgA and complement immunofluorescence in dermal papillae of uninvolved skin
4. Treatment: sulfapyridine, dapsone (and gluten-free diet in some)

mented macules, and hypopigmented scars exist at the same time. The general course of this disorder is chronic (often lasting five to ten years or more) with frequent exacerbations and remissions.

DIAGNOSIS.—The most useful diagnostic histologic changes in dermatitis herpetiformis are seen in the vicinity of new blisters. Whenever possible, cutaneous biopsy should include the newest vesicle and a piece of the surrounding erythematous portion of the lesion. The initial changes are first noted in the tips of the dermal papillae and consist of subepidermal microabscesses with accumulations of neutrophils and eosinophils. Immunofluorescent studies suggest the best criteria for diagnosis of dermatitis herpetiformis to be the finding of IgA and complement deposits at the tips of the dermal papillae in a speckled distribution (or, less frequently, in a linear pattern) along the basement membrane at the dermal-epidermal junction of normal appearing skin, without detectable circulating antibody to the basement membrane.[39, 40] Although dermatitis herpetiformis and bullous pemphigoid are distinct in most instances, on the basis of clinical and immunofluorescent features, it appears that mixed and overlapping cases of both disorders can occur.[41]

TREATMENT.—Clinical experience has shown that sulfapyridine and sulfones are effective in relieving the symptoms and suppressing the eruption of dermatitis herpetiformis in children as well as adults. Major relief from the use of these agents, frequently as early as 24 to 48 hours, is often helpful in the diagnosis of this disorder.

Sulfapyridine is generally considered the drug of choice. The initial dose of sulfapyridine is usually 100 to 200 mg/kg/per day for children, in four divided doses (with a maximum total of 2 to 4 grams a day). Once existing lesions have been suppressed, the dosage may be tapered at weekly intervals, with a maintenance level of 0.5 gm or less as the daily required dose for most patients. Nausea and vomiting are usually the first signs of sulfapyridine toxicity. Other side effects include anorexia, headache, fever, leukopenia, agranulocytosis, hemolytic anemia, serum sickness-type reactions, hepatitis, exfoliative dermatitis, and renal crystalluria.[42] A screening test for glucose-6-phosphate dehydrogenase (G6PD) deficiency should be performed prior to the initiation of therapy, and close observation of the patient with pretreatment and follow-up blood counts at monthly intervals is recommended. Patients should be encouraged to drink large quantities of fluid in order to avoid renal complication, and since the disease may remit spontaneously, gradual attempts at reduction of treatment should be attempted at intervals of three to six months.

Various sulfone derivatives of 4,4'-diaminodiphenyl sulfone (dapsone, DDS) are better tolerated and more economical than sulfapyridine. Their side effects, however, are more severe, and because of an increased tendency to hemolytic anemia in patients with glucose-6-phosphate dehydrogenase deficiency (G6PH), a screening test should be done prior to initiation of therapy. Available in 25 and 100 mg tablets as Avlosulfon (Ayerst), dapsone treatment may be initiated with 2 mg/kg/day, with an increase or decrease in dosage depending on the clinical response and the side effects. If side effects do not occur, a maximum of 400 mg a day may be reached, (the required dosage, however, is usually in the range of 50 mg three times daily).[42]

Since the disease has a tendency to remission after several years, as with sulfapyridine therapy, once a favorable response is achieved (usually within a week) the dose is decreased gradually to a minimum level (generally 25 to 50 mg daily). Unfortunately, in most patients, long-term therapy is generally the rule. In addition to hemolysis, side effects of dapsone therapy include methemoboglobinemia (manifested by bluish discoloration of the face, mucous membranes, and nails), nausea, vomiting, headache, giddiness, tachycardia, psychoses, anemia, fever, exfoliative dermatitis, liver necrosis, lymphadenitis, and peripheral neuropathy. Although leukopenia rarely occurs, complete blood counts and urinalyses should be checked at monthly intervals during the first year of therapy (after that, about three-month intervals appear to be adequate).

Since a high percentage of patients with dermatitis herpetiformis appear to have an associated gluten-sensitive enteropathy, it is recommended that patients have small-intestine studies for the possibility of this association. Although gluten-free diets (avoidance of foods containing wheat, rye, and barley flour) have been suggested in an attempt to reduce the symptoms of malabsorption, the conclusions of studies vary as to the efficacy of such diets on cutaneous lesions. Although the problems of maintaining a gluten-free diet make such therapy difficult for most patients, most investigators agree that a substantial number of patients will respond to a strict gluten-free diet over several months to two years, enabling them to reduce their dosage of sulfapyridine or sulfone substantially and, in some cases, to completely discontinue drug therapy.

Local applications of steroid creams of shake lotions such as Calamine lotion with menthol or phenol may diminish pruritus and permit control of the disorder with lower doses of systemic preparations. For patients who can neither tolerate sulfapyridine nor sulfone therapy, systemic corticosteroids (although not very effective) may be tried.

Epidermolysis Bullosa

Epidermolysis bullosa (EB) is a term applied to a group of inherited disorders characterized by bullous lesions that develop spontaneously or as a result of varying degrees of friction or trauma. Although the absence or presence of permanent scarring allows the disorder to be divided into two major groups, those that may result in healing without scarring and those that inevitably produce scars, current classifications of this complex and heterogeneous group of diseases depend to a large extent on the level of skin where the blistering occurs. Thus EB can now be divided into three major categories: (1) epidermolytic EB or EB simplex, where blister cleavage occurs within the epidermis and healing occurs without scarring; (2) junctional EB, where the skin separates in the lamina lucida of the dermoepidermal junction and blistering leads to mild atrophic changes; and (3) dermolytic or dystrophic (scarring) EB, where the blister forms below the basement membrane, in the papillary dermis, and healing results in dystrophy or scarring of the skin[42-46] (Table 9–3). Although the exact prevalence of epidermolysis bullosa is not known, mild variants have been estimated to occur as frequently as 1 in every 50,000 births and the more severe varieties are believed to occur in 1 per 500,000 population per year.[43]

Epidermolytic (nondystrophic, EB simplex)

Generalized EB simplex is an autosomal dominant disorder in which the bullae heal without scarring, mucosal involvement is mild, and the nails are rarely affected (if they are shed, they regrow without dystrophy or, on rare occasions, with longitudinal striations and/or brittleness). The disease often improves at puberty and patients usually have a normal lifespan (Fig 9–2). Electron microscopic examination in EBS shows cleavage through the basal layer (above the PAS-positive basement membrane of the epidermis), formation of vacuoles in the basal cells adjacent to areas of separation, and displacement of nuclei to the epidermal end of the involved cells. Although no specific histochemical abnormality has been delineated, the defect appears to be related to mechanical trauma and activation of temperature-

TABLE 9–3.—CLASSIFICATION OF HEREDITARY EPIDERMOLYSIS BULLOSA

TYPE	INHERITANCE	BLISTER LOCATION	STRUCTURAL DEFECT AND SPECIAL FEATURES
Simplex (Epidermolytic, nondystrophic)			
Generalized EB Simplex (Koebner)	AD*	Basal cells	Basal cell cytolysis
Localized EB Simplex (Weber-Cockayne)	AD	Basal and suprabasal cells	Basal and spinous cell cytolysis
Herpetiform (Dowling-Meara)	AD	Basal cells	Basal cell cytolysis preceded by clumping of tonofilaments and attachment to the hemidesmosomes
EB Simplex (Ogna variant, Gedde-Dahl)	AD	Intraepidermal	Basal cell cytolysis; bruising; linkage with glutamic pyruvic transaminase locus
Junctional (Atrophic)			
Junctional EB (Herlitz, lethal variant)	AR**	Lamina lucida	Reduced numbers and abnormal structure of hemidesmosomes
Generalized (nonlethal)	AR	Lamina lucida	
Dystrophic (Dermolytic)			
Recessive dystrophic (RDEB, generalized)	AD	Below basal lamina	Absence or decreased anchoring fibrils and collagenolysis
Recessive dystrophic (RDEB, localized)	AR	Below basal lamina	Reduced numbers of anchoring fibrils
Dominant dystrophic (DDEB)	AD	Below basal lamina	Anchoring fibrils decreased and abnormal in areas of blister-prone skin
Cockayne-Touraine variant	AD	Below basal lamina	Anchoring fibrils decreased
Pasini variant (albopapuloid)	AD	Below basal lamina	Anchoring fibrils decreased in all skin areas, abnormality of glycosaminoglycan synthesis

* Autosomal dominant; ** Autosomal recessive
(Modified from Briggaman R.A.: Ref. 46 and Eady R.A.J. and Tidman M.J.T.: Ref. 47.)

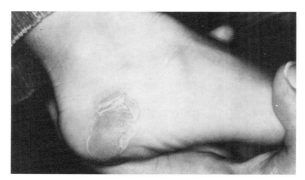

Fig 9–2.—Epidermolysis bullosa simplex. Blisters develop in areas of trauma and heal without subsequent scar formation. (From Hurwitz S., Epidermolysis bullosa, in Hurwitz S.: *Clinical Pediatric Dermatology.* W.B. Saunders Publishing Co., Philadelphia, 1981. Used by permission.)

sensitive cytolytic enzymes, defective structural proteins, or perhaps deficiencies of galactosylhydroxylysyl glucosyltransferase and gelatinase (enzymes involved in collagen degradation) in skin fibroblasts.[43]

Localized EB simplex (Weber-Cockayne, Bullous Eruptions of the Hands and Feet) is an autosomal dominant clinical variant that requires a higher threshold of frictional trauma to induce blister formation. Bullae are confined to the hands and feet (primarily the palms and soles) and are associated with hyperhidrosis and hyperkeratosis. Although blisters can occur in the first year or two of life, they frequently do not appear until adolescence or early adulthood. The blisters usually are associated with trauma, particularly in hot weather, and the disorder is usually not seriously debilitating. Lesions generally heal rapidly without scarring, nail involvement rarely occurs, and the teeth and mucous membranes are not involved. Although the pathophysiology of localized EB simplex is unknown, it appears to represent an exaggeration of the normal mechanism for production of friction blisters, possibly related to activation of a cytolytic enzyme (or enzymes) and an associated dyskeratosis of squamous cells in the epidermis.

As in generalized epidermolysis bullosa simplex, cytolysis of epidermal cells is the essential histologic feature of localized EB simplex. Epidermal cleavage usually appears in the mid-squamous area but may occur anywhere, from the suprabasal to the lower granular cell layers of the epidermis. In contrast to generalized EB simplex, the basal cells are spared.

EB herpetiformis (Dowling-Meara) is an autosomal dominant disorder characterized by blistering (often extensive) at birth or in early infancy. Herpetiform lesions on the trunk and proximal extremities, a distinctive feature of the disease, are commonly seen during childhood and hyperkeratosis of the palms and soles may occur after the age of 6.[44] Involvement of the mucosae and nails may occur during the neonatal period and although nails may shed they regrow without dystrophy. Blistering early in life may be accompanied by intense inflammation and milia formation. With extensive blistering, the disease may prove life-threatening, and there is significant morbidity and mortality during the neonatal period. After this period, the blistering is rarely a threat to life and the blistering tends to decrease during later childhood and adulthood.

EB simplex (Ogna variant) was originally recognized in a large pedigree from Ogna, Norway. It has its onset in infancy and is characterized by small hemorrhagic and serous blisters that occur on the hands and feet, and occasionally elsewhere, that heal without scarring. The distinguishing features of this disorder are onychogryphosis of the great toenails, an associated bruising tendency and genetic linkage to the glutamic pyruvic transaminase (GPT) locus.[44]

Junctional EB

Junctional EB (Herlitz variant) is a severe, often but not necessarily fatal, autosomal recessive disorder characterized by spontaneous bullae and large areas of erosion in which about 50% of patients die within the first two years of life. Healing frequently results in mild atrophic changes without scarring or milia formation. The oral mucous membranes are frequently affected, but pyloric atresia rarely occurs. The hands and feet are usually spared except for involvement of the nailfolds with blistering of the fingertips (an important if not diagnostic feature) and, at times, loss of nails. The teeth may be dysplastic, and a cobblestone appearance to the dental enamel is characteristic. Perioral involvement with sparing of the lips is said to be pathognomonic. Although patients who survive to adulthood do so without scars, severe growth retardation and recalcitrant anemia are common.

Generalized atrophic (benign) EB begins with serosanguineous blistering at birth and results in cutaneous atrophy and fragility but without scarring or milia formation. The nails may become dystrophic, hyperkeratosis of the palms and soles occurs frequently, mucous membrane involvement is mild, affected individuals generally have normal growth and lifespan, and atrophy of the scalp and alopecia are common.

Dystrophic (Dermolytic) EB

Recessive dystrophic epidermolysis bullosa (RDEB) may be mild and localized or a generalized severe distressing disorder characterized by widespread dystrophic scarring deformity and severe involvement of the mucous membranes. Although some blisters may appear to occur spontaneously, most seem to arise at sites of pressure or trauma (Fig 9–3). Bullae are often followed by atrophic scars that may fuse the fingers and toes with resulting pseudosyndactyly or mitten-like deformities (Fig 9–4). Blisters and erosions in the oral mucosa may limit eating and immobilize the tongue; esophageal webs, strictures, or pyloric atresia may occur and laryngeal bullae may produce respiratory stridor. The teeth are malformed and carious. Anemia due to chronic blood loss, poor nutrition and chronic disease is common. Cutaneous neoplasms may occur as a complication of this disorder,[50] and failure to thrive and secondary bacterial or candidal infection of the skin are frequently seen in individuals with this disorder.

Histopathologic examination of involved skin in dystrophic forms of epidermolysis bullosa reveals separation at the dermal-epidermal junction, fragmentation of collagen bundles in the floor of blisters, and a lymphohistiocytic infiltrate with extravasation of erythrocytes. Electron microscopy shows separation beneath the basal lamina (on the dermal side of the dermal-epidermal junction) and absence of anchoring fibrils in normal as well as blistered skin. The abnormality resides in the dermis.

The absence of anchoring fibrils (the apparent primary structural defect in recessive forms of dystrophic epidermolysis bullosa) allows disruption of

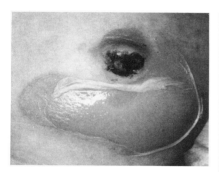

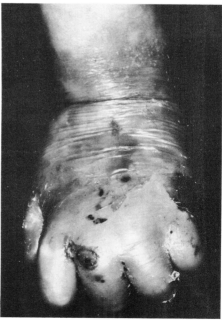

Fig 9–3 (above).—Recessive dystrophic epidermolysis bullosa. A large blister on the lower aspect of the abdomen of a newborn.

Fig 9–4 (right).—Pseudosyndactyly and fusion of the fingers in a flexed immobile position (mitten-like deformities) in a 3½-year-old child with recessive dystrophic epidermolysis bullosa (RDEB).

the structural integrity of the epidermal-dermal junction and subsequent blister formation.[51] Although anchoring fibrils are lacking in damaged skin of patients with dominant forms of dystrophic epidermolysis bullosa, studies of a large kindred revealed normal fibrils in the noninvolved skin of individuals with this disorder. This suggests a possible means of differentiating dominant from recessive forms of this disorder, but it requires confirmation.

The pathogenesis of recessive dystrophic epidermolysis is unknown. Two proposed mechanisms include: (1) destruction of dermal connective tissue by excessive amounts of a protease, and (2) abnormality of structural protein in the dermis which is ordinarily responsible for the integrity of the dermal-epidermal junction.[43] The most likely defect that would account for the pathologic alterations seen in dystrophic forms of epidermolysis bullosa therefore appears to be a structural abnormality of the dermal connective tissue, most probably the collagen, with an associated impaired function of anchoring fibrils. The role of collagenase in the pathophysiology of dystrophic epidermolysis bullosa has been suggested by observations of elevated collagenase levels in friction blisters of patients with the recessive form of this disorder.[52–54] Lazarus, however, has noted that elevated collagenase levels only appear in active lesions of dystrophic EB, without increased urinary hydroxyproline. He suggests that the increased collagenase activity in lesions of dystrophic epidermolysis bullosa may be secondary to tissue injury (rather than a primary abnormality) in individuals with this disorder.[55] Collagenase has also been found to be present in greater concentrations in fibroblast cultures of patients with recessive dystrophic epidermolysis bullosa than in control studies. Partially purified preparations of this enzyme display marked thermal lability and diminished affinity for $Ca++$, suggesting the existence of a mutant enzyme. These data suggest that three biochemical abnormalities (increased synthesis, decreased thermal stability, and diminished affinity for $Ca++$) may serve as in vitro markers for recessive dystrophic epidermolysis bullosa and may prove helpful in the prenatal diagnosis of this disorder.[56]

Dominant dystrophic epidermolysis bullosa (DDEB), a disorder of intermediate severity, usually begins in infancy. Also characterized by atrophic scarring, nail dystrophy and milia formation, in milder cases the onset of blisters may occur later in life. Although mucous membrane lesions appear in 20% of cases, they do not present the severe problems seen in patients with the recessive dystrophic disease. Bullae generally appear on the dorsal aspect of the extremities (Fig 9–5), milia are frequently present, and atrophic scars occur. The teeth generally are not affected, the hair is not affected, physical and mental development is normal, and the conjunctiva and cornea are less likely to be involved. In 80% of cases, the nails may

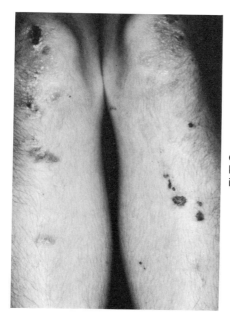

Fig 9–5.—Dominant dystrophic epidermolysis bullosa. Blisters over the knees and pretibial surface of the legs in an 11-year-old girl.

be thickened, dystrophic, or completely destroyed. The *albopapuloid form of dominant dystrophic EB*, although occasionally present in infancy, usually begins in later childhood, early adolescence, or adult life. This disorder is characterized by small, firm, ivory-white perifollicular papules that vary in size from several millimeters to a centimeter or more in diameter and normally occur on the lower back (Fig 9–6).

Milia characteristically are seen as 1 to 2 mm firm white globoid lesions at the sites of healed bullae. They are not specific for this disorder and often are present in recessive dystrophic EB and chronically traumatized skin (Fig 9–7). Also seen in porphyria and following dermabrasion, they appear to represent retention cysts caused by occlusion of pilosebaceous units. Although mutilating scars are rarely seen, soft, superficial, atrophic scars with wrinkled surfaces may develop as bullae heal. Erythematous plaques caused by mild trauma (insufficient to cause blistering) are also frequently seen. Hyperpigmentation or depigmentation may be found at healed blister sites, and hypertrophic and keloidal lesions occasionally occur.

Mucous membrane lesions appear in 20% of cases but do not present the severe problems seen in the recessive form of this disorder. The teeth generally are not affected, but oral milia resulting from detached islands of

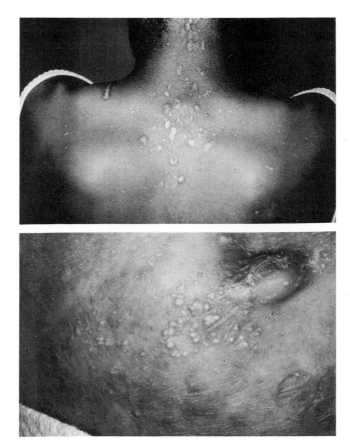

Fig 9–6 (top).—Albopapuloid form of epidermolysis bullosa. Small firm ivory-white perifollicular papules on the trunk of a patient with dominant dystrophic epidermolysis bullosa. (Courtesy of Robert A. Briggaman, M.D., from Hurwitz S.: Epidermolysis bullosa, in Hurwitz S.: *Clinical Pediatric Dermatology.* W.B. Saunders Co., Philadelphia, 1981. Used by permission.)

Fig 9–7 (bottom).—Erosions, superficial tissue-paper scars and milia on the abdomen of a 6-month-old infant with recessive dystrophic epidermolysis bullosa.

epithelium in areas of earlier bulla formation may be noted. The hair is not affected; physical and mental development are normal; and, in contrast to the recessive dystrophic disorder, the conjunctiva and cornea are never involved. However, in 80% of cases, the nails are thickened, dystrophic, and, at times, completely destroyed.

Other Forms of Epidermolysis Bullosa

Bart Syndrome.—In 1966, Bart and associates described a mechanobullous syndrome consisting of skin defects that affect the lower extremities, with blistering of the skin and mucous membranes and deformity of the nails.[57] Although the disorder appears to be autosomal dominant, isolated cases suggest the possibility of variable penetrance or spontaneous mutation.[58]

Some patients have only mouth erosions; others have deformed nails, recurrent blistering, or the complete syndrome, with characteristic localized, sharply marginated skin defects on the legs. Other skin defects, apparently due to mechanobullous phenomena induced by local shearing trauma, may appear as extensive erosions on the extensor aspects of the extremities, intertriginous areas, neck, and buttocks. Although skin and mucous membrane erosions heal without scarring, milia and occasional residual hypopigmentation may be noted.

Histologically, skin lesions show loss of the epidermis, an intact dermis with the basement membrane on the dermal side of the split, and normal adnexa and subcutaneous tissue. A tendency toward progressive spontaneous improvement without residual defects emphasizes the importance of early recognition and conservative management of individuals with this disorder.[58]

Acquired epidermolysis bullosa.—Acquired epidermolysis bullosa (epidermolysis bullosa acquisita) is a nonhereditary, late-onset bullous disorder that is first manifested in adolescence or adulthood and characterized by blister formation below the basement membrane. Ultrastructural findings are similar to those seen in the hereditary forms of dystrophic epidermolysis bullosa and most closely resemble those of the dominantly inherited disease. Patients with epidermolysis acquisita generally appear with a peculiar susceptibility to blister formation following trauma or pressure. The disorder is manifested by vesicles, bullae, and erosions over the pressure areas of the ears, elbows, knees, and particularly hands and feet. Scarring, milia, and nail dystrophy occur. Although the teeth are normal and mucous membrane erosions are frequently seen, the conjunctival, esophageal, and genitoanal mucous membranes are not involved.[59]

Diagnostic criteria of epidermolysis bullosa acquisita include bullae over the joints of hands, feet, elbows, and knees secondary to minor trauma; atrophic scars; milia; nail dystrophy; late-onset (adolescence or adulthood), and a negative family history of epidermolysis bullosa. The disorder has been seen in association with poison oak dermatitis, dermatitis herpetiformis, inflammatory bowel disorders (Crohn's disease), impetigo, scarlet fever, tuberculosis, porphyria, cutaneous amyloidosis, Ehlers-Danlos syndrome, and ingestion of sulfonamides, arsenic, and penicillamine.

TREATMENT.—As in any inherited disorder, it is the responsibility of the physician to inform parents of the risks associated with transmitting genetic abnormalities. When the condition is determined by a dominant gene (as in dominant dystrophic epidermolysis bullosa), if one parent is affected, there is a 50% risk that each child will be so afflicted. In a family in which a child manifests abnormalities due to a recessive gene (as in recessive dystrophic epidermolysis bullosa), parents must be prepared to risk a 25% possibility of this severe disorder occurring in future offspring.

The treatment of epidermolysis bullosa is palliative, with avoidance of trauma and control of secondary infection. Since blisters result from mechanical injury, measures should be taken to relieve pressure and prevent unnecessary trauma. A cool environment, avoidance of overheating, and lubrication of the skin to decrease the surface coefficient of friction are helpful in the reduction of blister formation. When blisters occur, extension may be prevented by aseptic aspiration of blister fluid. The roofs of blisters should be trimmed with a sterile scissors whenever feasible, and no ragged edges should be left under which organisms may flourish and lead to secondary infection.

A water mattress and a soft fleece covering will help to limit friction and trauma. Daily baths, saline soaks for crusted lesions followed by topical antibiotics, topical protective antibiotic dressings, or sterile Vaseline-impregnated gauze applied with sterile precautions may help reduce cutaneous bacterial infection and assist spontaneous healing of involved areas. Large denuded areas should be treated, whenever possible, by the open method (as in treatment of burns) with intravenous fluids, appropriate systemic antibiotics when indicated, and protection of injured areas by protective dressings and sterile Vaseline-impregnated gauze is helpful.

Although it has been stated that high concentration topical corticosteroid preparations may facilitate healing of chronically blistered areas,[60] this has not been verified. If sepsis is to be prevented or controlled, especially in the newborn and young infant, careful monitoring of the skin and mucosal florae is essential. In severe dystrophic forms of epidermolysis bullosa, prophylactic antibiotics such as penicillin and erythromycin are valuable. They lessen the tendency to local infection, sepsis, and severe scarring, and help prevent the risk of glomerulonephritis secondary to cutaneous streptococcal infection.

Oral vitamin E (DL-alpha tocopherol) has been suggested for the treatment of patients with epidermolysis.[61] Vitamin E is an antioxidant that enhances the activity of some enzymes and perhaps induces the synthesis of others. Although there are reports of favorable responses to oral vitamin

E in dosages of up to 2000 units per day, most studies do not confirm its value in the prevention of blistering and scarring.[62] However, vitamin, iron, and protein supplements are advisable if nutritional compromise exists.

Dysphagia is the major symptom of esophageal involvement in recessive dystrophic epidermolysis bullosa. It may result from a reversible inflammatory reaction or from a permanent stricture. Barium studies demonstrate esophageal lesions; endoscopy, however, is not recommended. Softening of the diet for several weeks may result in modest to marked improvement of symptoms. If conservative management fails to result in proper nourishment, bougienage, surgery, or both should be considered.[63, 64] Once bougienage has been initiated, however, some patients may require the procedure at frequent intervals. In those instances where surgery must be considered, colon transplant procedures have been successful.[65] With repeated blistering, ulceration, and scar formation, carcinomata may sometimes develop on the involved skin or mucous membrane. Although the cause of carcinoma is unknown, abnormal collagen formation in heavily scarred areas with continuous blistering activity appears to predispose to this complication.[50, 66]

Systemic steroids have been tried in all forms of epidermolysis bullosa. Although they appear to have value in the management of junctional bullous dermatosis (epidermolysis bullosa letalis, Herlitz disease), present studies do not substantiate reports that high dose systemic steroids prevent the scarring and mutilation in severe dystrophic forms of this disorder. Moynahan, however, feels that systemic steroids in high doses (140 to 160 mg of prednisone or its equivalent per day) may be life-saving in some cases of severe dystrophic forms during the neonatal periods.[60] Since high doses may be required for several weeks or months, if this form of therapy is initiated, it should be utilized only with recognition of the potential risks of associated complications, particularly sepsis. The value of systemic steroids in the long-term management of severe forms of epidermolysis bullosa remains controversial.

Oral diphenylhydantoin (Dilantin) has recently been suggested for the treatment of dystrophic and junctional forms of epidermolysis bullosa.[67–69] This form of therapy is based on the fact that diphenylhydantoin in pharmacological doses has been shown to cause significant inhibition of collagenolytic activity both in vivo and in vitro. Although large clinical trials are required before this can be accepted as an effective form of therapy, diphenylhydantoin (Dilantin) in dosages of 2.5 to 5.0 mg/kg of body weight per day, to a maximum dose of 200 mg per day (a dosage high enough to obtain serum levels of 5 to 12 mcg per milliliter), may prove helpful in the treatment of junctional and recessive dystrophic forms of this disorder.[68, 69]

The nursing care of the infant or child with severe epidermolysis bullosa is time-consuming and difficult. Dental hygiene is difficult in patients with severe oral and dental involvement. Attempts should be made to clean the teeth with a soft toothbrush and a pulsating device (such as the Water-Pik). Periodic care by a pediatric dentist is helpful. Restoration of function in severe fusion and flexion deformities of the hands and feet can often be helped by physiotherapy and appropriate plastic surgery. Mild cases of the dystrophic and nondystrophic types may be compatible with a nearly normal life. The severe dystrophic forms, however, remain a challenge and require cooperation by patient, parents, and physician.

Parental support and information groups are beneficial to many families who have children with epidermolysis bullosa. The Dystrophic Epidermolysis Bullosa Research Association (D.E.B.R.A.) is a national and international group dedicated to research and support for patients with all forms of epidermolysis and their families. In the United States, information regarding this organization may be obtained from Ms. Arlene Pessar, R.N.: D.E.B.R.A. of America, Inc.; 2936 Avenue W; Brooklyn, New York 11229.

Peutz-Jeghers Syndrome

The syndrome of mucocutaneous pigmentation and gastrointestinal polyposis constitutes a unique autosomal dominant disorder designated by the names of the physicians who first described the disorder in 1921 and 1949 respectively.[70]

CLINICAL MANIFESTATIONS.—The characteristic features of the Peutz-Jeghers syndrome are dark brown pigmented macules of the skin that clinically resemble lentigines and hamartomatous polyps of the gastrointestinal tract (Table 9–4). The cutaneous marker of this syndrome usually appears

TABLE 9–4.—PEUTZ-JEGHERS SYNDROME

1. Autosomal dominant
2. Cutaneous lesions usually first appear within first two years of life
   a. Flat dark brown or black pigmented macules
     (1) Usually oval, elliptical or rod-shaped
     (2) Less than 5 mm in diameter
   b. Most common on lips, perioral and perianal regions, and distal aspects of limbs
3. Gastrointestinal polyps (benign hamartomas)
   a. 96% of cases in small bowel
   b. A low incidence of malignancy (2% to 6%)
   c. Most common symptoms are recurrent attacks of colicky pain, intussusception, hematemesis, and/or melena
4. Conservative management with careful follow-up examinations (elective major resection generally not indicated)

during the first year or two of life and increases during childhood. These flat, darkly pigmented lesions are irregularly oval, elliptical, or rod-shaped, usually measure less than 5 mm in diameter, and are most commonly seen on the lips, perioral regions, the buccal mucosa, nasal and periorbital regions, elbows, dorsal aspects of the fingers and toes, palms, soles, and perianal or labial regions; occasionally the gums and hard palate, and, on rare occasion, even the tongue may be involved. The pigmented lesions on the skin and lips frequently fade after puberty; those on the buccal mucosa, palate, and tongue, however, persist.

Although some authors classify the pigmentary lesions of Peutz-Jeghers syndrome with freckles, histologic demonstration of increased melanocytes in the basal layer of the skin and mucous membranes suggest them to be either lentigines or a separate and distinct form of melanosis.

The gastrointestinal polyps seen in this disorder may be found from the gastroesophageal junction down to the anal canal; the small bowel represents the most frequently involved portion of the intestinal tract (96% of cases). The polyps represent benign hamartomas and have a low malignant potential (2% to 6%).[71, 72] The polyps may vary in size from minute pinhead lesions to those measuring several centimeters in diameter. They may occur in early childhood, but frequently develop during the second decade of life.

Symptoms in the pediatric patient frequently consist of abdominal pain, melena, or intussusception. The most common symptom, recurrent attacks of colicky abdominal pain, is believed to result from recurring transient episodes of incomplete intussusception. Hematemesis, although less common, may occur owing to involvement of the stomach, duodenum, or upper jejunum. Carcinoma rarely develops in the gross polyps of this disorder, but has been associated with micropolyposis of the mucosa of the colon or gastroduodenal area.[71–77] Death in young individuals is generally attributed to intestinal obstruction. In older individuals, however, neoplastic disease is an important cause of death.

DIAGNOSIS.—The diagnosis of Peutz-Jeghers syndrome is usually made by the finding of characteristic pigmented macules of the skin and mucous membranes, gastrointestinal symptoms, a history of multiple abdominal surgical procedures, or both. In patients where there is a positive family history, the diagnosis is more easily made. Some patients may have only skin pigmentation or pigmentation limited to the buccal mucosa with only vague abdominal symptoms. In such cases the diagnosis is more difficult and gastrointestinal x-rays, sigmoidoscopy, gastroscopy, and biopsy may be necessary to determine the presence of gastrointestinal polyps.

TREATMENT.—The therapeutic management of polyposis in Peutz-Jeghers syndrome is limited to the relief of symptoms rather than radical multiple resections that may lead to malabsorption.[73–75] Multiple individual poly-pectomis are the treatment of choice when small bowel lesions become symptomatic and elective major resection of benign polyps is not indicated. After initial evaluation, such patients can be followed by barium contrast studies, gastroscopy, and gastric cytology. When the colon or rectum is involved, however, the possibility of an independently developing malig-nancy suggests careful inspection and prophylactic resection, just as if the Peutz-Jeghers syndrome did not exist.[73]

Dyskeratosis Congenita

Dyskeratosis congenita is a rare genetic disorder characterized by a triad of congenital atrophy, reticulated hyperpigmentation and telangiectasia of the skin; nail dystrophy; and whitish thickening (leukokeratosis) of the oral and, at times, anal mucosa (Table 9–5). Almost all reported cases have been males, and available pedigrees suggest it to be an X-linked recessive disorder.[77]

CLINICAL MANIFESTATIONS.—Nail changes are usually the first to make their appearance (Fig 9–8). Between the ages of 5 and 13, they become thin and dystrophic. In mild cases they develop ridging and longitudinal grooving; in severe forms they are shortened and, at times, almost nonex-istent. Cutaneous changes may develop simultaneously or in a few years following the onset of nail changes and reach their full development within three to five years. A fine reticulated grayish-brown hyperpigmentation (surrounding hypopigmented and atrophic patches of uninvolved skin) on the face, neck, shoulders, upper back, and thighs is characteristic of this disorder. Other cutaneous changes may include telangiectasia of the trunk, redness and atrophy of the face with irregular macular hyperpigmentation, palmoplantar hyperkeratosis, hyperhidrosis of the palms and soles, and a diffuse atrophic, transparent, and shiny appearance on the dorsal aspects of the hands and feet. There may be associated atrophic changes of the muscles and bones of the hands and feet, giving the palms a "cupped" appearance. Bullae frequently occur on the palms and soles (these are be-lieved to be induced by trauma); eyebrows and eyelashes may be absent,

TABLE 9–5.—DYSKERATOSIS CONGENITA

1. A rare X-linked disorder (affects mostly males)
2. A triad of poikilodermatous lesions (atrophy, hyperpigmentation and telangiectasia); nail dystrophy, and leukoplakia (leukokeratosis of oral and, at times, anal mucosa)
3. Cutaneous malignancy (predominantly epidermoid carcinoma) and carcinoma in areas of leukoplakia (usually between third and fifth decades)

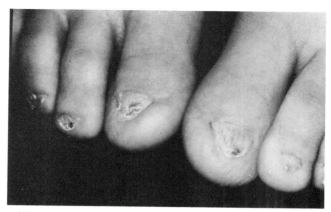

Fig 9–8.—Dyskeratosis congenita. Thin dystrophic nails with longitudinal grooving.

and the hair of the scalp, eyebrows, and eyelashes are lusterless and frequently sparse.[77–79]

Mucous membrane changes consist of small blisters, erosions, and subsequent leukoplakia of the oral and anal mucosa (Fig 9–9), esophagus, and urethra. Similar changes of the tarsal conjunctiva may result in atresia of the lacrimal ducts, excessive lacrimation, chronic blepharitis, conjunctivitis, and ectropion. The teeth tend to be defective and subject to early decay. Peridontitis may develop, and affected individuals have an increased incidence of cutaneous malignancy (predominantly epidermoid carcinoma) and a high incidence of carcinoma in the areas of leukoplakia.[78, 80, 81] The latter complication has been noted in up to one-third of reported cases and usually appears between the third and fifth decades of life.

In some patients a severe hematologic disease resembling Fanconi's anemia has been reported. In these patients, there is severe anemia with leukopenia (especially neutropenia), thrombocytopenia terminating in a severe

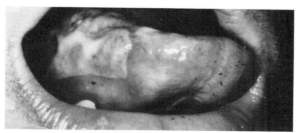

Fig 9–9.—Dyskeratosis congenita. Erosions and leukoplakia of the tongue.

pancytopenia, splenomegaly, and, at times, hemorrhagic diatheses.[78, 83] Other features include prenatal and postnatal growth retardation, mental retardation, elevated immunoglobulin levels, gastrointestinal hemorrhage from mucosal ulceration, intracranial calcification, and nutmeg-like cirrhotic changes of the liver.[84] Opportunistic infection, sepsis, leukemia, gastrointestinal bleeding, and generalized debilitation are common. Patients seldom survive beyond 50 years of age, with death generally being attributed to cancer, leukemia, hemorrhage, or sepsis.[77]

DIAGNOSIS.—The diagnosis of patients with dyskeratosis congenita is dependent upon the clinical history and characteristic features, with nearly all patients eventually manifesting the diagnostic triad of cutaneous pigmentation, nail dystrophy, and leukoplakia. There are no consistent laboratory abnormalities available to confirm the diagnosis, but approximately 50% of the patients manifest an anemia or pancytopenia secondary to bone marrow hypoplasia. Cultured cells of patients with dyskeratosis congenita grow poorly and have a reduced culture life-span. Chromosomes of cells of patients show a greater increase in sister chromatid exchanges after exposure to psoralens plus ultraviolet light than do cells of normal persons.[80] Cells of affected patients also show delayed excision of psoralen-DNA cross-linking photoadducts, suggesting a defect in the repair of DNA cross-links in patients with this disorder.[82]

Histopathologic examination of cutaneous lesions reveal a poikilodermatous picture with thinning of the epidermis. The epidermis is thin and some of the basal cells have vacuolization of the cytoplasm.[79] The dermal collagen is edematous with fragmentation of the elastic tissue. The areas of mucous membrane leukoplakia may reveal hyperkeratosis, and cellular atypia. At times, squamous cell carcinoma may be present.

TREATMENT.—The management of patients with dyskeratosis congenita consists of bougienage for esophageal stenosis, fulguration, curettage, and surgical excision of leukokeratosis of the buccal and anal mucosae, and regular supervision for early detection of mucosal or cutaneous carcinomata.

Pyoderma Gangrenosum

Pyoderma gangrenosum is a severe, chronic, inflammatory disorder of the skin characterized by a painful sloughing ulceration with purulent base and an elevated dusky blue or purple undermined border surrounded by a red areola. Although the disorder may be seen without associated disease, it frequently develops in patients with a variety of systemic disorders, namely ulcerative colitis, regional enteritis, a rheumatoid arthritis-like disorder, chronic hepatic disease, hematologic disorders (myelogenous leukemia, acute lymphoblastic leukemia, myeloid metaplasia, and polycythemia vera), and various paraproteinemias, including multiple myeloma.[85] Despite many hypotheses, the cause of pyoderma gangrenosum remains unknown. On the basis of recent histologic, clinical and immunologic data, however, it appears to have an immunogenic etiology, perhaps a cell-mediated hypersensitivity or a vasculitis triggered by a variety of predisposing factors[85-87] (Table 9-6).

CLINICAL MANIFESTATIONS.—Pyoderma gangrenosum is characterized by single or multiple cutaneous ulcerations with an irregular purulent base and an elevated dusky blue or purplish-red ragged undermined border surrounded by a red areola. The ulcers begin as pustules or as fluctuant tender nodules which break down leaving moist, necrotic, red granular ulcerations occasionally covered by a yellow exudate. Although usually seen in adults, the disorder has also been seen in infants and children (particularly adolescents).[88]

DIAGNOSIS.—The diagnosis of pyoderma gangrenosum is based upon clinical features and the elimination of other causes of cutaneous ulceration simulating this condition. The histologic appearance of lesions is not diagnostic. Early lesions show areas of necrosis with edema and infiltration of polymorphonuclear leukocytes and lymphocytes; older lesions show epidermal proliferation, acanthosis, fibroblastic activity and, on occasion, multinucleated giant cells.[89]

TREATMENT.—Since the pathogenesis of pyoderma gangrenosum remains unknown, the treatment is empirical and relies on various systemic and topical approaches in conjunction with a vigorous attempt to control the underlying disease. Topical therapy is directed toward debridement of the underlying base of lesions, continuous soaks with 0.25% acetic acid, wet dressings with potassium permanganate, whirlpool baths, silver sulfadiazine cream, benzoyl peroxide, pigskin dressings, hyperbaric oxygen, topical steroid creams, and intralesional steroids. Systemic steroids are usually the drug of choice for patients resistant to topical therapy. If pathogenic organism can be cultured from lesions, specific antibiotic therapy may be instituted. Other therapeutic modalities include dapsone, sulfapyridine, minocycline, clofazimine, rifampin, thalidomode and immunosup-

TABLE 9–6.—PYODERMA GANGRENOSUM

1. A painful ulceration with purulent base, undermined elevated border and a surrounding red areola
2. An immunologic abnormality (cell-mediated hypersensitivity or vasculitis)?
3. May be seen in association with ulcerative colitis, regional enteritis, chronic hepatitis, arthritis, various paraproteinemias and hematologic disorders
4. Treatment: topical therapy, intralesional steroids, systemic steroids, dapsone, sulfapyridine and perhaps rifampin, thalidomide, clofazimine or immunosuppressive therapy

pressive agents, but their efficacy requires further investigation and evaluation.[90-92]

Gardner's Syndrome

Gardner's syndrome is a rare autosomal dominantly transmitted disorder with an estimated incidence of 1 in 14,000 births. The main features of this disorder include: (1) intestinal polyposis; (2) epidermal cysts (especially on the face and scalp); (3) osteomas with a predilection for the membranous bones of the head; and (4) fibrous tumors located in the skin, subcutaneous tissue, or abdominal cavity, or desmoid tumors that invade adjacent muscles[93, 94] (Table 9–7). Oldfield's syndrome, a familial condition of multiple sebaceous cysts associated with premalignant polyposis of the colon, may be a distinct entity or may merely represent a variant of Gardner's syndrome.

CLINICAL MANIFESTATIONS.—Skin lesions and bony abnormalities are generally the first sign of Gardner's syndrome. Epidermoid cysts, the most common skin lesions seen in Gardner's syndrome, are present in 63% of cases. Although they may occur anywhere on the cutaneous surface, they have a predilection for the face and scalp. They may be present at birth or early infancy, increase in size and number for a period of years, and then stabilize. Osteomas occur in over 50% of patients. Although they may occur anywhere on the body, they have a predilection for the membranous bones of the face and head and have been noted in children as young as eight years of age. Other skin lesions include fibromas, desmoid tumors, and fibrosarcomas.[93] Other benign skin tumors less commonly seen are lipomas, leiomyomas, trichoepitheliomas and neurofibromas. Fibromas may occur intracutaneously, subcutaneously, in the mesentery, or retroperitonally. Desmoid tumors may develop spontaneously or at incision sites following surgery (probably from the muscle aponeuroses).

Intestinal polyps, rarely seen in children prior to the age of 10, appear gradually and increase in number during the second decade of life. By age 20, about 50% of patients with Gardner's syndrome will have demonstrable

TABLE 9–7.—GARDNER'S SYNDROME

1. A rare autosomal dominant disorder
2. Intestinal polyposis, epidermal cysts, osteomas, and fibrous or desmoid tumors
3. Periodic proctoscopic examination and x-ray of colon recommended for patients with multiple epidermal cysts (particularly if seen with osteomas)
4. Since there is a high risk of cancer, genetic counseling and early prophylactic colectomy is recommended for patients with polyposis in this area

polyps. Carcinomatous degeneration, rare before the age of 20, is common in patients between 20 and 30 years of age. If patients do not die of other causes, the potential for malignant change appears to be 100%.[94]

DIAGNOSIS.—The combination of osteomas and sebaceous cysts occurs in no other entity. Patients with multiple sebaceous or epidermal cysts, particularly if seen in association with osteomas, therefore. should be carefully investigated for the possibility of intestinal polyposis. Examination should include periodic proctoscopic examination and x-ray examination of the colon. Carcinoma of the small intestine has also been noted. Roentgenologic studies of the upper gastrointestinal tract are also indicated for individuals affected with this disorder.

TREATMENT.—Since this is an autosomal dominant disorder with a high risk of cancer, genetic counseling and early, prophylactic total or subtotal colectomy with careful follow-up is recommended as the treatment of choice for patients with Gardner's syndrome. This may not be curative, however, since small intestinal polyps also have a small but definite premalignant potential. In patients with familial polyposis, there have been occasional reports of carcinoma of the stomach and small intestine.[95, 96]

Familial Mediterranean Fever

Familial Mediterranean fever (benign paroxysmal peritonitis, familial paroxysmal peritonitis, recurrent polyseritis, Armenian disease) is an autosomal recessive disorder of unknown etiology seen almost exclusively in individuals of Armenian or Arabic origin and individuals of Jewish descent from central and eastern Europe (Table 9–8). Characterized by acute febrile attacks with peritonitis, pleuritis, synovitis, abdominal, chest and articular pain and an insidious development of amyloidosis, it occurs one to one-and-a-half times more frequently in men than in women.[97–102]

CLINICAL MANIFESTATIONS.—There appear to be two phenotypes of familial Mediterranean fever. Type 1 (the common variant) is characterized

TABLE 9–8.—FAMILIAL MEDITERRANEAN FEVER

1. An autosomal recessive disorder
2. Generally seen in Armenians, Arabs, and Ashkenazic Jews
3. Acute febrile attacks with peritonitis, pleuritis, synovitis, and abdominal, chest and articular pain
4. Cutaneous lesions in 10% of cases (urticaria, erythematous papules, vesicles, subcutaneous nodules and erysipelas—or cellulitis-like lesions)
5. Amyloidosis in 25% (with eventual death in 90% of patients with renal amyloidosis)
6. Fat-free diet, aspirin, and bed rest; colchicine for those unresponsive to dietary management

by recurrent attacks of fever and short, self-limiting episodes of peritonitis, pleuritis, arthritis, and erysipelas-like cutaneous lesions, with renal amyloidosis manifesting as the nephrotic syndrome eventually developing in at least one-quarter of affected patients. Type 2 (a more rare variant) is characterized by amyloidosis as the initial or sole manifestation of the disorder.[99] Principally involving the kidneys, this complication is particularly common in non-Ashkenazic (Sephardic) Jews and Arabs.[98, 99, 103]

The disorder may appear as short attacks that occur at irregular unpredictable intervals or it may have a more chronic protracted course. Although not present at birth, attacks of familial Mediterranean fever usually begin in early childhood (during the first decade in 67% of cases and by the second decade in 90%) and continue throughout life. Most attacks are self-limiting and may be followed by prolonged asymptomatic intervals, sometimes lasting several years. Attacks of peritonitis and pleuritis begin suddenly and subside spontaneously within 72 hours. Symptoms of joint inflammation persist longer, sometimes for several months, but they rarely leave residual damage. As a rule, single joints (usually a knee or ankle) are involved and reports of chronic irreversible arthritic changes are almost exclusively confined to the hip and sacroiliac joints. Breathing may be painful in patients with pulmonary serositis and arthritic symptoms may be severe. Acute appendicitis is frequently difficult to differentiate from the peritonitis of familial Mediterranean fever manifesting right lower quadrant pain. Patients with frequent recurring attacks of the disorder are particularly prone to narcotic addiction.

Cutaneous lesions, seen in approximately 10% of cases, may be seen as urticaria, erythematous papules, vesicles, subcutaneous nodules histologically resembling periarteritis nodosa, or painful tender erythematous lesions usually appearing on the calves, around the ankles, and on the dorsal aspects of the feet (Fig 9–10). These erysipelas- or cellulitis-like lesions, the most frequently seen cutaneous manifestations, may occur as the only manifestation of an attack or may accompany the arthritic symptoms and, like the arthritis, the cutaneous lesions may be precipitated by trauma.

Amyloidosis occurs in about 25% of patients and causes death in 90% of individuals affected with this complication before the age of forty. There appears to be no relationship between the age of onset and the type, frequency, or severity of attacks, but renal amyloidosis appears to be more common in Sephardic Jews. Ashkenazic Jews and Californians of Armenian descent have a better prognosis than Sephardic Jews.[101, 104]

DIAGNOSIS.—The diagnosis of familial Mediterranean fever is dependent upon the above constellation of clinical features in individuals of certain ethnic backgrounds. Rectal biopsy appears to be the diagnostic procedure of choice. Histopathologic examination reveals acute inflammation of

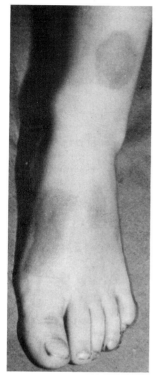

Fig 9–10.—Painful erysipelas-like erythematous nodules on the dorsal aspect of the feet and above the ankles in a child with familial Mediterranean fever. (Courtesy of J.E. Rasmussen, M.D., Ann Arbor, Michigan.)

the involved serosa (and amyloidosis in those individuals affected with this complication).

TREATMENT.—Familial Mediterranean fever is a severe, chronic, incurable disorder with an unpredictable and often fatal course in a significant number of patients (those with renal amyloidosis). Although there is no completely effective therapy, a fat-free diet, aspirin, and bed rest are beneficial, and colchicine (0.6 mg two or three times daily) has been reported to be effective in preventing attacks in approximately 70% of patients.[105, 106] However, this use is not listed in the manufacturer's official directive, and it is currently suggested that this form of therapy be reserved for those children who are incapacitated by frequent and severe attacks and do not respond to dietary fat restriction.

REFERENCES

1. Danbolt N., Closs K.: Acrodermatitis enteropathica. *Acta Derm. Venereol.* 23:127–169, 1942.

2. Wells B.T., Winkelmann R.K.: Acrodermatitis enteropathica—report of 6 cases. *Arch. Dermatol.* 84:90–102, 1961.
3. Moynahan E.J.: Acrodermatitis enteropathica: a lethal inherited human zinc-deficiency disorder. *Lancet* 2:399–400, 1974.
4. Moynahan E.J., Barnes P.M.: Zinc deficiency and a synthetic diet for lactose intolerance. *Lancet* 1:676–677, 1973.
5. Evans G.W., Johnson P.E.: Zinc-binding factor in acrodermatitis enteropathica. *Lancet* II:1310, 1976.
6. Hurley L.S., Duncan J.R., Sloan M.D., et al.: Zinc-binding ligands in milk and intestine: a role in neonatal nutrition. *Proceedings of the National Academy of Sciences in U.S.A.* 74:3547–3559, 1977.
7. Cousins R.J.: Zinc-thionein and heritable disorders associated with aberrant zinc metabolism. *Lancet* II:686–687, 1976.
8. van Vloten W.A., Bos L.P.: Skin lesions in acquired zinc deficiency due to parenteral nutrition. *Dermatologica* 156:175–183, 1978.
9. Arlette J.P., Johnston M.M.: Zinc deficiency dermatitis in premature infants on prolonged parenteral alimentation. *J. Am. Acad. Dermatol.* 5:37–42, 1981.
10. Wolman S.L., Anderson H., Marliss E.B.: Zinc in total parenteral nutrition: requirements and metabolic effects. *Gastroenterology* 76:458–467, 1979.
11. Ecker R.I., Schroeter A.L.: Acrodermatitis and acquired zinc deficiency. *Arch. Dermatol.* 114:937–939, 1978.
12. Weismann K., Wadskov S., Mikkelson H.I., et al.: Acquired zinc deficiency in man. *Arch. Dermatol.* 114:1509–1511, 1978.
13. Herson V.C., Phillips A.F., Zimmerman A.: Clinical memoranda. Acute zinc deficiency in a premature infant after bowel resection and intravenous alimentation. *Am. J. Dis. Child.* 135:968–969, 1981.
14. Aggett P.J., Atherton D.J., More J., et al.: Symptomatic zinc deficiency in a breast-fed preterm infant. *Arch. Dis. Child.* 55:547–550, 1980.
15. Parker P.H., Helinek G.L., Meneely P.H.: Clinical memoranda. Zinc deficiency in a premature infant fed exclusively human milk. *Am. J. Dis. Child.* 136:77–78, 1982.
16. Lepow M.L., Greenberg R.D., Stover M.L., et al.: Acrodermatitis in breastfed premature infants: evidence for a defect of mammary zinc secretion. *Pediatrics* 69:176–183, 1982.
17. McClain C., Soutor C., Zieve L.: Zinc deficiency: a complication of Crohn's disease. *Gastroenterology* 78:272–279, 1980.
18. Freeland-Graves J.H., Bodzy P.W., Eppright M.A.: Zinc status of vegetarians. *J. Amer. Dietet. Assoc.* 77:655–661, 1980.
19. Brazin S.A., Johnson W.T., Abramson L.J.: The acrodermatitis enteropathica-like syndrome. *Arch. Dermatol.* 115:597–599, 1979.
20. Michie D.O., Wirth F.H.: Plasma zinc levels in premature infants receiving parenteral nutrition. *J. Pediatr.* 92:798–800, 1978.
21. Hirsh F.S., Michel B., Strain W.H.: Gluconate zinc in acrodermatitis enteropathica. *Arch. Dermatol.* 112:475–478, 1976.
22. Dillaha C.J., Lorincz A.L., Aavik O.R.: Acrodermatitis enteropathica—review of the literature and a report on a case successfully treated with diodoquin. *J.A.M.A.* 152:509–512, 1953.
23. Weston W.L., Huff J.C., Humbert J.R., et al.: Zinc correction of defective chemotaxis in acrodermatitis enteropathica. *Arch. Dermatol.* 113:422–425, 1977.

24. Neldner K.H., Hagler L., Wise W.R., et al.: Acrodermatitis enteropathica—a clinical and biochemical survey. *Arch. Dermatol.* 110:711–721, 1974.

25. Neldner K.H., Hambidge K.M.: Zinc therapy of acrodermatitis enteropathica. *N. Engl. J. Med.* 292:879–882, 1975.

26. Michaelssohn G.: Zinc therapy in acrodermatitis enteropathica. *Acta Derm. Venereol.* 54:377–381, 1974.

27. Hambidge K.M., Walravens P.A.: Acrodermatitis enteropathica. *Int. J. Dermatol.* 17:380–387, 1978.

28. Marks J., Shuster S., Watson A.J.: Small bowel changes in dermatitis herpetiformis. *Lancet* 2:1280–1282, 1966.

29. Marks J., Shuster S.: Dermatitis herpetiformis: the role of gluten. *Arch. Dermatol.* 101:452–457, 1970.

30. Menzel E.J., Pehamberger H., Holubar K.: Demonstration of antibodies to wheat gliadin in dermatitis herpetiformis using ^{14}C-radioimmunoassay. *Clin. Immunol. Immunopathol.* 10:193–201, 1978.

31. Zone J.J., LaSalle B.A., Provost T.T.: Induction of IgA circulating immune complexes after wheat feeding in dermatitis herpetiformis patients. *J. Invest. Dermatol.* 78:375–380, 1982.

32. Katz S.I., Hertz K.C., Rogentine G.N., et al.: The association between HLA-B8 and dermatitis herpetiformis in patients with IgA deposits in skin. *Arch. Dermatol.* 113:155–156, 1977.

33. Katz S.I., Strober W.: The pathogenesis of dermatitis herpetiformis. *J. Invest. Dermatol.* 70:63–75, 1978.

34. Marks J., Birkett D., Shuster S., et al.: Small intestinal mucosal abnormalities in relatives of patients with dermatitis herpetiformis. *Gut* 11:493–497, 1970.

35. Leonard J., Haffenden G., Tucker W., et al.: Gluten challenge in dermatitis herpetiformis. *N. Engl. J. Med.* 308:816–819, 1983.

36. Frödin T., Gotthard R., Hed J., et al.: Gluten-free diet for dermatitis herpetiformis: long-term effect on cutaneous, immunologic, and jejunal manifestations. *Acta Derm. Venereol.* (Stockh.) 61:405–411, 1981.

37. Fry L., Leonard J.N., Swain F., et al.: Long-term follow-up of dermatitis herpetiformis with and without gluten withdrawal. *Br. J. Dermatol.* 107:631–640, 1982.

38. Ackerman A.B., Tolman M.M.: Papular dermatitis herpetiformis in childhood. *Arch. Dermatol.* 100:286–290, 1969.

39. Hertz D.C., Katz S.I., Aaronson C.: Juvenile dermatitis herpetiformis: an immunologically proven case. *Pediatrics* 59:945–948, 1977.

40. Seah P.P., Fry L.: Immunoglobulins in the skin in dermatitis herpetiformis and their relevance in diagnosis. *Br. J. Dermatol.* 92:157–166, 1975.

41. Jablonska S., Chorzelski T.P., Beutner, E.H., et al.: Dermatitis herpetiformis and bullous pemphigoid: intermediate and mixed forms. *Arch. Dermatol.* 112:45–48, 1976.

42. Bauer E.A.: Epidermolysis bullosa, in Blandau R.J. (Editor): *Morphogenesis and Malformation of the Skin.* Alan R. Liss, Inc., New York, 1981, pp. 173–190.

43. Cooper T.W., Bauer E.A.: Epidermolysis bullosa: a review. *Pediatric Dermatology* 1:No. 3, 181–188, 1984.

44. Briggaman R.A.: Hereditary epidermolysis bullosa with special emphasis on newly recognized syndromes and complications, in Jegosathy B.V. and Lazarus G.S. (Guest Editors); Symposium on Blistering Diseases, *Dermatologic*

Clinics. W.B. Saunders Publishing Co., Philadelphia, Vol. 1, No. 2 (April 1983), pp. 263–280.

45. Eady R.A.J., Tidman M.J.T.: Diagnosing epidermolysis bullosa. *Br. J. Dermatol.* 108:621–626, 1983.
46. Gedde-Dahl T., Jr.: Sixteen types of epidermolysis bullosa: on the clinical discrimination, therapy and prenatal diagnosis. *Acta Dermato-venereologica Supplement* 95:74–87, 1981.
47. Hillemeier C., Touloukian R., McCallum R., et al.: Esophageal web: a previously unrecognized complication of epidermolysis bullosa. *Pediatrics* 67:678–682, 1981.
48. Bull M.J., Norins A.L., Weaver D.D., et al.: Epidermolysis bullosa—pyloric atresia: an autosomal recessive disorder. *Am. J. Dis. Child.* 137:449–451, 1983.
49. Moynahan E.J.: Epidermolysis bullosa affecting the buccal and pharyngeal mucosae. *Proc. Royal Soc. Med.* 56:885–887, 1963.
50. Reed W.B., College J., Jr., Frances M.J.V.: Epidermolysis bullosa dystrophica with epidermal neoplasms. *Arch. Dermatol.* 110:894–902, 1974.
51. Briggaman R.A., Wheeler C.Z., Jr.: Epidermolysis bullosa dystrophica-recessive: a possible role of anchoring fibrils in the pathogenesis. *J. Invest. Dermatol.* 65:203–211, 1975.
52. Eisen A.Z.: Human skin collagenase: localization and distribution in normal human skin. *J. Invest. Dermatol.* 52:442–448, 1969.
53. Eisen A.Z.: Human skin collagenase: relationship to the pathogenesis of epidermolysis bullosa dystrophica. *J. Invest. Dermatol.* 52:449–453, 1969.
54. Bauer E.A.: Recessive dystrophic epidermolysis bullosa. Evidence for an altered collagenase in fibroblast cultures. *Proc. Natl. Acad. Sci. USA* 74:4646–4650, 1977.
55. Lazarus G.: Collagenase and connective tissue metabolism in epidermolysis bullosa. *J. Invest. Dermatol.* 58:242–249, 1972.
56. Bauer E.A.: Abnormalities in collagenous expression as *in vitro* markers for recessive dystrophic epidermolysis bullosa. *J. Invest. Dermatol.* 79 (Supplement 1):105s–108s, 1982.
57. Bart B.J., Gorlin R.J., Anderson V.E., et al.: Congenital localized absence of the skin, blistering and abnormality of nails. *Arch. Dermatol.* 93:296–304, 1966.
58. Smith S.Z., Cram D.L.: A mechanobullous disease of the newborn—Bart's syndrome. *Arch. Dermatol.* 114:81–84, 1978.
59. Raab B., Fretzin D.F., Bronson D.M., et al.: Epidermolysis bullosa acquisita and inflammatory bowel disease. *J.A.M.A.* 250:1746–1748, 1983.
60. Moynahan E.J.: Epidermolysis bullosa. in Maddin S. (Ed.): *Current Dermatologic Management.* C.V. Mosby Co., St. Louis, 1970, pp. 110–111.
61. Smith E.G., Michener W.M.: Vitamin E treatment of dermolytic bullous dermatosis. *Arch. Derm.* 108:254–256, 1973.
62. Pearson R.W.: Advances in the diagnosis and treatment of blistering diseases: A selective review, in Malkinson F.D., Pearson R.W., (Eds.): *Yearbook of Dermatology,* 1977, pp. 7–52.
63. Katz J., Gryboski J.P., Rosenbaum H.M., et al.: Dysphagia in children with epidermolysis bullosa. *Gastroenterol.* 52:259–262, 1967.
64. Orlando R.C., Bozymski E.M., Briggaman R.A., et al.: Epidermolysis bullosa: gastrointestinal manifestations. *Ann. Int. Med.* 81:203–206, 1974.

65. Absolon K.B., Finney L.A., Waddill G.M., Jr., et al.: Esophageal constriction—colon transplant—in two brothers with epidermolysis bullosa. *Surgery* 65:832–836, 1969.
66. Schwartz R.: Squamous cell carcinoma in dominant type epidermolysis bullosa dystrophica. *Cancer* 47:615–620, 1981.
67. Eisenberg M., Stevens L.H., Schofield P.J.: Epidermolysis bullosa: new therapeutic approaches. *Australian J. Dermatol.* 19:1–8, 1978.
68. Bauer E.A., Cooper T.W., Tucker D.R., et al.: Phenytoin therapy of recessive dystrophic epidermolysis bullosa. *N. Engl. J. Med.* 303:776–781, 1980.
69. Guill M.F., Wray B.B., Rogers R.B., et al.: Junctional epidermolysis bullosa. Treatment with phenytoin. *Am. J. Dis. Child.* 137:992–994, 1983.
70. Jeghers H., McKusick V.A., Katz K.H.: Localized intestinal polyposis and melanin spots of the oral mucosa, lips and digits. *N. Engl. J. Med.* 241:993–1005, 1031–1033, 1946.
71. Dozois R.R., Judd E.S., Dahlin D.C., et al.: The Peutz-Jeghers syndrome. Is there a predisposition to the development of intestinal cancer? *Arch. Surg.* 98:509–517, 1969.
72. Schwabe A.D., Lewin K.J.: Gastrointestinal polyposis syndrome. *Viewpoints on Digest. Dis.* 12:1–4, 1980.
73. McKittrick J.E., Lewis W.M., Doane W.A., et al.: The Peutz-Jeghers syndrome. *Arch. Surg.* 103:57–62, 1971.
74. Beck A.R., Jewett T.C.: Surgical implications of the Peutz-Jeghers syndrome. *Ann. Surg.* 165:229–302, 1967.
75. Wenzl J.E., Bartholomew L.G., Hallenbeck G.A., et al.: Gastrointestinal polyposis with mucocutaneous pigmentation in children (Peutz-Jeghers syndrome). *Pediatrics* 28:655–661, 1961.
76. Ryo U.Y., Roh S.K., Balkin R.B., et al.: Extensive metastases in Peutz-Jeghers syndrome. *J.A.M.A.* 239:2268–2269, 1978.
77. Sirihaven C., Trowbridge A.A.: Dyskeratosis congenita: clinical features and genetic aspects: report of a family and review of the literature. *J. Med. Gen.* 12:339–354, 1975.
78. Steier W., Van Voolen G.A., Selmanowitz V.: Dyskeratosis congenita: relationship to Fanconi's anemia. *Blood* 39:510–521, 1972.
79. Rider J.: Dyskeratosis congenita, in Demis D.J., Dobson R.L., McGuire J.: *Clinical Dermatology,* Harper & Row Publishers, Philadelphia, ed. 10. 1983, Unit 1–34, 1–4.
80. Carter D.M., Gaynor A., McGuire J.: Sister chromatid exchanges in dyskeratosis congenita after exposure to trimethyl psoralen and UV light, in Hanawalt P.C., Friedberg E.C., Fox C.F.: DNA repair mechanisms. *ICN-UCLA Symposium on Molecular and Cellular Biology,* IX. Academic Press, Inc., New York, 1978, pp. 671–674.
81. Cannell H.: Dyskeratosis congenita. *Br. J. Oral Surg.* 9:8–20, 1971.
82. Carter D.M., Pan M.S., Gaynor A., et al.: Psoralen-DNA cross-linking photoadducts in dyskeratosis congenita: delay in excision and promotion of sister chromatid exchange. *J. Invest. Dermatol.* 79:97–101, 1979.
83. Gutman A., Frumkin A., Adam A., et al.: X-linked dyskeratosis congenita with pancytopenia. *Arch. Dermatol.* 114:1667–1671, 1978.
84. Womer R., Clark J.E., Wood P., et al.: Dyskeratosis congenita: two examples of this multisystem disorder. *Pediatrics* 71:603–609, 1983.
85. Hickman J.G., Lazarus G.S.: Pyoderma gangrenosum: new concepts in etiol-

ogy and treatment, in Moschella S.L. (editor-in-chief): *Dermatology Update.* Reviews for physicians, 1979 edition, Elsevier, New York, 1979, pp. 325–342.

86. Samitz M.H.: Cutaneous vasculitis in association with ulcerative colitis. *Cutis* 2:283–287, 1966.
87. Holt P.J.A., Davies M.G., Saunders K.C., et al.: Pyoderma gangrenosum. *Medicine* (Baltimore) 59:114–133, 1980.
88. Dick D.C., Mackie R.M., Patrick W.J.A., et al.: Pyoderma gangrenosum in infancy. *Acta Dermatovener.* 62:348–350, 1982.
89. Percival G.H.: Pyoderma gangrenosum: the histology of the primary lesion. *Br. J. Dermatol.* 69:130–136, 1957.
90. Jennings J.L.: Pyoderma gangrenosum: successful treatment with intralesional steroids. *J. Am. Acad. Dermatol.* 9:575–580, 1983.
91. Lynch W.S., Bergfeld W.F.: Pyoderma gangrenosum responsive to minocycline hydrochloride. *Cutis* 21:535–538, 1978.
92. Kark E.C., Davis B.R., Pomeranz J.R.: Pyoderma gangrenosum treated with clofazimine. *J. Am. Dermatol.* 4:152–159, 1981.
93. Weary P.E., Linthicum A., Cowley E.P., et al.: Gardner's syndrome: a family group study and review. *Arch. Dermatol.* 90:20–30, 1964.
94. Golitz L.E.: Heritable cutaneous disorders which affect the gastrointestinal tract, in Callen J.P. (Guest Editor), Symposium on cutaneous signs of systemic disease, *The Medical Clinics of North America.* W.B. Saunders Co., Philadelphia, 1980, Vol. 64, Number 5, pp. 829–846.
95. Jones T.R., Nance F.C.: Periampullary malignancy in Gardner's syndrome. *Ann. Surg.* 185:565–573, 1977.
96. Coli R.D., Moor J.P., LaMarche P.H., et al.: Gardner's syndrome. A revisit to a previously described family. *Am. J. Dig. Dis.* 15:551–568, 1970.
97. Shapiro T.R., Ehrenfeld E.N.: Recurrent polyserositis ("periodic disease," "familial Mediterranean fever") in children. *Pediatrics* 30:443–449, 1962.
98. Siegel S.: Familial paroxysmal polyserositis: analysis of fifty cases. *Am. J. Med.* 36:893–918, 1964.
99. Sohar E., Gafni J., Pras M., et al.: Familial Mediterranean fever: a survey of 470 cases and review of the literature. *Am. J. Med.* 43:227–253, 1967.
100. Ehrenfeld E.N., Eliakim M., Rachmilewitz M.: Recurrent polyserositis (familial Mediterranean fever; periodic disease): a report of fifty-five cases. *Am. J. Med.* 31:107–123, 1961.
101. Schwabe A.D., Peters R.S.: Familial Mediterranean fever in Armenians: analysis of 100 cases. *Medicine* 53:453–462, 1974.
102. Cozzetto J.J.: Familial Mediterranean fever. *Am. J. Dis. Child.* 101:52–59, 1961.
103. Sturtz G.S., Burke E.: "Periodic peritonitis." *Am. J. Dis. Child.* 92:390–394, 1956.
104. Braverman I.M.: Diseases of the gastrointestinal tract, in Braverman I.M.: *Skin Signs of Systemic Disease.* W.B. Saunders Co., Philadelphia, 1981, pp. 577–580.
105. Dinarello C.A., Wolff S.M., Goldfinger S.E., et al.: Colchicine therapy for familial Mediterranean fever: a double-blind trial. *N. Engl. J. Med.* 291:934–937, 1974.
106. Wright D.G., Wolff S.M., Fauci A.S., et al.: Efficacy of intermittent colchicine therapy in familial Mediterranean fever. *Ann. Int. Med.* 86:162–165, 1977.

10 / Vascular Lesions With Systemic Significance

Cutaneous Hemangiomas

OCCURRING IN ABOUT 10% OF ALL INFANTS, there are basically three types of congenital cutaneous hemangioma: (1) strawberry hemangiomas, (2) port-wine stains (nevus flammeus), and (3) cavernous hemangiomas (Table 10–1). Strawberry and cavernous hemangiomas are usually not present at birth but become apparent during the first three to five weeks of life. In a few instances, strawberry hemangiomas present at birth as pink macules or as demarcated vascular lesions surrounded by an area of pallor. During the first few weeks of life, this area becomes vascularized and progresses into the classic purplish-red, lobulated vascular lesion with well-defined borders and minute capillaries that protrude from its surface; hence the strawberry-like appearance and its name. Of developmental origin and apparently derived as a result of angioblastic tissue that fails to establish normal communication with the adjacent vascular system during fetal life, the rapid enlargement and clinical appearance of the strawberry hemangioma results from canalization and establishment of blood flow in these areas.[1, 2]

Strawberry Hemangiomas

The strawberry hemangioma, reported to occur in 2.6% of newborns[1] and 10% of all babies under one year of age,[3, 5] is frequently referred to as a "capillary hemangioma" or "strawberry nevus" and consists of greatly dilated capillaries engorged with blood (Fig 10–1). Since cavernous spaces may also be present in such lesions, the term "capillary" hemangioma is inappropriate and probably should be discarded.[2, 3]

Strawberry hemangiomas are characterized by two phases—a proliferative and an involuting phase. During their period of growth, they are characterized by hyperplasia of their endothelial cells. In maturing lesions, the capillary lumina are wider and the endothelial cells lining them appear flatter; in the involuting phase, deposits of hyaline appear to lead to narrowing and occlusion of the capillary lumina. This is followed by involution of the capillaries and their replacement by edematous collagen.[4]

Strawberry hemangiomas become solid, bright red in color and elevated, and enlarge quite rapidly reaching full size during the proliferative phase, often reaching full size by four to six months of age.[3] Between 6 to 18

TABLE 10–1.—INCIDENCE
OF VASCULAR NEVI

1. Salmon patches (40% of neonates)
2. Strawberry hemangiomas
   a. 2.6% of newborns
   b. 10% of babies under one year of age
3. Cavernous hemangiomas (one-tenth the incidence of strawberry hemangiomas)
4. Nevus flammeus (0.3% of newborns)
5. More common in prematures
6. More common in girls than boys (60%–70%)

months, the lesions become quiescent and grow at the same rate as the child, and involution generally starts after 12 to 18 months of age.[5] At least 90% of strawberry angiomata undergo partial or complete resolution, frequently involuting completely by the fifth or sixth years of life. In 50% of cases, the hemangiomas disappear by age 5, in 70% they disappear by age 7, and in 90% they disappear by age 9, leaving little residual scar or evidence that they ever existed.[6] Superficial lesions generally resolve completely without trace or only with slight atrophy of the involved area. In the large hemangiomas with deep elements, a relatively loose, atrophic, pale scar is the only residual clinical defect unless extensive ulceration and infection supervened during its course.[3] Accordingly, fewer than 10% of strawberry hemangiomas constitute any cosmetic handicap, and less than 2% require active therapy.[7]

Port-Wine Stains (Nevus Flammeus)

Port-wine stains (nevus flammeus), in contrast to strawberry hemangiomata, represent a congenital vascular malformation involving mature cap-

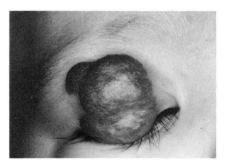

Fig 10–1.—Strawberry hemangioma of the upper eyelid with occlusion of the eye. Following therapy with systemic steroids the hemangioma involuted rapidly (without ocular defect).

illaries. Seen in 0.3% of newborns, they are present at birth, reddish-purple, flat or barely elevated above the surface of the surrounding skin, and do not fade appreciably with age. Composed of dilated mature capillaries in the dermis with no evidence of cellular proliferation, port-wine stains appear to be the result of a congenital weakness of the capillary walls, and thus represent a telangiectasia rather than a true angioma.[5] The cosmetic management of nevus flammeus is discussed later in the section on Sturge-Weber syndrome.

Cavernous Hemangiomas

Cavernous hemangiomas represent basically the same pathological process as strawberry nevi but are composed of larger mature vascular elements in a delicate fibrous stroma that involves the dermis and subcutaneous tissue. Seen less frequently than strawberry hemangiomas by about tenfold,[7] they are present at birth, grow in proportion to the growth of the individual, and are generally seen as bluish-red masses with less distinct borders (Fig 10–2). Occasionally a combination of strawberry and cavernous hemangioma may occur. Although the natural history of cavernous hemangiomas parallels that of the strawberry hemangioma, cavernous hemangiomas have a lesser growth rate, and regression is not as complete as that of the strawberry lesions, but the eventual cosmetic appearance is generally quite satisfactory.

TREATMENT.—Except for port-wine stains, most hemangiomas regress completely, or almost completely, and except for special cases, generally require no therapy, the final result in untreated lesions generally being far

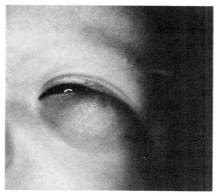

Fig 10–2.—Cavernous hemangioma of the lower eyelid in a 3-month-old infant. Systemic steroids induced rapid resolution of the hemangioma without ocular defect.

superior to that obtained from most forms of therapeutic intervention. Office management, accordingly, of both strawberry and cavernous hemangiomas generally consists of judicious observation; avoidance, whenever possible, of active therapy; and constant reassurance to the parents of affected children. Hemangiomas that require intervention are those that by their size and growth compromise vital structures such as the eyes, nares, auditory canals, pharynx, or larynx; those that have an alarming rate of growth, tripling or quadrupling in size within a period of a few weeks; large, usually cavernous lesions that have an associated thrombocytopenia (Kasabach-Merritt syndrome); or lesions that by their size or location are particularly susceptible to trauma, hemorrhage, or secondary infection.

The complication rate of patients with hemangiomas of the eyelids and orbit followed over a period of five years has been described to be as high as 80% (Figs 10–1, 10–2). These include amblyopia 60%, skin problems (discoloration and irregularities) 50%, strabismus 34%, residual proptosis 30%, orbital-palpebral asymmetry 16%, ptosis 10%, keratitis 4%, and optic atrophy 2%.[8] For such cases, systemic corticosteroids or intralesional injection have been recommended. Because of the proximity to the eye, this author prefers the use of systemic corticosteroids to the intralesional form of therapy often recommended in the ophthalmological literature.[8–11]

When intervention is required, intralesional injection of sterile triamcinolone acetonide suspension (Kenalog-10 Injection, Squibb), in a dosage of 1 to 3 mg/kg two or three times at three-week intervals, may result in involution within several months,[2] or a course of oral prednisone may be used in a dosage of 2 to 3 mg/kg per day (or its equivalent) for four weeks, followed by alternate-day therapy using the same or doubled dosage for periods of four to six weeks, with gradual tapering of the dosage as the condition warrants.[11–15] Involution usually begins about the second or third week and continues during the second month. Within 3 to 21 days of institution of prednisone therapy, the enlarging hemangioma will stop growing in 90% of patients and the lesion will shrink if treatment is continued for 30 to 90 days. If rebound occurs, a second or third course may be necessary.[2, 12, 13]

The Kasabach-Merritt Syndrome

The Kasabach-Merritt syndrome (thrombocytopenia reputedly caused by platelet sequestration in giant cavernous hemangiomas) is a disorder that generally affects infants three months of age or younger. Although most cavernous hemangiomata associated with thrombocytopenia are exceedingly large, excessive size is not necessarily a prerequisite of this disorder. Lesions as small as 5 or 6 cm in diameter have had confirmed thrombocytopenia.[2] Thrombocytopenia, frequently with blood platelet levels as low as 10,000 to 40,000, may be detected during the first few days of life. Children with rapidly expanding cavernous lesions (with or without ecchymoses) should be checked for platelet entrapment with thrombocytopenia.

The danger of the Kasabach-Merritt syndrome is the development of acute hemorrhage or possible compression of vital structures during a period of rapid growth. Nearly one-fourth of reported infants with this complication died from bleeding disorders, respiratory distress, infection, or malignant transformation. Hence, infants with large cavernous hemangiomas and thrombocytopenia should be hospitalized and promptly treated.

Treatment consists of fresh whole-blood or platelet transfusion as needed, compression bandages over the hemangioma site whenever possible, a short intensive course of systemic steroids, cautious use of anticoagulants in the presence of disseminated intravascular coagulopathy, and surgical removal of the hemangiomatous lesions whenever feasible. Although surgery is relatively safe (if fresh whole-blood transfusions are used and the surgeon is experienced), surgical excision is almost never justified unless the characteristics of the hemangioma itself warrant this approach.[16-18] Although this procedure can at times be successfully accomplished, the hazards are often great, and most patients require treatment with corticosteroids or judicious radiation because of poor surgical risk or the size of the hemangioma.

The Sturge-Weber Syndrome

The Sturge-Weber syndrome (encephalofacial or encephalotrigeminal angiomatosis) is a syndrome characterized by a nevus flammeus (port-wine stain) in the distribution of the first branch of the trigeminal nerve associated with a vascular malformation of the ipsilateral meninges and cerebral cortex (Table 10–2). Although there have been reports of Sturge-Weber syndrome in the absence of a facial nevus, these do not fulfill the criteria for Sturge-Weber syndrome and are termed meningeal angiomatosis.[19, 20]

Alexander and Norman, in their survey of 787 cases of nevus flammeus, found 257 cases of Sturge-Weber syndrome. All cases showed part of the facial nevus involving the forehead and/or upper eyelid to some extent.

TABLE 10–2.—STURGE-WEBER SYNDROME

1. First branch of trigeminal nerve
2. Ipsilateral meninges and cerebral cortex
3. Must involve upper eyelid and/or forehead
4. Seizures (80%), retardation (60%), hemiplegia (30%)
5. 45% with glaucoma (with involvement of both ophthalmic and maxillary divisions of trigeminal)

(From Hurwitz S.[2])

When the nevus occurred exclusively below the palpebral fissure, the cerebral angiomatosis was not found.[19] From this observation it may be inferred that if the vascular nevus does not involve the upper eyelid or forehead, one probably need not worry about the possible association of central nervous system involvement (Fig 10–3).

The oral mucous membranes may show telangiectatic hypertrophy, and ocular involvement occurs in 40% to 50% of patients with the Sturge-Weber syndrome. Studies suggest that if the vascular nevus involves both the ophthalmic and maxillary divisions of the sensory branch of the trigeminal nerve, childhood glaucoma appears in 45% of patients; involvement of one branch alone does not seem to be associated with glaucoma.[21]

In 50% of patients, the earliest symptoms of the intracranial lesions of Sturge-Weber syndrome develop during the first year. Although extensive meningeal lesions may remain silent throughout life, onset of symptoms after age 20 is unusual. Seizures, reported in 80% of affected individuals, often as early as 3 weeks of age, frequently present as the initial symptom of this disorder. Hemiplegia has been reported in up to 30%, and mental retardation may be seen in 60% of affected individuals.[22]

The association of a conspicuous nevus flammeus with epilepsy or hemiplegia establishes the diagnosis. If the port-wine stain does not involve the upper eyelid or forehead, then Sturge-Weber syndrome is not present. Electroencephalography shows unilateral depression of cortical activity with or without spike discharges.[23] X-ray of the skull reveals characteristic calcifications in two-thirds of patients. These calcifications follow the con-

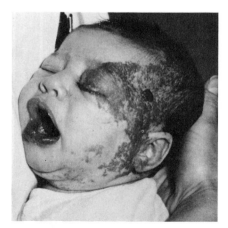

Fig 10–3.—Sturge-Weber syndrome. Nevus flammeus in the distribution of the fifth (trigeminal) nerve. Sturge-Weber syndrome is unlikely if the vascular nevus occurs exclusively below the palpebral fissure and does not involve the upper eyelid or forehead.

volutions of the cerebral cortex and are characterized by sinuous parallel streaks (called "tramlines"). Calcification can be detected as early as four or five months but are more commonly seen after the first or second year of life and become more extensive up to the second decade, after which time they remain stable. X-ray of the skull is rarely helpful in the diagnosis before the age of one or two years.

Surgical treatment of the intracranial lesion is occasionally successful. Accordingly, neurosurgical consultation should be sought as soon as the diagnosis has been established, preferably, if possible, before the onset of seizures. Palliative measures for the control of gingival overgrowth include surgical excision of excess tissue, injection of sclerosing solutions, and radiation therapy.[23] Regular supervision by an ophthalmologist and control of glaucoma by goniotomy is an important aspect of therapy for these patients.

Lesions of nevus flammeus show little tendency toward involution, and treatment for cosmetic purposes heretofore has generally been unsatisfactory. Treatments with thorium X, cryosurgery, and Grenz rays have been disappointing. Tattooing with skin-colored pigment is tedious, and since the secondary skin color changes with age, seasons, and tanning, results have not been very successful. However, Covermark, a tinted opaque waterproof cream (manufactured by Lydia O'Leary) is useful and can do much to alleviate the cosmetic appearance of such lesions.

Recent studies on the use of argon laser beam therapy are encouraging. Although this technique may not completely eliminate the lesion, it can induce lightening of the hemangioma. Those that are deep purple may become light violet; those that are deep red become light pink; and the sponginess and irregularity of the skin that may appear during life is frequently improved, thus allowing easier application of readily available makeups. Although results to date remain preliminary and future clinical and laboratory investigation will be necessary before argon laser therapy can be recommended as the treatment of choice for all such vascular deformities, it appears that this approach allows a more optimistic outlook for the future management of such disorders.[24–26]

Argon laser beam therapy is not recommended for children under 9 years of age. In general, darker lesions with more pronounced vascular ectasia on biopsy as well as more numerous vessels occupying a larger area of the dermis are most responsive to this form of therapy. Since these changes are more pronounced with aging, older patients seem to obtain a more successful result.

The Klippel-Trenaunay-Parkes-Weber Syndrome

The Klippel-Trenaunay-Parkes-Weber syndrome (nevus vasculosus hypertrophicus) is a vascular malformation characterized by local overgrowth of bone and soft tissue of an extremity or portion of the trunk associated with phlebectasia, arteriovenous aneurysms, cutaneous telangiectasia resembling a port-wine stain, and, often, varicosities. More often of an upper rather than a lower extremity and on the left rather than the right side of the body, the hypertrophy involves the length as well as the circumference of the extremity, and boys are more frequently affected than girls (Fig 10–4).

The hemangioma may be capillary or cavernous in nature and is often complicated by arteriovenous shunts and lymphangiomatous anomalies. At birth it usually is associated with a port-wine stain. Later in infancy, cavernous hemangiomas, ectasias, venous varicosities and arteriovenous shunts may also appear.[3] Treatment is generally unsatisfactory. Compression of dilated veins by support bandages has some merit, and surgery may be effective in the prevention of severe limb hypertrophy in occasional patients. Surgery is not indicated for superficial venous varicosities resulting from hypoplasia or atresia of the deep venous system and can produce disastrous results. Appropriate radiographic studies, therefore, are advisable prior to any attempts at surgical correction.[27] Although radiation therapy has been advocated for some individuals, to date this approach has not met with enthusiastic support and should be used judiciously or rarely, if at all.

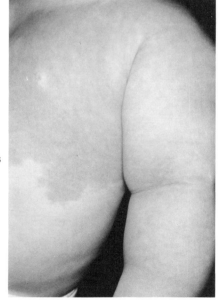

Fig 10–4.—Klippel-Trenaunay-Parkes-Weber syndrome. Local hypertrophy of the bone and soft tissue associated with a port-wine stain (nevus flammeus) in a 3-month-old infant.

Maffucci's Syndrome

Maffucci's syndrome (dyschondroplasia with hemangiomata) is characterized by vascular hamartomas (hemangiomas, phlebectasias, and lymphangiomas) and associated dyschondroplasia. Two-thirds of reported patients have been males.

Individuals with this disorder are usually normal at birth (only rarely are they born with visible hemangiomas or skeletal nodules). During the prepubertal years (the first twelve years of life), the multiple hemangiomata and dyschondroplasias, usually manifested clinically by hard nodules on the fingers or toes followed by other nodular lesions elsewhere on the extremities, become apparent. Subsequently, other progressive skeletal abnormalities due to defects of ossification (marked bony deformities complicated by pathologic fractures) may be seen.

The vascular lesions consist of dilated veins and soft bluish cavernous hemangiomata, which occur on the affected limb or elsewhere. The distribution of vascular lesions does not correspond to that of the skeletal lesions. Some 30% of patients with this disorder develop some type of associated malignant disease (chondrosarcoma or angiosarcoma). The management of this disorder, accordingly, consists of surgery, when indicated, and periodic evaluation to detect and extirpate any lesions suggestive of neoplastic degeneration.

Blue Rubber-bleb Nevus Syndrome

The blue rubber-bleb nevus is a variant of a cavernous hemangioma that presents as a soft compressible blue to purple rubbery protuberance of the dermis and subcutaneous tissue. Some lesions may be spontaneously painful and tender to palpation. In this syndrome, the vascular lesions are sometimes present at birth or early childhood (occasionally in adult life) and, with time, frequently increase in size or number. The importance of this type of lesion lies in its frequent association with angiomas of the gastrointestinal tract. The gastrointestinal hemangiomas are found most frequently in the small intestine or colon but may occur anywhere throughout the gastrointestinal tract. They tend to bleed readily and frequently cause anemia.

The cutaneous lesions are blue and raised, their surfaces are wrinkled, and they vary in size from 0.1 to 5.0 cm in diameter. They may present as large cavernous hemangiomas, blue rubber blebs, or irregular blue marks on the cutaneous surface. They may be solitary or may number in the hundreds and can occur anywhere on the cutaneous surface (usually the trunk or arms) or the mucous membranes of the nose and mouth. One of the diagnostic features is the fact that blood can be expressed from the lesions with pressure, leaving an empty wrinkled sac. The treatment of this disorder is mainly symptomatic with resection of bowel, when indicated, to control excessive bleeding and anemia.[28, 29]

Diffuse Neonatal Hemangiomatosis

Cases of infants with multiple hemangiomas of the visceral organs, the gastrointestinal tract, liver, central nervous system, and lungs (diffuse neonatal hemangiomatosis, multinodular hemangiomatosis) have been reported. Although most cases of diffuse neonatal hemangiomatosis are complicated by visceral involvement, some may have multiple cutaneous hemangiomas without visceral complications (benign neonatal hemangiomatosis).[30] Although infants with diffuse neonatal hemangiomatosis may not present with cutaneous involvement, most affected children display widely disseminated small, red to bluish-black papular cutaneous hemangiomata (usually present at birth or developing during the first few weeks of life) numbering in the hundreds (Fig 10–5). Despite supportive therapy, affected infants often die of high output cardiac failure, from hepatic complications, gastrointestinal hemorrhage, respiratory tract obstruction, thrombocytopenia with bleeding, or severe neurologic deficit due to compression of neural tissue.[31–33]

When seen in association with multinodular hemangiomatosis, cardiac

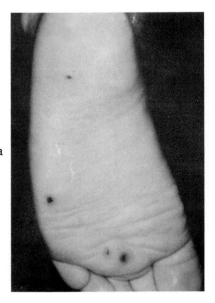

Fig 10–5.—Diffuse neonatal hemangiomatosis. Multiple bluish-black cutaneous hemangiomata on the foot of a 4½-year-old girl with visceral hemangiomatosis.

failure is believed to be the result of arteriovenous shunts in hepatic hemangiomas, which ultimately lead to increased venous return and increased cardiac output. When present, this complication occurs early in life (usually at 2 to 9 weeks of age). Hepatic hemangiomas, when present, may be delineated by liver and spleen scan or hepatic angiography or both. Recognition of the cutaneous component, which may be minimal in some patients, frequently permits early diagnosis and helps prevent confusion with cardiac failure seen in association with congenital heart disease. Surgical management of this complication, by lobectomy or selective ligation of hepatic vessels, can frequently be avoided by therapy with systemic corticosteroids and digitalis (particularly when initiated early).[32, 33]

Gorham's Syndrome

Gorham's syndrome (disappearing bones, vanishing bone disease, angiomatous nevi with osteolysis) is a rare disorder that consists of cutaneous hemangiomas in association with massive osteolysis and complete or partial replacement of bone by extensive fibrosis. The skin and soft tissue involvement in this disorder is usually confined to areas near the bony lesions. Although the cause of increased bone resorption is not known, it has been theorized that this phenomenon may be due to localized hyperemia associated with the hemangiomas.

Usually a disorder of young children, involving single or multiple bones, Gorham's disease is believed to be a slowly developing, probably self-limiting condition and does not progress to neoplastic formation. Numerous methods of therapy have been employed, but none has proved of value. The only reported deaths associated with this disorder are those that resulted from hemorrhage into serous cavities.[34, 35]

Riley-Smith Syndrome

The Riley-Smith syndrome (macrocephaly with unusual cutaneous angiomatosis) is presumably an autosomal dominant disorder characterized by multiple cavernous hemangiomata, macrocephaly, and pseudopapillomata. Recently this disorder has been expanded to include individuals with the Klippel-Trenaunay-Parkes-Weber syndrome, a combination of Sturge-Weber and the Klippel-Trenaunay-Parkes-Weber syndrome, cutis marmorata telangiectatica congenita, and macrocephaly with multiple lipomas and hemangiomas.[36, 37] Because normal central nervous system function is frequently seen in association with this syndrome, awareness of the benign nature of the macrocephaly should help avoid unnecessary concern or intervention, except in patients who also manifest signs of increased intracranial pressure or central nervous system dysfunction.

The Cobb Syndrome

The Cobb syndrome consists of a cutaneous vascular nevus (angiolipoma, cavernous hemangioma, port-wine stain, or angiokeratoma) and an associated angioma in the spinal cord corresponding within a segment or two to the involved dermatome.[38, 39] Males slightly outnumber females in most cases reported to date, and in the majority of patients, the neurologic problems occur during childhood or adolescence. In most patients, lateral thoracic and lumbar spine radiograms may show early bone erosion.

Treatment, as well as diagnosis, may be aided by spinal angiography. Spinal angiomas fed by the posterior spinal artery are often juxtamedullary and can be extirpated surgically without appreciable damage to the spinal cord. Those fed by the anterior spinal artery, however, are often intramedullary and supply critical motor pathways and neurons. Surgical removal of such lesions is often technically impossible.

Angiokeratomas

The term *angiokeratoma* is applied to a group of disorders characterized by ectasia (dilation of the superficial vessels of the dermis) and hyperkeratosis of the overlying epidermis. All have in common the presence of asymptomatic vascular lesions, seen as firm, dark-red to black papules that measure from 1 to 10 mm with varying degrees of secondary hyperkeratosis.

There are six recognized forms of angiokeratoma. Four represent cosmetic problems only. These include solitary or multiple angiokeratomas, angiokeratoma circumscriptum, angiokeratoma of Mibelli, and angiokeratoma of the scrotum and vulva (angiokeratoma of Fordyce). The fifth and sixth forms are diffuse diseases of systemic significance. They are known as angiokeratoma corporis diffusum or Fabry's disease (a sex-linked disorder characterized by storage of a neutral glycolipid, ceramidetrihexoside, in many types of cells in the body) and fucosidosis (an autosomal recessive disease characterized by the abnormal intracellular accumulation of a fucose-containing glycosphingolipid).[2]

Angiokeratoma Corporis Diffusum (Fabry Syndrome)

In 1898, Fabry in Germany and Anderson in England independently described a form of angiokeratoma now known as angiokeratoma corporis diffusum or Fabry syndrome. The disorder appears to be an X-linked recessive disease with complete penetrance and variable clinical expressivity in homozygous males and occasional mild penetrance in the heterozygous female[40–42] (Table 10–3). The disorder is characterized by systemic intracellular accumulation of glycosphingolipid (trihexosyl ceramide) in the skin

TABLE 10–3.—Fabry Syndrome

1. X-linked recessive
   a. Complete penetrance in homozygous males
   b. Occasional mild penetrance in heterozygous females
2. Alpha-galactosidase (ceramide trihexosidase) deficiency
3. Angiokeratomas
   a. Usually before puberty (between 5 and 13 years)
   b. Clusters of individual punctate macular or papular angiectases
4. Pain and paresthesias of hands and feet, pedal and ankle edema, paralyses, hypohidrosis and scant body hair
5. Spoke-like posterior capsular corneal opacities (pathognomic when present)

and viscera, particularly in the cardiovascular-renal system. The primary metabolic defect is the deficient activity of a specific alpha-galactosidase (ceramide trihexosidase) which normally catabolizes the accumulated glycosphingolipid.

CLINICAL FEATURES.—The cutaneous vascular lesions characteristic of this disorder are telangiectases. They usually appear before puberty, generally between 5 and 13 years of age. Occasionally they occur during infancy, and in some instances, onset may be as late as age 20. The lesions generally appear as clusters of individual punctate macular or papular dark red angiectases that do not blanch with pressure. The eruption is usually symmetrical, and the lesions generally increase progressively in size and number with age. Despite their name, they generally show little to no hyperkeratosis.

Angiokeratomas of Fabry usually appear in the area between the umbilicus and knees. They may number into the thousands and cluster in the ileosacral areas, about the umbilicus, and over the scrotum, buttocks, posterior thorax, and thighs. The first lesions frequently appear in the scrotum and must be differentiated from those of angiokeratoma of Fordyce. Lesions seldom occur on the hands or feet, have not been reported on the scalp, ears, or face, except for a small area on the chin, and are permanent unless they become thrombosed, after which they disappear (which is rare). A majority of patients have pinpoint macular purplish spots on the lips, particularly near the vermilion border of the lower lip. These lesions are smaller than those on the skin. The tongue is not affected, but hemoptysis and epistaxis have been reported with involvement of the buccal and nasal mucosae. In addition to the typical cutaneous lesions, fine telangiectases have been described in the axillae on the upper chest. In heterozygous females, angiomas appear in only 20% of cases and, when present, are less numerous and more limited in extent than in males.[43]

Attacks of pain and paresthesias of the hands and feet often accompany the eruption. Although often spontaneous or elicited by exertion, they are apparently associated with vasomotor disturbances and usually occur subsequent to temperature changes. Edema of the ankles, paralyses, scant body hair, and hypohidrosis are often present. Pedal and ankle edema are present in most cases and may result in stasis ulcers. Edema, when present, is presumably due to increased vascular permeability and is more prominent in summer than winter.

Patients with angiokeratoma corporis diffusum are often hypertensive and, with advancing age, are particularly susceptible to cerebrovascular accidents, coronary artery disease, and renal disease. Neurologic complications are common and include asphasia, paresis, tremors, paralyses, loss of consciousness, and psychotic disturbances. Other systemic manifestations include diarrhea, colitis and proctitis, an unusual arthritis of the distal interphalangeal joints with some loss of motion, cataracts, corneal opacities, and tortuosity of the conjunctival blood vessels with characteristic sausage-like constriction and dilatation.

The corneal opacities are usually present during childhood; they are found in all affected males as well as most female carriers with this disorder. Of particular diagnostic importance is the fact that the posterior capsular cataracts have a characteristic spoke-like appearance. This spoke-like feature, when present, is pathognomonic of this disorder.

Most men with angiokeratoma of Fabry die between ages 30 to 50 as the result of renal failure with uremia and hypertension, cerebrovascular accidents, or congestive heart failure. The course in female heterozygotes is more benign. Afflicted women have skin lesions (in 20% of cases), cataracts, and relatively normal longevity. Although the disorder is generally asymptomatic in women, some have hypohidrosis, attacks of pain in the extremities, arthritis, urinary tract infection, and renal failure.

DIAGNOSIS.—The diagnosis of angiokeratoma corporis diffusum is made by the presence of cutaneous angiomas, a positive family history, corneal opacities on slit-lamp examination, and the presence of trihexosyl ceramide in the urine, plasma, or cultured fibroblasts. Hemizygotes and heterozygotes may also be diagnosed by hair root analysis.[44] Early in the course of the disease, casts, red cells, fat-laden epithelial cells (mulberry cells), and lipid inclusions with characteristic birefringent "Maltese crosses" appear in the urinary sediment. Proteinuria, gradual deterioration of renal function, and azotemia occur in the second to fourth decade of life. Biopsy of the skin or kidney is confirmatory if intracellular birefringent lipoid deposits can be demonstrated, and prenatal detection can be accomplished by the demonstration of deficient alpha galactosidase activity in cultured fetal cells obtained by amniocentesis.[45]

TREATMENT.—Unfortunately, there is no specific therapy to correct the biochemical defect of Fabry's disease. Treatment, therefore, is generally supportive in nature. Although diphenylhydantoin in dosages of 100 to 300 mg daily has been reported to be helpful for the treatment of acroparesthesias in patients with this disorder, the therapeutic response has been at best inconsistent. Replacement transfusion and periodic infusion with normal plasma, however, provide ceramide trihexosidase to patients with this inherited metabolic disease and have resulted in a temporary decrease in plasma levels of ceramide trihexoside.[46]

Fucosidosis

Disseminated angiokeratomas may also be seen in patients with fucosidosis, an autosomal recessive disease characterized by absence or deficiency of the lysosomal enzyme alpha-L-fucosidase (Fig 10–6) (Table 10–4). The disorder, first described by Durand in 1966, is associated with tissue accumulation of polysaccharides, mucopolysaccharides, and glycolipids and is characterized by mental retardation, weakness, spasticity, and growth retardation, with or without angiokeratomas.[47, 48]

CLINICAL FEATURES.—Three variants of fucosidosis have been described but only type III is associated with cutaneous lesions.[49] The first occurs in infancy and is characterized by progressive neurologic degeneration, mental retardation, weakness, spasticity, marked growth retardation, enlarged heart, repeated respiratory infection, hypoplastic lumbar vertebrae, and

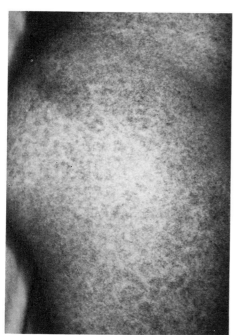

Fig 10–6.—Disseminated angiokeratomas on the hip and upper thigh of a child with fucosidosis. (Courtesy of Benjamin K. Fisher, M.D., from Hurwitz S.: *Clinical Pediatric Dermatology.* W.B. Saunders Co., Philadelphia, 1981. Used by permission.)

TABLE 10–4.—FUCOSIDOSIS

1. Autosomal recessive
2. Absence or deficiency of alpha-L-fucosidase (with tissue accumulation of polysaccharides, mucopolysaccharides and glycolipids)
3. Mental retardation, weakness, growth retardation and spasticity with or without angiokeratomas
4. Three variants:
    a. Type 1—progressive neurologic degeneration, mental and growth retardation, weakness, spasticity, enlarged heart, hypoplastic lumbar vertebrae, hyperhidrosis and thickening of skin, repeated respiratory infection, and death usually within first few years of life
    b. Type 2 (lysosomal bone disease)—normal intelligence, moderate growth retardation, spondyloepiphyseal dysplasia
    c. Type 3—mental retardation, weakness, seizures, spasticity, coarse facies, mild spondyloepiphyseal dysplasia, growth retardation, decreased sweating, purple nail bands (in some), and cutaneous lesions

death, generally within the first few years of life. Cutaneous signs of type I fucosidosis include hyperhidrosis, thickening of the skin, and increased levels of sodium chloride in sweat.

The second, a milder form of fucosidosis described in 1971, is referred to as lysosomal bone disease. This unusual form is associated with normal intelligence, moderate growth retardation, and spondyloepiphyseal dysplasia.[50]

The third type of fucosidosis (type III disease) is compatible with life, at least until adolescence. It is associated with central nervous system involvement (mental retardation, weakness, spasticity, and, at times, seizures), coarse facies, mild spondyloepiphyseal dysplasia, retardation of growth, frequent respiratory infections, decreased sweating, purple nail bands in some patients, and cutaneous lesions similar to those seen in patients with angiokeratoma corporis diffusum.[50] In typical patients with type III disease, psychomotor regression is first noted at the age of 12 to 18 months and is associated with spasticity and seizures. Ectasia of the cutaneous vessels develops earlier than in Fabry's disease (usually between 6 months and 8 years of age).[49, 51]

DIAGNOSIS.—Patients with all three types of fucosidosis have markedly decreased or absent alpha-L-fucosidase activity, which results in increased levels of fucose-containing compounds in all tissues. Asymptomatic carriers of this autosomal recessive trait have also been found to have abnormally low alpha-L-fucosidase activity in cells and serum. Patients with Fabry disease may be confused with those with type III fucosidosis. Those with fucosidosis, however, do not have hypertensive cardiovascular disease, cerebral hemorrhage, or renal failure, and fat stains of histologic material from patients with fucosidosis do not show lipids, as seen in the cytoplasmic inclusions of Fabry disease.

TREATMENT.—There is, to date, no effective form of therapy for fucosidosis. However, efforts at enzyme replacement, as in other lysosomal diseases, show promise.

Disorders Associated With Vascular Dilatation

Livedo Reticularis

Livedo reticularis is a mottled or reticulated bluish-red discoloration of the skin that occurs chiefly on the trunk, legs, and forearms of children and adults. The etiology of livedo reticularis is not completely understood, but exposure to cold usually intensifies the vascular pattern of this disorder. Most investigators attribute its reticulated appearance to vasospasm of the arterioles in response to cold, with subsequent hypoxia and dilatation of capillaries and venules. This results in sluggish blood flow through the subpapillary venous plexuses and a mottled livid or cyanotic appearance to the involved areas. The blotchy discoloration persists even after the skin has been warmed. This contrasts to the physiologic livid mottling of skin (cutis marmorata) produced by cold in infants and young children.

Livedo reticularis is usually normal when it affects the trunk or limbs of girls and young women in a continuous or persistent pattern. When it develops in a blotchy or interrupted asymmetrical distribution, however, it often represents an early sign of systemic disease, such as rheumatoid arthritis, rheumatic fever, lupus erythematosus, idiopathic thrombocytopenia, thrombotic thrombocytopenic purpura, leukemia, neurologic disorders (cerebrovascular accidents), periarteritis nodosa, or cryoglobulinemia.[52] In rare cases, recurrent small ulcerations may develop on the lower legs and feet in adults with idiopathic livedo reticularis. Mild hypertension and edema of the skin of the ankles, feet, and legs have been described in such cases. This form of the disease has been termed livedo vasculitis, livedoid vasculitis, or livedo reticularis with summer or winter ulcerations. It now appears that there is a spectrum of disease that starts with livedo reticularis and ends with livedoid vasculitis.[52] Although there is no specific treatment for livedo reticularis, vasodilatating and anticoagulant drugs have been used with moderate success in patients with severe ulceration.[53]

Cutis Marmorata Telangiectatica Congenita (congenital generalized phlebectasia)

Cutis marmorata telangiectatica congenita (congenital generalized phlebectasia, CMTC) is an uncommon disorder of infants and children characterized by a reticulated bluish mottling of the skin that resembles an exaggerated form of cutis marmorata. Seen in males as well as females (contrary to many statements in current textbooks and literature), the disorder is seen as dilated reticulated venous and capillary channels measuring 3 to 4 mm or more in diameter (Table 10–5) (Fig 10–7). Usually present at birth, the vascular pattern generally extends somewhat during the first few weeks of life and, in most patients, eventually improves substantially during childhood. In some cases the cutaneous marbling pattern persists on into adulthood.[54–57] In most patients the vascular pattern of cutis marmorata telangiectatica congenita is distributed in a generalized manner over the trunk and extremities. In some, however, the involvement may be segmental or localized to one extremity or a limited portion of the trunk.

The etiology is unknown, but it appears to represent a developmental ectasia involving both capillaries and veins. In some patients, little or no histopathologic abnormality can be seen. In others, however, microscopic examination of a cutaneous biopsy may reveal dilated capillaries, capillary and venous lakes, and large dilated veins in all layers of the dermis and subcutaneous tissue.[54, 56] Since histopathologic features are variable, diagnosis is best made on clinical criteria.

Ulcerations over the reticulated vascular pattern have been seen in a few patients with this disorder. In general, cutis marmorata telangiectatica congenita has a benign course and requires no specific therapy. It may be associated, however, with other abnormalities in up to 50% of cases[58] and should not be confused with diffuse phlebectasia (Brockenheimer's syndrome), a rare hamartomatous malformation of the deeper venous channels of a limb or part of a limb that assumes bizarre patterns with tumor-like vascular swellings of the involved area. Other abnormalities seen in asso-

TABLE 10–5.—CUTIS MARMORATA
TELANGIECTATICA CONGENITA

---

1. Reticulated bluish mottling of skin
   a. Dilated venous and capillary channels
   b. Usually generalized distribution over trunk and extremities (occasionally segmental or localized)
   c. Usually present at birth (or first few weeks of life)
   d. Although some persist, most improve during childhood
2. 50% of cases manifest other abnormalities (ulceration, varicosities, or other vascular abnormalities; patent ductus arteriosus, congenital glaucoma with mental retardation, branchial cleft cysts, atrophy or hypertrophy of soft tissue or bone, aplasia cutis congenita)

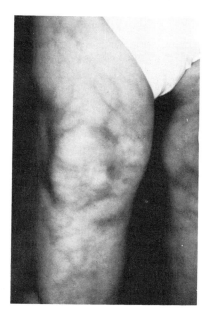

Fig 10–7.—Cutis marmorata telangiectatica congenita (congenital generalized phlebectasia) on the leg of a one-year-old male. This disorder must be differentiated from cutis marmorata, a normal physiologic response to chilling in the newborn.

ciation with cutis marmorata telangiectatica congenita include hemangiomatous abnormalities and varicosities, telangiectatic capillary nevi, patent ductus arteriosus, congenital glaucoma with mental retardation, branchial cleft cysts, atrophy or hypertrophy of soft tissue or bone, hemiatrophy, hemihypertrophy, and aplasia cutis congenita suggesting a possible developmental defect of the mesoderm. Patients with this disorder should be examined and followed carefully for the possibility of other associated malformations.[55, 56]

Hereditary Hemorrhagic Telangiectasia

Hereditary hemorrhagic telangiectasia (Osler's disease, Osler-Rendu-Weber disease) is an autosomal dominant disorder characterized by the presence of numerous telangiectases on the skin and mucous membranes of the nose and mouth, recurrent nosebleeds, and a family history of the disorder (Table 10–6) (Fig 10–8). Recurrent epistaxis, the usual presenting symptom of this disorder, may begin in early childhood (generally at about 8 or 10 years), or early in infancy, but more commonly does not begin until puberty or adult life. The characteristic mucocutaneous lesions, however, are rarely observed in children and generally do not become evident until the third decade of life, or later, and significant gastrointestinal bleeding generally does not begin until after the fourth decade of life.

TABLE 10–6.—Hereditary
Hemorrhagic Telangiectasia

1. Autosomal dominant
2. Multiple telangiectases of skin and mucous membranes
   a. Slightly elevated, ill-defined border and "legs" radiating
      from an eccentrically placed punctum
   b. May also effect pharynx, larynx, bronchi, liver, brain, retina,
      urinary bladder and g.i. tract
3. Recurrent epistaxis (usually first presenting symptom)
4. Hemorrhages may occur from cutaneous, mucosal or internal
   lesions (pulmonary a-v fistulae are seen in adults but are rare in
   children)

True lesions of this disorder tend to be slightly elevated with an ill-defined border and one or more legs radiating from an eccentrically placed puncta.[52] They develop primarily on the lips, tongue, palate, nasal mucosa, conjunctiva, ears, palms, under the nails, on the plantar surfaces of the feet, and occasionally the trunk and toes. Similar lesions may also occur in the pharynx, larynx, bronchi, liver, brain, retina, urinary bladder, and gastrointestinal tract. Hemorrhages may occur from any site, and their severity and frequency determine the clinical manifestations and course of the disorder. Pulmonary arteriovenous fistulae are present in some cases, and occur in certain families, but are rare in children. When present, associ-

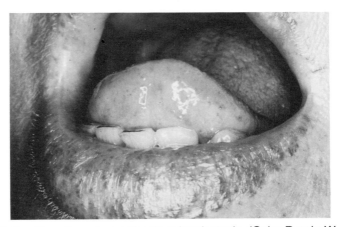

Fig 10–8.—Hereditary hemorrhagic telangiectasia (Osler-Rendu-Weber disease). Multiple 1 to 4 mm slightly elevated bright red to purple telangiectatic vessels with one or more legs radiating from an eccentrically placed punctum on the lips and tongue of a patient with Osler-Rendu-Weber disease. (From Hurwitz S.: *Clinical Pediatric Dermatology.* W.B. Saunders Co., Philadelphia, 1981. Used by permission.)

ated signs and symptoms include dyspnea, cyanosis, polycythemia, and clubbing of the fingers and toes in adolescence.

Diagnosis is dependent upon the history and morphologic configuration of individual telangiectatic lesions. Microscopic examination reveals a subepidermal tortuous mass of dilated vessels with a markedly thin wall composed almost entirely of a single layer of endothelium.

Treatment of mild cases is not necessary. Individual lesions may be cauterized, and iron supplements may help control secondary anemia. In severe disorders, systemic estrogens have been advocated but, when used in small dosages (as in contraceptive pills) actually may aggravate the disorder. Resection of pulmonary arteriovenous shunts and involved segments of the gastrointestinal tract may be necessary, and for severe epistaxis, dermoplasty may be beneficial for some individuals.

Ataxia Telangiectasia

Ataxia telangiectasia (Louis-Bar syndrome) is an autosomal recessive syndrome characterized by progressive cerebellar ataxia, oculocutaneous telangiectasia, and combined immunodeficiency that predisposes to recurrent respiratory tract (sinopulmonary) infection and lymphoreticular malignancy (Table 10–7). The frequency of this disorder has been estimated at 1 in 40,000. It also has been estimated that 1% of the unaffected population is heterozygous for this disorder with carriers of the trait having a higher incidence of malignant disease than the general population.[57] An associated thymic defect and immunologic defect in some cases has led some to classify this as a disturbance of defective thymic development, generalized lymphoreticular abnormalities, immunologic deficiency, and an unusual

TABLE 10–7.—ATAXIA TELANGIECTASIA
(LOUIS-BAR SYNDROME)

1. Autosomal recessive (incidence 1 in 40,000)
2. Usually develops between 3 and 5 years of age
    a. Oculocutaneous telangiectasia (bulbar conjunctiva, ears, eyelids, cheeks and "V" area of chest)
    b. Progressive cerebellar ataxia
    c. Immunologic defects
        (1) Recurrent sinopulmonary infection
        (2) IgA and IgE deficiencies, impaired lymphocyte transformation and lymphopenia
        (3) A tendency to lymphoreticular malignancy
3. Most patients die in childhood or adolescence (of pulmonary insufficiency or overwhelming pulmonary infection)

susceptibility to lymphoreticular malignancy estimated to be 1,200 times that of normal individuals.[58, 59]

The underlying cause of ataxia telangiectasia is unknown, but the disorder is considered to be a progressive degenerative immunodeficiency disease with faulty mesodermal-endodermal interaction and an increased sensitivity to specific intrinsic agents known to damage DNA.[59, 60]

The high incidence of malignancy may be the result of faulty immune surveillance, chromosomal instability,[61] or a molecular deficiency in DNA repair which results in easily induced breakage following exposure to x-rays and chemical mutagens[62, 63] The presence of a fetal-like thymus and elevated alpha-fetoprotein levels in patients with this disorder also suggests suppressed mesodermal development as a factor in this disease.[64] Since fetal protein is produced by immature hepatocytes, the high concentrations of this substance appear to support the concept that the liver is poorly differentiated in these patients. The finding of a deficiency of hydroxylysine content in collagen in two siblings also supports this hypothesis, the biochemical abnormality of collagen accounting for many of the clinical manifestations observed in individuals with this disorder.[65]

CLINICAL MANIFESTATIONS.—Children affected with ataxia telangiectasia are usually small and appear to be normal until the ataxia and clumsiness become apparent (this usually occurs between the ages of 12 and 18 months). In addition to the ataxia, affected individuals develop choreoathetosis, drooling, peculiar ocular movements, and a sad mask-like facies, and by the age of 12 the ataxia generally becomes so severe that patients are unable to walk without assistance.

The telangiectasia usually develops between the ages of 3 and 5 (occasionally as early as the second year of life). The fine symmetrical bright red telangiectases characteristically involve the temporal and nasal aspects of the bulbar conjunctiva (sparing the superior and inferior portions), and the cutaneous telangiectases appear later (at about 5 or 6 years of age) and affect the ears, eyelids, butterfly areas of the cheeks, the neck, and the V area of the upper chest (areas receiving the greatest sun exposure). With time they extend to the popliteal and antecubital fossae and the dorsal aspect of the hands and feet. With continued sun exposure and aging, the skin becomes sclerodermatous, with a mottled pattern of hyperpigmentation and hypopigmentation. Other cutaneous findings include café au lait spots, diffuse graying of the scalp hair, eczema (in 40% to 60% of patients), and hirsutism of the arms and legs.

Recurrent sinopulmonary infections, varying from acute rhinitis with infections of the ears to chronic bronchitis, recurrent pneumonia, and bronchiectasis, occur in 75% to 80% of affected patients. Death, when it occurs, is generally associated with bronchiectasis and pneumonia. Immunologic deficiencies include defects in both antibody and cell-mediated immune mechanisms. Among the immunologic defects seen in association with this disorder are deficiencies of immunoglobulin A (IgA) and immunoglobulin E (IgE), structural anomalies of the thymus and lymph nodes, impaired lymphocyte transformation, and lymphopenia.[58, 66]

About 30% of patients with ataxia telangiectasia have mild to moderate intellectual deficits. Associated immunologic deficiencies have been implicated in the severe sinopulmonary infections that shorten the lives of children with this disorder. Immunodeficiency and recurrent sinopulmonary infections, however, are not necessarily components of the syndrome since formes frustes of the disease occur. Most patients die in childhood or adolescence of pulmonary insufficiency or overwhelming pulmonary infection. Those surviving beyond adolescence develop peripheral neuropathy and progressive spinal muscle atrophy.[61] Of those individuals who survive to the late teens, about 10% develop lymphoreticular malignancy (lymphosarcoma, Hodgkin's disease, reticular cell sarcoma, or leukemia); other associated disorders include ovarian dysgerminoma, medulloblastoma, glioma, and adenocarcinoma.

DIAGNOSIS.—The development of telangiectasia on the bulbar conjunctivae, ears, eyelids, butterfly areas of the cheeks, and other areas receiving a high incidence of sun exposure in a child with cerebellar ataxia is highly suggestive of this disorder. This tendency, however, is not a true photosensitivity. A recently described rapid diagnostic test for ataxia telangiectasia consists of a simple two-day culture of peripheral lymphocytes grown in phytohemagglutinin which can distinguish normal cells from ataxia telangiectasia cells by their sensitivity to radiation. Although this test can be used for prenatal diagnosis (on amniotic fluid cells) of affected individuals, it does not detect carriers of this disorder.[67, 68]

TREATMENT.—No specific therapy is known for patients with ataxia telangiectasia. Affected individuals generally go progressively downhill, with death usually occurring in the second decade of life. Antibiotic therapy of the recurrent sinopulmonary infections is only of temporary benefit, and long-term prophylaxis is generally ineffective. The parents of affected children should receive genetic counseling (since there is a 25% risk of an affected child with each pregnancy) and prenatal diagnosis is now available.[69] Children with ataxia telangiectasis should have a complete blood count with each physical examination. Starting in late adolescence, annual physical examinations should include sigmoidoscopy, tests for occult blood in the stool, and breast and pelvic examination with Papanicolaou smears in an effort to detect possible malignancy at an early stage.[70]

Purpura Fulminans

Purpura fulminans and disseminated intravascular coagulation are terms used to describe a form of nonthrombocytic purpura characterized by an acute, severe, often rapidly fatal hemorrhagic infarction and necrosis of the skin. Usually occurring in children, the disease is triggered by a preceding infectious process such as scarlet fever or other streptococcal infection, meningococcal and other septicemias, chickenpox, measles, vaccinia, or rickettsial disorders such as Rocky Mountain spotted fever (Fig 10–9).

The etiology has not been firmly established, but purpura fulminans usually has its onset within 3 to 30 days after a resolving infection. The cause represents a nonimmunologic hypersensitivity reaction similar to that of an induced Schwartzman phenomenon. The primary pathology is a consumptive coagulopathy (disseminated intravascular coagulation) characterized by intravascular consumption of plasma coagulation factors (fibrinogen, factors II, V, and VIII), with low-normal to severely reduced platelet counts, hypofibrinogenemia, and hypoprothrombinemia associated with microthrombosis and a hemorrhagic diathesis[71, 72] (Table 10–8).

CLINICAL FEATURES.—The disorder is characterized by symmetrically distributed localized cutaneous ecchymoses, often with sharp irregular borders on the extremities, particularly in the areas of pressure. Lesions are tender, enlarge rapidly, coalesce, and develop central necrosis, with hemorrhagic blebs and a raised edge with surrounding erythema. They spread to the trunk and may occasionally involve the lips, ears, and nose. Chills, fever, tachycardia, anemia, and prostration are common. Visceral involvement with hematuria or gastrointestinal bleeding may occur, and shock, coma, and death frequently develop. When hemorrhage and necrosis of

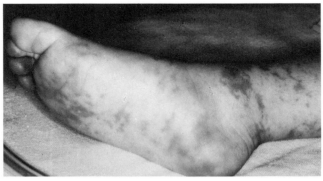

Fig 10–9.—Purpura fulminans on the foot and lower leg of a 4-year-old boy with Rocky Mountain spotted fever.

TABLE 10–8.—Purpura Fulminans (Disseminated
Intravascular Coagulation)

1. A nonthrombocytic purpura triggered by a preceding infection
2. Usually in children (a Schwartzman-like phenomenon)
    a. Consumptive coagulopathy with intravascular consumption of
       fibrinogen, factors II, V, and VIII
    b. Characterized by symmetrical localized ecchymoses with
       sharp borders on extremities
3. Hemorrhagic infarction and necrosis of skin
4. Chills, fever, tachycardia, anemia, and prostration are common
5. Visceral involvement; hematuria, gastrointestinal bleeding,
   shock, coma and death in 18% to 35% (previously 90%)

the adrenal glands are present, the designation Waterhouse-Friderichsen syndrome has been applied to this disorder.

DIAGNOSIS.—Since current studies support the concept that purpura fulminans is usually the result of disseminated intravascular coagulation, the presence of a consumptive coagulopathy should be confirmed prior to the institution of therapy.[73] However, disseminated intravascular coagulation is more difficult to diagnose in premature infants because of the normal prolonged coagulation value in prematures.[74] Usually the number of platelets is markedly reduced, coagulation factors I (fibrinogen), II (prothrombin), V, and VIII are usually decreased in number, and histopathologic studies show small vessel occlusion and hemorrhagic necrosis of the skin, subcutaneous tissue, and often the underlying fascia and muscle.

TREATMENT.—Although the outlook is grave and death frequently occurs within 48 to 72 hours (until recently the mortality was over 90%), prompt initiation of therapy improves the prognosis for most patients with current estimates of mortality in the range of 18% to 35%. Treatment consists of early recognition of this disorder, prompt identification and therapy of any associated infection, correction of clotting factor deficiencies due to intravascular coagulation, and general supportive measures. In view of its rapid onset of action, heparin, 50 to 150 units (0.5 to 1.5 mg) per kg of body weight, given intravenously immediately and repeated every four hours, with periodic adjustment according to clinical progress is generally the treatment of choice. Dextran, 6% solution in saline or water (600 mg/ kg over a period of two to four days and then every two or three days), or low molecular weight dextran (Dextran 40), 10 ml of the 10% solution per kg every 12 hours for the first two days and then daily until adequate healing has occurred, and the replacement of the consumed clotting factors with fresh whole blood or frozen plasma is often necessary. General supportive measures, treatment of shock, anemia, infection, renal failure, debridement, skin grafting, and, on occasion, amputation may also be performed, if necessary, depending upon the clinical picture.[2]

REFERENCES

1. Jacobs A.H., Walton R.G.: The incidence of birthmarks in the neonate. *Pediatrics* 58:218–222, 1976.
2. Hurwitz S.: Vascular disorders of infancy and childhood, in Hurwitz S.: *Clinical Pediatric Dermatology*. W.B. Saunders Publishing Co., Philadelphia, 1981, pp. 190–213.
3. Jacobs A.H.: Vascular nevi, in Rasmussen J.E. (editor), *Pediatric Clinics of North America, Symposium on Pediatric Dermatology (Part I)*. W.B. Saunders Co., Philadelphia, 1983, pp. 465–482.
4. Nakayama H.: Clinical and historical studies of the classification and the natural course of the strawberry mark. *J. Dermatol.* (Tokyo) 8:277–291, 1981.
5. Levy R.S., Fisher M.: Hemangiomas, in Demis D.J., Dobson R.L., McGuire J.: *Clinical Dermatology*, ed. 10. Harper & Row, Philadelphia, 1983, Unit 7–63, pp. 1–7.
6. Bowers R.E., Graham E.A., Tomlinson K.M.: The natural history of the strawberry nevus. *Arch. Dermatol.* 82:667–680, 1960.
7. Margileth A.M., Museles M.: Cutaneous hemangiomas in children. *J.A.M.A.* 194:523–526, 1965.
8. Robb R.M.: Refractive errors associated with hemangiomas of the eyelids and orbit in infancy. *J. Ophthal.* 83:52–58, 1977.
9. Nelson L.B., Melick J.E., Harley R.D.: Intralesional corticosteroid injections for infantile hemangiomas of the eyelid. *Pediatrics* 74:241–245, 1984.
10. Haik B.G., Jakobeic F.A., Ellsworth R.M., et al.: Capillary hemangiomas of the lids and orbit: an analysis of the clinical features and therapeutic results in 101 cases. *Ophthalmol.* 86:760–789, 1979.
11. Kushner B.J.: Local steroid therapy in adnexal hemangioma. *Am. J. Ophthalmol.* 11:1005–1009, 1979.
12. Fost N.C., Esterly N.B.: Successful treatment of juvenile hemangiomas with prednisone. *J. Pediatr.* 72:351–357, 1968.
13. Zarem H.A., Edgerton M.T.: Cavernous hemangiomas and prednisolone therapy. *Plast. Reconstr. Surg.* 39:76–83, 1976.
14. Edgerton M.T.: The treatment of hemangiomas with special reference to the role of steroid therapy. *Ann. Surg.* 183:517–532, 1976.
15. Grabb W.C., Dingman R.O., Oneal R.M., et al.: Facial hamartomas in children: neurofibroma, lymphangioma, and hemangioma. *Plastic Reconst. Surg.* 66:509–527, 1980.
16. Martins A.G.: Hemangioma and thrombocytopenia. *J. Pediatr. Surg.* 5:641–648, 1970.
17. Esterly N.B.: Kasabach-Merritt syndrome in infants. *J. Am. Acad. Dermatol.* 8:504–513, 1983.
18. Hagerman L.J., Czapek E.E., Donnellan W.L., et al.: Giant hemangioma with consumption coagulopathy. *J. Pediatr.* 87:766–768, 1975.
19. Alexander G.L., Norman R.M.: The Sturge-Weber syndrome without port-wine nevus. *Pediatrics* 60:785, 1977.
20. Jacobs A.H.: Response to a letter: Sturge-Weber syndrome without port-wine nevus. *Pediatrics* 60:785, 1977.

21. Stevenson R.F., Thomson H.G., Marin J.D.: Unrecognized ocular problems associated with port-wine stain of the face in children. *Can. Med. Assoc. J.* 111:953–954, 1974.
22. Rook A.: Naevi and other developmental defects, in Rook A., Wilkinson D.S., Ebling F.J.G.: *Textbook of Dermatology*, ed. 2. Blackwell Scientific Publications, London, 1972, 126–167.
23. Solomon L.M., Esterly N.B.: Vascular disorders and malformations, in *Neonatal Dermatology*. W.B. Saunders Publishing Co., Philadelphia, 1973, pp. 68–80.
24. Goldman L.: Laser treatment of extensive mixed cavernous and port-wine stains. *Arch. Dermatol.* 113:504–505, 1977.
25. Apfelberg D.B., Maser M.R., Lash H.: Argon laser treatment of cutaneous vascular abnormalities. *Ann. Plast. Surg.* 1:14–18, 1978.
26. Noe J.M., Barsky S.H., Geer D.E., et al.: Port wine stains and the response to argon laser therapy: successful treatment and the predictive role of color, age, and biopsy. *Plast. Reconstruct. Surg.* 65:130–136, 1980.
27. Phillips G.N., Gordon D.H., Martin E.C., et al.: The Klippel-Trenaunay syndrome: clinical radiologic aspects. *Radiology* 128:428–434, 1978.
28. Fine R.M., Derbes V.J., Clark W.H., Jr.: Blue rubber bleb nevus. *Arch. Dermatol.* 84:802–805, 1961.
29. Morris S.J., Kaplan S.R., Ballan K., et al.: Blue rubber-bleb nevus syndrome. *J.A.M.A.* 239:1887, 1978.
30. Stern J.K., Wolfe J.E., Jr., Jarratt M.: Benign neonatal hemangiomatosis. *J. Am. Acad. Dermatol.* 4:442–445, 1981.
31. Holden K.R., Alexander F.: Diffuse neonatal hemangiomatosis. *Pediatrics* 46:411–421, 1970.
32. Wishnick M.M.: Multinodular hemangiomatosis with partial biliary obstruction. *J. Pediatr.* 92:960–962, 1978.
33. Keller L., Bluhm J.F. III: Diffuse neonatal hemangiomatosis. A case with heart failure and thrombocytopenia. *Cutis* 23:295–297, 1979.
34. Frost J.I., Caplan R.M.: Cutaneous hemangiomas and disappearing bones with a review of cutaneo-visceral hemangiomatosis. *Arch. Dermatol.* 92:501–508, 1965.
35. Gellis S.S., Feingold M.: Picture of the month. Contributed by Ryan M.E., Spahr R.C.: Hemangioma with osteolysis (Gorham's disease, vanishing bone disease). *Am. J. Dis. Child.* 132:715–716, 1978.
36. Stephan M.J., Hall B.D., Smith D.W., et al.: Macrocephaly in association with unusual cutaneous angiomatosis. *J. Pediatr.* 87:353–359, 1975.
37. Zonana J., Rimoin D.L., David D.C.: Macrocephaly with multiple lipomas and hemangiomas. *J. Pediatr.* 89:600–603, 1976.
38. Jessen R.T., Thompson S., Smith E.B.: Cobb syndrome. *Arch. Dermatol.* 113:1587–1590, 1977.
39. Zala L., Mumenthaler M.: Cobb syndrome. *Dermatologica* 163:417–425, 1981.
40. Danehower C.C., Moyer D.G.M.: Angiokeratoma corporis diffusum. *Arch. Dermatol.* 94:628–631, 1966.
41. Gorlin R.H., Pindborg J.J., Cohen M.M., Jr.: Fabry Syndrome, in *Syndromes of the Head and Neck*. McGraw-Hill Book Co., New York, 1976, pp. 295–299.
42. von Gemmingen G., Kierland R.R., Opitz J.M.: Angiokeratoma corporis diffusum (Fabry's disease). *Arch. Dermatol.* 91:206–218, 1965.
43. Burda C.D., Winder P.R.: Angiokeratoma corporis diffusum universale (Fa-

bry's disease) in female subjects. *Am. J. Med.* 42:293–301, 1967.
44. Beaudet A.L., Caskey C.T.: Detection of Fabry's disease heterozygotes by hair root analysis. *Clin. Genet.* 13:251–258, 1978.
45. Brady R.O.: Fabry's disease. *Science* 172:174–175, 1971.
46. Mapes C.A., Anderson R.L., Sweeley C.C.: Enzyme replacement in Fabry's disease, an inborn error of metabolism. *Science* 169:987–989, 1970.
47. Durand P., Borrone C., Della Cella G.: A new mucopolysaccharide lipid-storage disease? *Lancet* 11:1313–1314, 1966.
48. Smith E.B., Graham J.L., Ledman J.A., et al.: Fucosidosis. *Cutis* 19:195–198, 1977.
49. Dvoretzky I., Fisher B.K.: Fucosidosis. *Int. J. Dermatol.* 18:213–216, 1979.
50. Schafer I.A., Powell D.W., Sullivan J.C.: Lysosomal bone disease. *Pediatr. Res.* 5:391–392, 1971.
51. Epinette W.W., Norins A.L., Drew A.L., et al.: Angiokeratoma corporis diffusum with alpha-L-fucosidase deficiency. *Arch. Dermatol.* 107:755–757, 1973.
52. Braverman I.M.: Blood vessels, in Braverman I.M.: *Skin Signs of Systemic Disease.* W.B. Saunders Co., Philadelphia, 1970, pp. 287–311.
53. Feldaker M., Hines E.A., Jr., Kierland R.R.: Livedo reticularis with summer ulcerations. *Arch. Dermatol.* 72:31–42, 1955.
54. Lynch P.J., Zelickson A.S.: Congenital phlebectasia—a histopathologic study. *Arch. Dermatol.* 95:98–101, 1967.
55. Miller J.Q.: Cutis marmorata telangiectatica congenita. *J. Assoc. Milit. Dermatol* 1(2):33–35, 1975.
56. Petrozzi J.W., Rahn E.K., Mofenson H.: Cutis marmorata telangiectatica congenita. *Arch. Dem.* 101:74–77, 1970.
57. Taylor A.M.R., Harndin D.G., Arlett C.F., et al.: Ataxia telangiectasia: a human mutation with abnormal radiation sensitivity. *Nature* 258:427–429, 1975.
58. Peterson R.D.A., Cooper M.D., Good R.A.: Lymphoid tissue abnormalities associated with ataxia-telangiectasia. *Am. J. Med.* 41:342–359, 1966.
59. Dwyer J.M.: Cutaneous manifestations of immunogenetic deficiency disorders, in Blandau R.J. (editor): *Morphogenesis and malformation of the Skin.* Alan R. Liss, Inc., New York, 1981, pp. 92–115.
60. Paterson M.C., Smith T.J.: Ataxia telangiectasia. an inherited human disorder involving hypersensitivity to ionizing radiation and related DNA-damaging chemicals. *Am. Rev. Genet.* 13:291–318, 1979.
61. Boder E.: Ataxia telangiectasia: some historic, clinical and pathological observations. *Birth Defects* 11:255–270, 1975.
62. Paterson M.C., Smith B.P., Loman P.H.M., et al.: Defective excision repair of gamma-ray-damaged DNA in humans (ataxia-telangiectasia) fibroblasts. *Nature* 260:444–447, 1976.
63. Hoar V.I., Sargent P.: Chemical mutagen hypersensitivity in ataxia-telangiectasia. *Nature* 261:590–592, 1976.
64. Richkind K.E., Boder E., Teplitz R.L.: Fetal proteins in ataxia-telangiectasia. *J.A.M.A.* 248:1346–1347, 1982.
65. McReynolds E.W., Dabbous M.K., Hanissian A.S., et al.: Abnormal collagen in ataxia telangiectasia. *Am. J. Dis. Child.* 130:305–307, 1976.
66. Amman A.J., Cain W.A., Ishizaka K., et al.: Immunoglobulin E deficiency in ataxia-telangiectasia. *N. Engl. J. Med.* 281:469–472, 1969.
67. Jason J.M., Gelfand E.W.: Diagnostic considerations in ataxia-telangiectasia. *Arch. Dis. Child.* 54:682–686, 1979.

68. Jaspers N.G.J., Scheres J.M.J.C., de Wit J., et al.: Rapid diagnostic test for ataxia telangiectasia. *Lancet* 2-1:473, 1981.
69. Shaham M., Voss R., Becker Y., et al.: Prenatal diagnosis of ataxia telangiectasia. *J. Pediatr.* 100:134–137, 1982.
70. Swift M., Sholman L., Perry M., et al.: Malignant neoplasms in the families of patients with ataxia-telangiectasia. *Cancer Res.* 36:209–215, 1976.
71. Dudgeon D.L., Kellogg D.R., Gilchrist G.S., et al.: Purpura fulminans. *Arch. Surg.* 103:351–358, 1971.
72. Antley R.M., McMillan C.W.: Sequential coagulation studies in purpura fulminans. *N. Engl. J. Med.* 276:1287–1290, 1967.
73. Esterly N.B.: Purpura fulminans, in Demis D.J., Dobson R.L., McGuire J. (Eds.): *Clinical Dermatology, Vol. 2.* Harper and Row, Hagerstown, Md., 1977, 7–24, 1–3.
74. Woods W.G., Corman Lubin N.L., Hilgartner M.G., et al.: disseminated intravascular coagulation in the newborn. *Am. J. Dis. Child.* 133:44–46, 1979.

11 / Photosensitivity Disorders and Systemic Disease in Children

REACTIONS TO THE SUN'S RAYS have become increasingly common in recent years, owing not only to the ever-expanding number of photosensitizers in our environment, but also to the public's ever-increasing obsession with sunbathing. Although photosensitivity in childhood is relatively uncommon, when present, it is frequently associated with a serious or potentially serious condition.[1] Frequently genetic in origin, the photosensitivity disorders of particular significance in children include xeroderma pigmentosum, the Bloom syndrome, Rothmund-Thomson syndrome, Cockayne syndrome, Hartnup disease, Kwashiorkor, and the erythropoietic and hepatic porphyrias. Although lupus erythematosus may also be classified as a disease associated with photosensitivity, this condition is discussed in the section on collagen vascular (connective tissue) disorders.

Xeroderma Pigmentosum

Xeroderma pigmentosum is a severe, rare, autosomal recessive disease characterized by cutaneous photosensitivity, a decreased ability to repair deoxyribonucleic acid (DNA) damaged by ultraviolet radiation, and a tendency toward early development of cutaneous malignancies. The cardinal features of the disorder include sensitivity to light in the middle ultraviolet (UVB) spectrum with wave lengths of 290 and 320 nm; premature aging of the skin accompanied by dystrophy, pigmentary changes, and development of ephithelial neoplasms; severe eye involvement; and usually early death from malignancy.[1-4]

The basic abnormality in xeroderma pigmentosum is attributed to a defect in endonuclease, an enzyme that recognizes ultraviolet light-damaged regions in DNA and excises damaged thymine dimers so that other enzymes (DNA polymerase and polynucleotide ligase) may initiate DNA recovery.[5] Recent techniques have led to the discovery of a multitude of different genetic defects. Although not seen as distinct clinical entities, each of the variants is caused by mutation at a different locus. Thus, the xeroderma pigmentosum phenotype is the result of at least eight different genetic defects (termed A to G in the classic form, plus the XP variant).[1]

CLINCIAL FEATURES.—Occurring about once in every 250,000 births, children with xeroderma pigmentosum develop erythema, excessive freckling on sun-exposed skin, increased pigmentation after exposure to sunlight giving the skin an appearance similar to that of chronic radiodermatitis, and other evidence of chronic actinic damage at an early age. Most cases begin in early childhood. In 75% of cases, the first symptoms appear between 6 months and 3 years of age and reach the tumor stage (basal cell carcinoma, angiosarcoma, fibrosarcoma, actinic keratoses, keratoacanthoma, squamous cell carcinoma, and in about 3% of patients, malignant melanoma, often before the age of 20) (Table 11–1).

In the acute form, the first manifestations appear very early, sometimes shortly after birth or during the first few weeks of life, after the first exposure to sun. Initial clinical findings include photophobia (in over 90% of patients), erythema (which sometimes progresses to vesiculation and bulla formation), freckled hyperpigmentation of exposed parts, and subsequent papillomatous or verrucous lesions followed by degenerative and eventual malignant changes (Fig 11–1). When present at an early age, xeroderma pigmentosum usually presents a relentless course with irreversible skin damage. Although the severity of the disease varies, those individuals with severe forms frequently expire before the age of 10 years, and two-thirds of affected children die before the age of 20.[6] Although rigid protection from exposure to the sun in recent years has reduced the incidence of malignant skin disease, death still occurs at an early age from metastatic malignant disease.[1]

Many authors have reported the presence of neurologic complications in patients with xeroderma pigmentosum. In addition to their cutaneous manifestations, those with the most severe form of this disorder (termed the *DeSanctis-Cacchione* syndrome) have microcephaly with mental deficiency, premature closure of the sutures, retarded growth and sexual development, choreoathetosis, cerebellar ataxia, shortening of the achilles tendons, and, at times, sensorineural deafness.[3, 7]

DIAGNOSIS.—Xeroderma pigmentosum can now be diagnosed prenatally by testing amniotic cells for the ability to perform excision repair of damaged DNA.[8] Postnatally, tests for excision repair of DNA in skin fibroblasts coupled with observation of cutaneous reactivity to ultraviolet light allows

TABLE 11–1.–XERODERMA PIGMENTOSUM

1. Rare, autosomal recessive (1 in 250,000 births)
2. An inability to repair UVB damaged DNA
3. Photophobia, erythema, vesiculation, bulla formation, freckled hyperpigmentation, irreversible skin damage and malignant change
4. Ophthalmic changes (conjunctivitis, keratitis, corneal opacities, symblepharon and ectropion)

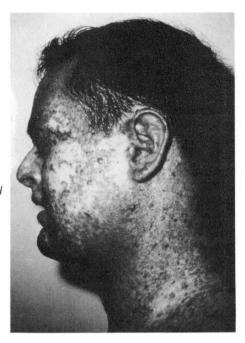

Fig 11–1.—Xeroderma pigmentosum. Freckled hyperpigmentation, papillomatous and verrucous lesions on the face and neck. (From the Department of Dermatology, Yale University School of Medicine, from Hurwitz S.: *Clinical Pediatric Dermatology.* W.B. Saunders Co., Philadelphia, 1981. Used by permission.)

early diagnosis in infants before the cutaneous features of the disorder become apparent. Once the possibility of xeroderma pigmentosum is suspected, however, the clinical features are so distinctive that diagnosis is usually obvious. The characteristic clinical features usually develop between the ages of 2 and 8 years. These include erythema, freckling, both hyperpigmentation and depigmentation, an appearance of premature aging, telangiectases, hyperkeratoses, ulcerations, keratoacanthomas, and, after a relatively short period of time, skin cancer. Conjunctivitis, keratitis, corneal opacities of the eyelids, symblepharon (adhesion of lids to the eyeball), and ectropion are highly characteristic and said to occur in 60% to 90% of individuals with this disorder. Most children will also have a history of adverse reaction to sunlight from early infancy, with marked solar erythema or sunburn following short exposures to sunlight.[9] Areas of skin ordinarily protected by clothing, however, remain normal or may eventually show similar features, but to a lesser degree.

TREATMENT.—The treatment of xeroderma pigmentosum consists of genetic counseling, avoidance of ultraviolet light exposure, the use of protective clothing and opaque sunscreen preparations, destruction of individual premalignant and malignant tumors by topical antimetabolite agents such as 5-fluorouracil, early excision of small cutaneous neoplasms and, at times, resurfacing of severely damaged skin by dermabrasion or with homografts from less severely involved cutaneous surfaces.[10]

Although effective treatment for the defect of xeroderma pigmentosum is not yet available, the information obtained from amniocentesis can be reassuring to the parents if the baby is free of chromosomal aberrations, or it can afford them the chance to decide on termination of pregnancy if abnormalities are found. It is usually impossible to detect a heterozygous fetus by amniocentesis, but this is of little clinical importance since xeroderma pigmentosum is an autosomal recessive disease and heterozygotes are phenotypically normal.[8, 11]

Bloom Syndrome (Congenital Telangiectatic Erythema)

Bloom syndrome (congenital telangiectatic erythema) is a rare autosomal recessive disorder characterized by a triad of telangiectatic erythema, photosensitivity, and severe intrauterine and postnatal growth retardation.[12] In this disorder, photosensitivity with erythema of the cheeks (often resembling lesions of lupus erythematosus) appears between the second and third week of life, and typically spreads with exposure to sunlight to involve the nose, eyelids, forehead, ears, and lips (Table 11–2). Eighty per cent of affected children are males and 50% are Jewish.

CLINICAL MANIFESTATIONS.—Affected patients are born at term with reduced body weight and size. They have small narrow faces with prominent features. Although physical growth is stunted, intellectual and sexual development is normal. The cutaneous changes include facial erythema in a butterfly distribution that develops after exposure to sunlight. Although this light sensitivity eventually disappears, erythema, telangiectasia, mottled pigmentation, scarring, and atrophy of these sites remain as prominent features (Fig 11–2). Other findings may include café au lait spots, defective dentition, prominent ears, polydactyly, clinodactyly, syndactyly, cryptor-

TABLE 11–2.—BLOOM SYNDROME

1. Rare, autosomal recessive
2. Triad of telangiectatic erythema, photosensitivity, low birth weight and growth retardation
3. 80% are males, 50% are of Jewish descent
4. Café au lait spots, clinodactyly, syndactyly, cryptorchidism
5. Normal intellect and sexual development
6. Reduced immunoglobulins (especially IgA and IgM), frequent gastrointestinal and respiratory infections, and predisposition to neoplastic disease

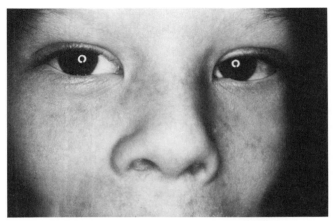

Fig 11–2.—Bloom syndrome. Facial erythema and telangiectasia on cheeks in a young male. (From the Department of Dermatology, Yale University School of Medicine.)

chidism, shortened lower extremities, clubbed feet, reduced immunoglob-ulins (especially IgA and IgM), a high incidence of nonspecific chromo-somal breakage, and increased predisposition to neoplastic disease, particularly leukemia, lymphoma and carcinomas of the alimentary tract during the second and third decades of life.[13] Patients also develop serious and sometimes fatal gastrointestinal and respiratory tract bacterial infec-tions early in life as a result of defects in both humoral and cellular immune function. With increasing age, however, resistance to infection becomes more normal.

DIAGNOSIS.—The diagnosis of Bloom syndrome may be suggested by a history of low birth weight, the presence of facial telangiectasia and pho-tosensitivity in a child of small stature of Ashkanazi Jewish heritage and can be confirmed by the demonstration of chromosomal abnormalities.

TREATMENT.—Although there is no specific treatment for patients with Bloom syndrome, avoidance of sun exposure and protection by sunscreens may help prevent some of the cutaneous eruptions associated with photo-sensitivity. Immunologic abnormalities of Bloom syndrome are diffuse and involve both B cell and T cell function with impairment of both cellular and humoral immunity.[14, 15] Appropriate antibiotics for gastrointestinal and respiratory tract bacterial infections are frequently helpful in the manage-ment of patients with this disorder and, since life expectancy may be short-ened by malignancy, periodic evaluation for possible neoplastic disease is advisable.

Rothmund-Thomson Syndrome (Poikiloderma Congenitale)

Poikiloderma congenitale (Rothmund-Thomson syndrome) is a rare inherited condition transmitted as an autosomal recessive disorder characterized by atrophy, pigmentation and telangiectasia of the skin in association with juvenile cataracts, shortness of stature, partial or total alopecia, defects of the nails and teeth, and hypogonadism[16] (Table 11–3). About 70% of affected individuals are females.

CLINICAL FEATURES.—Although the skin may be involved at birth, cutaneous changes generally make their appearance between the third and sixth months of life. Cutaneous features include diffuse erythema and, at times, edema and vesiculation on the cheeks, forehead, chin, ears, buttocks, and extensor surfaces of the arms and legs. As the erythema resolves, the skin begins to show a reticulated pattern of telangiectasia and alterations in pigmentation (both hypopigmentation and hyperpigmentation) with areas of atrophy. Although photosensitivity is a feature of many cases and exposure to sunlight may extend the distribution of the eruption, it probably is not responsible for the poikilodermatous appearance that develops on unexposed as well as light-exposed areas.

Patients are frequently short in stature and some have a characteristic facies with saddle nose, frontal bossing, wide forehead, and narrow chin giving a triangular configuration to the face. Hypotrichosis with sparse or absent eye-brows or eyelashes (and sometimes involvement of the scalp, face, and body) occurs in 50% of patients. Hypogonadism occurs in one-fourth of patients (females may be amenorrheic, males may have undescended testes), and affected individuals may exhibit prematue greying and loss of hair.[17]

Cataracts occur in about 40% of reported cases, and defective bone development, which predominantly involves long bones, and occurs in about two-thirds of affected individuals (absence, hypoplasia or other dysplasias of bones is most common at the distal portions of the limbs). Other deformities include absence or shortening of digits, cleft hand or foot, an asymmetry in length of limbs, and cystic lesions, osteoporosis and sclerotic areas on x-ray examination of the long bones and pelvic areas. Nail changes

TABLE 11–3.—ROTHMUND-THOMSON SYNDROME

1. Rare, autosomal recessive (70% are females)
2. Atrophy, pigmentation and telangiectasia of skin (poikiloderma), juvenile cataracts, short stature, defective bone development, alopecia, hypogonadism and defects of teeth and nails
3. Normal life span

(rough, ridged, heaped-up, small or atrophic nails) and dental abnormalities (microdontia, malformation and failure of teeth to erupt) may be seen,[18] and, as in patients with radiodermatitis, carcinomatous changes may develop in some adults with this disorder.

TREATMENT.—Individuals with Rothmund-Thomson syndrome have a normal life span and there is no effective treatment except for the use of sunscreens, prophylactic avoidance of sunlight and surgical attention to keratoses and carcinomas of the skin.

Cockayne Syndrome

Cockayne syndrome (trisomy 10) is a rare recessively inherited disorder, generally seen in individuals of English lineage, characterized by dwarfism, bird-like facies with disproportionately large extremities, sunken eyes, large eyes and nose, a "senile" appearance in childhood due to diffuse loss of subcutaneous fat, telangiectasia, photosensitivity, intracranial calcification, hypertension and renal disease in some individuals, cold extremities, unsteady gait, quick bird-like movements, and a 4 to 1 male preponderance[19-27] (Table 11–4).

Since there is a wide range of clinical severity among patients with this disorder, it has been suggested that Cockayne disease, as xeroderma pigmentosa, may be a genetically heterogeneous disorder.[25] Renal studies in some individuals have demonstrated glomerular lesions with thickened basement membrane, increased mesangial matrix, tubular atrophy and interstitial fibrosis.[26] Immunologic studies of tissue obtained by renal biopsy have demonstrated deposits of immunoglobulin and complement in the vessels and glomeruli in some patients with this disorder. IgG, IgA, IgM and C_3 in glomerular basement membranes in one patient suggest an immune mechanism in this degenerative disorder,[24] and studies of cultured fibroblasts suggest an enzymatic defect in the repair of ultraviolet light-induced damage.[28, 29]

CLINICAL MANIFESTATIONS.—Children with Cockayne syndrome appear to be normal during infancy and begin to develop signs of the disorder

TABLE 11–4.—COCKAYNE SYNDROME

---

1. Rare, autosomal recessive (4 to 1 male preponderance)
2. Dwarfism, bird-like facies, telangiectasia, photosensitivity, ataxia, growth retardation, disproportionately long extremities, large hands and feet, contractures of joints and large protruding ears with a "Mickey Mouse"-like appearance
3. Mental retardation, retinal atrophy, cataracts, deafness
4. Photosensitivity diminishes with age
5. Hypertension and deafness may occur, and death from atheromatous vascular disease (usually during second or third decade of life)

during the second year of life. The cutaneous changes include facial erythema in a butterfly distribution that develops after exposure to sunlight. Although this light sensitivity eventually disappears, erythema with telangiectasia characteristic of photosensitivity, mottled pigmentation, scarring, and atrophy of these sites remain as prominent features. Loss of subcutaneous fat produces a "bird-like" facies and a tendency toward progressive ataxia and long limbs (the upper extremities are long in proportion to body length), disproportionately large hands and feet, progressive contractures of the joints and large protruding ears suggest a "Mickey Mouse"-like appearance. Affected individuals are generally below the tenth percentile for height, and other abnormalities include thickened skull bones, retinal pigmentation, optic atrophy, cataracts, deafness, and mental retardation. The skin of patients with this disorder becomes atrophic and develops striae, scalp and body hair are sparse, and victims usually die from atheromatous vascular disease during the second or third decade of life.

At the time of the first skin eruptions, growth retardation becomes apparent. Other features include premature aging and abnormalities of the skeleton such as microcephaly, prognathism, ankylosis, and contractures of the joints. The premature aging results in retinal atrophy and cataracts, deafness, and progressive mental deficit (with full development of the condition by the time the child reaches the age of 5).

DIAGNOSIS.—The clinical features of the Cockayne syndrome (dwarfism, photosensitivity, a "bird-like" facies, ataxia, disproportionately large hands and feet, and large protruding ears (the "Mickey Mouse"-look) should suggest the diagnosis of this disorder. Although prenatal diagnosis of Cockayne disease should be possible, the length of time required to measure colony-formation ability after ultraviolet light radiation has been a problem.

TREATMENT.—There is no effective treatment for patients with Cockayne syndrome and most patients die in the second or third decade of life as a result of arteriosclerotic vascular disease.

Hartnup Disease

Hartnup disease, first described in 1956[30] and named after a family in which the disorder was first reported, is a rare, autosomal, recessive light-sensitive disorder characterized by a pellagra-like cutaneous eruption, neurologic abnormalities, and a specific aminoaciduria (due to a defect in the cellular transport of a group of monoamino-monocarboxylic amino acids) (Table 11–5). The basic defect appears to be a failure in the absorption of tryptophan from the gastrointestinal tract and a renal tubular defect causing inadequate reabsorption of amino acids, including tryptophan. This results in reduced levels of available tryptophan and, accordingly, decreased synthesis of nicotinic acid. Some believe that this lack of nicotinic acid may be

TABLE 11–5.—Hartnup Disease

---

1. Autosomal recessive
2. A defect in tryptophan absorption and renal reabsorption of amino acids resulting in decreased synthesis of nicotinic acid
3. Photosensitive pellagra-like eruption, cerebellar ataxia, and mental retardation
4. Treatment: high doses (40 to 200 mg) of nicotinic acid or nicotinamide

---

responsible for the pellagra-like photosensitivity. As yet, however, there is no proof that the photosensitivity in pellagra nor that the pellagra-like symptoms in patients with Hartnup disease are caused by a lack of nicotinic acid.[32–34]

CLINICAL MANIFESTATIONS.—Aminoaciduria is a constant feature of Hartnup disease. Clinical manifestations, however, are intermittent, recurrent, and quite variable. The cutaneous eruption usually appears in the spring and summer. It may be present in early childhood (in children between 3 and 9 years) and occasionally during infancy, with symptoms generally becoming milder with age. The cutaneous manifestations consist of a symmetrical distribution of inflammatory macules that tend to coalesce and eventuate in well-marginated red scaly lesions. They tend to appear over areas of the face and neck, uncovered areas of the arms, inframammary and perineal folds, elbows, knees, the dorsal aspects of the hands and wrists, and the lower legs, and once they appear they usually persist for weeks or months.

Acute dermatitis and blistering with secondary crusting and scarring frequently occur following sun exposure. These changes (together with marked hyperpigmentation) are similar to the findings seen in pellagra. Malnutrition and intercurrent infections frequently aggravate the dermatitis and glossitis, and angular stomatitis, vulvovaginitis, diffuse hair loss and fragility, and nail abnormalities (longitudinal streaking) may also be seen. In many patients, the cutaneous manifestations become milder with subsequent sun exposure, and some individuals may occasionally tolerate the sun without any difficulty. The reason for this inconsistency is not known.

Cerebellar ataxia is the predominant neurologic feature of Hartnup disease. Seen in over two-thirds of those afflicted with this disorder, it usually occurs during periods when the rash is most prominent or following acute episodes of febrile illness.[33, 35] The gait is broad-based and unsteady, and patients have both nystagmus and an intention tremor. Ocular abnormalities include diplopia and ptosis, and several patients are mentally retarded, have emotional lability or frank psychosis.[36]

DIAGNOSIS.—The diagnosis of Hartnup disease is based upon the clinical picture and demonstration of specific amino acid and indole excretion patterns (not the total amino acid excretion).

TREATMENT.—Treatment consists of avoidance of sunlight exposure and prolonged oral administration of high doses (40 to 200 mg) of nicotinic acid or nicotinamide. Since nicotinamide does not cause the flushing generally associated with administration of nicotinic acid, the former is generally the drug of choice. Although the eruption and ataxia seem to improve when patients are on this regimen, assessment of therapy is difficult since the natural history of the disorder is one of spontaneous remission and exacerbation.[36, 37]

Pellagra

Pellagra is a systemic disturbance caused by a cellular deficiency of niacin due to inadequate dietary intake of nicotinic acid or its precursor (tryptophan) or the ingestion of certain antinicotinic substances such as hydantoin derivatives used in the therapy of epilepsy or the antituberculosis drug isoniazid.[39, 40] Dietary deficiency as a cause of pellagra can be seen in all ages, but as a result of current nutritional standards and vitamin supplementation, the disorder has become very rare in infancy and relatively uncommon in children in most parts of the world. In adults, however, it still occurs frequently as a result of dietary deficiency in chronic alcoholics.

CLINICAL FEATURES.—Pellagra is characterized by seasonal recurrences and a classic triad of three Ds—dermatitis, diarrhea, and dementia (Table 11–6). At the onset of the disorder, there is weakness, loss of appetite, abdominal pain, mental depression and photosensitivity. In the latter stages, nervous symptoms may predominate to such a degree that the cutaneous lesions may be overlooked. The most prominent cutaneous lesions of pellagra are precipitated by the sun and, although not always pesent, begin as asymptomatic or pruritic symmetrical erythematous eruptions on areas exposed to sunlight, heat, friction, or pressure. The usual sites of

TABLE 11–6.—PELLAGRA

1. Etiology:
   a. Inadequate intake of niacin or its precursor (tryptophan)
   b. Ingestion of antinicotinic sustance (hydantoin, isoniazid)
2. Dermatitis, diarrhea, and dementia (the three Ds)
3. Treatment: appropriate diet (meat, vegetables, milk and eggs) and nicotinic acid or nicotinamide supplements (50 to 400 mg of niacin daily)

involvement include the face, neck, dorsal surface of the hands, arms and feet, the inguinal region, and, particularly in infants and small children, the diaper area. The eruption begins as well-marginated erythema and superficial scaling on sun-exposed areas (resembling sunburn, with or without vesiculation or blister formation) that gradually subsides, leaving a dusky, brown-red discoloration (Figs 11–3, 11–4). In acute cases, the lesions may progress to vesiculation, ulceration, exudation, cracking, and, at times, secondary infection. With chronicity, lesions become more livid, thickened, scaly, and ultimately fissured, atrophic, deeply pigmented, and, at times sclerotic. About the lower neck, the eruption may appear as a broad collarette of dermatitis known as *Casal's necklace.* In cases in which the "necklace" is incomplete, the lesions maintain their symmetrical and otherwise characteristic appearance.

The nose has a fairly characteristic appearance with a dull erythema of the nasal bridge with slight scaling with a powdery appearance. Except for its location, this scaly appearance frequently resembles seborrheic dermatitis. Mucous membrane involvement, when present, consists of painful fissures and ulceration. The lips and cheeks are thin and pale, the mouth

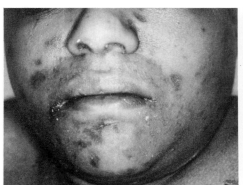 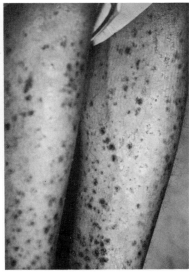

Fig 11–3 (left).—Pellagra. Symmetrical erythematous eruptions on the face precipitated by sun exposure. (From the Department of Dermatology, Yale University School of Medicine.)

Fig 11–4 (right).—Pellagra. Well-marginated symmetrical erythematous scaly eruptions on the sun exposed aspect of the legs. (Courtesy of Charles Samuel Fulk, M.D., Fort Bragg, N.C.)

is dry, the tongue is red, swollen, and, at times, darkened (the so-called "black tongue"). Aphthous ulcers, fissuring, and angular cheilitis are also common.

Neurologic manifestations may appear with or without involvement of the skin and digestive tract. In mild cases they consist of weakness, anorexia and depression. In more severe cases, delirium, amentia, posterolateral spinal cord degeneration, and pyramidal and peripheral nerve involvement may be noted. The disease tends to be progressive and, if untreated, may eventuate in death within several years.

DIAGNOSIS.—The characteristic skin lesions, with or without gastrointestinal and neurologic manifestations, should suggest the diagnosis. This can be aided by an abnormal dietary history or a history of therapy with antinicotic substances such as hydantoin or isoniazid. When the diagnosis is suspected, measurement of the urinary excretion of N_1-methylnicotinamide and/or pyridone (metabolites of niacin) are helpful. Histopathologic examination of cutaneous lesions of pellagra are non-specific. Early lesions present a chronic inflammatory infiltrate in the upper dermis and, at times, subepidermal or intraepidermal vesicles or bullae. Older lesions are characterized by hyperkeratosis, parakeratosis and a moderate degree of acanthosis. Melanin is increased in the basal layer of the epidermis and the dermis may show fibrosis in addition to the chronic inflammatory infiltrate. Although the histologic picture of pellagra is frequently not diagnostic and may merely present as a chronic dermatitis, in the end stages of the disease, atrophy of the stratum malpighii can help differentiate this disorder from other forms of chronic dermatitis.

TREATMENT.—The recommended daily allowance of niacin is 4 mg for infants and 6 to 12 mg for older children. Treatment of pellagra consists of appropriate dietary management in the form of meat, vegetables, eggs, and milk, supplemented by nicotinic acid or nicotinamide in dosages of 50 to 400 mg of niacin daily. As in the treatment of Hartnup disease, nicotinamide appears to be the drug of choice.

Kwashiorkor

Kwashiorkor, a clinical syndrome that results from a severe deficiency of protein (and less than aequate caloric intake), is the most serious and prevalent form of malnutrition in the world today. Seen primarily in industrially underdeveloped countries, the inadequate protein intake results in amino acid (phenylalanine and tyrosine) deficiency, pellagrous cutaneous changes, hair abnormalities, impaired growth, mental and gastrointestinal features, and in the absence of proper dietary treatment, a high mortality rate[41] (Table 11–7).

TABLE 11–7.—Kwashiorkor

1. Generally in children between 6 months and 5 years of age
2. Inadequate protein intake with phenylalanine and tyrosine deficiency
3. Pellagra-like skin lesions, hair abnormalities, impaired growth, mental and gastrointestinal features
4. Edema, xerosis with mosaic "cracked" appearance, reddish or coffee-colored skin ("red children")
5. Treatment: high protein diet, vitamin supplementation, and correction of dehydration and electrolyte imbalance

Clinical manifestations.—The clinical picture generally occurs in children between 6 months and 5 years of age and consists of a conspicuous dermatosis that begins as an erythema that blanches on pressure, rapidly followed by small dusky purple patches that do not blanch. The eruption has a sharply marginated edge raised above the surrounding skin, much as enamel paint that is lifting up and about to peel off. In contrast to lesions of pellagra, the dermatosis seldom appears on areas exposed to sunlight and tends to spare the feet and dorsal areas of the hands. Photosensitivity, purpura, and excessive bruisability may also be present.

In mild cases, the cutaneous eruption is associated with a superficial desquamation; in severe cases, there are large areas of erosion. As the disease progresses, the entire cutaneous surface develops a reddish or coffee-colored hue, hence the term "red children." Other associated features include circumoral pallor, loss of pigmentation (especially after minor trauma), depigmentation of the hair from its normal black color in African children to a reddish-yellow, gray or straw color. Edema, xerosis, fine branny desquamation, dyschromia with hypopigmentation (perhaps due to phenylalinine deficiency), with cracking along Langer's lines that produces a "mosaic" or "cracked" appearance of the skin, complete the cutaneous picture.

Apathy and dejection are almost universal, particularly when the disorder is well established. Affected children whimper rather than cry when disturbed and appear indifferent to their surroundings. Other associated features include changes in mental behavior, anorexia, irritability, growth retardation, fatty infiltration of the liver with hypoproteinemia and, as a result, edema of the face, feet and abdomen with a characteristic pot-belly appearance.

Treatment.—Children afflicted with Kwashiorkor are extremely ill, and untreated cases carry a mortality rate of 30% or more. Prevention consists of an appropriate diet containing essential nutrients, including adequate amounts of good quality protein.[41–43] In areas where Kwashiorkor is common, breast-feeding should be encouraged and continued for a longer period of time than is customary, since even small amounts of milk will provide the necessary nutriments lacking in the local diet. Treatment of affected individuals consists of administration of a high protein diet, vitamin supplementation, and correction of dehydration and electrolyte imbalance when present.

The Porphyrias

The porphyrias are a group of genetically determined or acquired disorders of porphyrin, the chemical precursor for hemoglobin synthesis. Porphyrins are the only well-established photosensitizers made by the human body. These are substances that produce photodynamic types of phototoxic reactions with a primary action spectrum in the 400 nanometers range.[44–46] There are two main categories of porphyric disease in man. Based upon the tissue in which the biochemical lesion is localized, they are classified into erythropoietic or hepatic forms. The erythropoietic porphyrias are divided into erythropoietic or hepatic forms. The erythropoietic porphyrias are divided into erythropoietic porphyria (EP) and erythropoietic protoporphyria (EPP) ; the hepatic porphyrias include acute intermittent porphyria (AIP), acquired hepatic porphyria (porphyria cutanea tarda, PCT) and porphyria variegata, a combination of AIP and PCT (Table 11–8).

Erythropoietic Porphyrias

Erythropoietic Porphyria (Günther's Disease, EP)

Erythropoietic porphyria (Günther's disease, EP), an extremely rare autosomal recessive disorder (approximately 200 cases have been reported in the literature), is characterized by the appearance of red urine during infancy, severe photosensitivity that occurs in the first two or three years of life, splenomegaly, and hemolytic anemia. The biochemical disturbance in this disease appears to be a deficiency of normal enzyme controlling mechanisms in the formation of hemoglobin at a step prior to the formation of uroporphyrin resulting in marked overproduction of uroporphyrin I and coporporphyrin I in circulating erythrocytes and bone marrow cells.[46]

CLINICAL MANIFESTATIONS.—Photosensitivity is frequently absent in the neonatal period but generally becomes apparent during the first years of life as exposure to sun increases. Recurrent vesiculobullous eruptions on sun-exposed areas of the skin eventually result in mutilating ulceration and scarring. These may lead to loss of acral tissue (the ears, tip of the nose, nails, and distal phalanges) with marked limitation of functional ability of the hands. Other common clinical features include hypertrichosis manifested as fine blond lanugo hair over the face and extremities, conjunctivi-

TABLE 11–8.—CLASSIFICATION OF THE PORPHYRIAS

TYPE AND HEREDITY	MANIFESTATIONS	ONSET	DIAGNOSIS
Erythropoietic Porphyrias			
Erythropoietic Porphyria (EP) Autosomal recessive	Extremely rare, blistering and severe scarring with loss of acral tissue, brown-stained teeth that fluoresce, urine pink to port-wine color, hemolytic anemia and splenomegaly	Infancy	Fluorescence of teeth, hemolytic anemia, splenomegaly, elevated uroporphyrin I
Erythropoietic Protoporphyria (EPP) Autosomal dominant	Mild photosensitivity, burning with red edematous plaques and thickening of skin with cobblestone appearance	Childhood	Fluorescence of erythrocytes (but not teeth and nails), high protoporphyrin level
Hepatic Porphyrias			
Acute Intermittent Porphyria (AIP) Autosomal dominant	No photosensitivity or skin lesions, abdominal pain, vomiting, neuropathy, psychoses (may be provoked by various medications)	Young adults, never before puberty	Elevated ALA and PBG, urine darkens on standing
Porphyria Cutanea Tarda (PCT) Autosomal dominant	Vesicles, blisters, erosions, ulcerations, milia, and thickening of skin on sun exposed areas (can be precipitated by estrogens)	Middle age (a few cases in childhood)	Fluorescence of urine, elevated uro- and coproporphyrins in urine and feces
Porphyria Variegata Autosomal dominant	A combination of AIP and PCT	Young adults	Elevated protoporphyrins (ALA and PBG during attacks)

tis, keratitis, brown-stained teeth that fluoresce under exposure to Wood's light, hyperpigmentation, hemolytic anemia, loss of fingernails, growth retardation and bone fragility due to encroachment of the hyperplastic marrow on the cortex. The legendary werewolves of the middle ages with fluorescent teeth and nails, mutilated and deformed ears, nose, and eyelids, and nocturnal habits due to their sensitivity to light may indeed have been persons afflicted with congenital erythropoietic porphyria.

The prognosis of EP is poor, with few patients surviving into the fourth or fifth decade. Death, when it occurs, is frequently associated with the hemolytic anemia, sequelae of iron-overload associated with repeated transfusion therapy, and cirrhosis of the liver and its complications (hematemesis or hepatorenal failure).

DIAGNOSIS.—The diagnosis of erythropoietic porphyria can be made by the clinical features that appear early in life: flourescence of the teeth under black light examination, and sharply elevated levels of uroporphyrin I in erythrocytes, plasma, urine, and feces. Splenomegaly, an almost constant feature of this disorder, may remain undetected during the neonatal period only to appear as a child grows older. In the majority of reported cases, hemolytic activity is indicated by normochromic anemia, elevated reticulocyte levels, circulating normoblasts, normoblastic hyperplasia of the bone marrow, and increased excretion of fecal urobilinogen. The anemia is thought to be due to hemolysis secondary to an intra-corpuscular defect and ineffective erythropoiesis. The color of the urine of patients may vary from faint pink to burgundy or port-wine, depending upon the concentration of uroporphyrin derived from the oxidation of uroporphyrinogen. When the diagnosis is suspected on clinical grounds, screening tests with the aid of a Wood's light may reveal porphyrin fluorescence in urine or aqueous suspensions of feces and red fluorescence in a thin smear of peripheral erythrocytes examined under a fluorescent microscope.[46]

Skin biopsy may be helpful but cannot be relied on for a definitive diagnosis since the skin lesions are the same in all types of porphyria with cutaneous lesions, and differences are based on the severity rather than the type of porphyria. Histopathologic examination may reveal subepidermal bullae and an atrophic epidermis with destruction of adnexal glands and fibrosis in patients with advanced disease. Other features include varying degrees of inflammatory change and PAS-positive staining hyaline material around capillaries and other small blood vessels in the papillary dermis.[47]

TREATMENT.—In families with a history of congenital erythropoietic porphyria, genetic counseling should be given. Treatment of affected patients includes avoidance of sun exposure and trauma, frequently with resolution of cutaneous manifestations, anemia, and splenomegaly. Splenectomy has had variable success. Window glass and ordinary sunscreen preparations provide little protection from the ultraviolet spectrum to which these patients are sensitive. Therefore, appropriate clothing and wide-spectrum sun protectants at wave lengths greater than 400 nm (such as those containing zinc oxide or titanium dioxide, or zinc oxide ointment or RVPaque) should be used for appropriate topical protection. Oral beta-carotene, available as Solatene (Roche), in doses of 30 to 150 mg a day, also appears to be an effective photoprotective agent.[48]

Erythropoietic Protoporphyria (EPP)

Erythropoietic protoporphyria (EPP), the most common form of porphyria seen by the practicing dermatologist in many parts of the world, is among the more recently recognized of the porphyrias. Approximately 300 cases have been reported to date, but the relative subtlety of clinical signs and the absence of increased levels of protoporphyrin in urine (due to the insolubility of this porphyrin in water) predispose toward this failure of recognition.[46] The incidence of EPP, however, continues to increase as physicians' awareness increases and more appropriate biochemical testing procedures are employed.[49] An autosomal dominant disorder characterized by mild photosensitivity, slight eczematization and inflammation of exposed skin and high concentrations of protophorphyrin in erythrocytes, plasma, and feces, the primary biochemical defect of EPP appears to be related to a deficiency of ferrochelatase, the enzyme that accelerates the incorporation of iron into protoporphyrin.

CLINICAL MANIFESTATIONS.—EPP usually becomes symptomatic between the ages of 2 and 5 years. It may present clinically as burning, tingling, or itching of the exposed skin (often manifested by the child's crying when placed in sunshine) following short periods of sunlight exposure. This burning sensation may be followed by pruritic reddened edematous plaques that return to normal within 24 hours, occasionally papulovesicular and petechial eruptions that may persist for longer periods, and chronic changes such as hypopigmentation, hyperpigmentation, and a papular thickening that gives a cobblestone appearance to the skin. In a few patients, hypersplenism with associated hemolytic anemia (which responds favorably to splenectomy) has been reported. Liver biopsies of patients with EPP reveal portal and periportal fibrosis and deposition of pigment in bile canaliculi and bile ducts with terminal hepatic failure (in a small number of patients).[50–52] Cholecystitis and cholelithiasis have also been reported (in up to 12% of patients) with gallstones consisting of almost pure protoporphyrin IX.[53–55] It now appears that this disease is much more common than previously suspected and may account for many undiagnosed light-sensitive reactions.

DIAGNOSIS.—Laboratory findings in patients with EPP are those of abnormally high protoporphyrin levels in circulating erythrocytes, bone marrow cells, and plasma. Fluorescence of the erythrocytes can be demonstrated by Wood's light or fluorescence microscopy. In contrast to erythropoietic porphyria, fluorescence of teeth and nails is not present, and there is no increase in fecal or urinary uroporphyrins. Diagnosis has been facilitated by a rapid microfluorometric assay readily available to most well-equipped hospitals.[56]

TREATMENT.—The management of erythropoietic protoporphyria is dependent upon limited exposure to sunlight, the use of opaque sunscreens, and perhaps the administration of betacarotene (Solatene).[57–59] As in erythropoietic protoporphyria (EP), window glass does not protect patients with this disorder.

Hepatic Porphyrias

Acute Intermittent Porphyria (AIP)

Acute intermittent porphyria (AIP) is a rare autosomal dominant disorder characterized by overproduction of porphyrin precursors (aminolevulinic acid and porphobilinogen), episodes of abdominal pain associated with vomiting, constipation, peripheral paresis or paralysis, psychologic manifestations or psychoneuroses provoked by barbituates, sulfonamides, dapsone, griseofulvin, anticonvulsive agents, sulfonylurea compounds, and estrogens. Although the disease never manifests itself before puberty, the disorder is included here as a matter of completeness. Women seem to have a greater predisposition than men, and photosensitivity is not seen in association with this disorder. Freshly voided urine may be colorless and only darkens on standing and, except for possible laparotomy scars from previous abdominal surgery, cutaneous lesions are absent.

The fundamental problem of diagnosis is the differentiation of acute intermittent porphyria (AIP) from medical or surgical cases of an acute abdomen and from other organic, psychiatric, or neurologic disease. The classic triad of abdominal pain, urine that darkens on standing, and neuropsychiatric symptoms, particularly when associated with multiple laparotomy scars from previous surgery, should raise suspicion of this disorder. Diagnosis can be made by the demonstration of elevated aminolevulinic acid (ALA) and porphobilinogen (PBG) during attacks and by the demonstration of porphobilinogen in the urine by the Watson-Schwartz test.

There is no effective treatment for acute intermittent porphyria. Drugs that are known to precipitate porphyric attacks should be avoided. Bromides have been used with success, propoxyphene (Darvon) is tolerated well, chlorpromazine (Thorazine) is useful for the treatment of acute abdominal pain, and, for severe pain, meperadine (Demerol) is effective.

Porphyria Cutanea Tarda (PCT)

Porphyria cutanea tarda (PCT) is the most common form of porphyria seen in dermatologic practice in the United States. With an estimated incidence of $1:25,000$, it appears to be an inborn error of metabolism characterized by the excretion of excessive uroporphyrin and coproporphyrin in both urine and feces. Although most common in adults during the third and fourth decades of life, this disorder has also been seen in children (three cases have been reported in children below 15 years of age, one as young as 2 years of age) and it has a high incidence among the Bantus in Africa where home-brewed alcohol or beer with high iron content is ingested.[60]

Porphyria cutanea tarda can also be precipitated by estrogen therapy, alcoholic cirrhosis, and accidental ingestion of the fungicide hexachlorobenzene (C_6Cl_6). This should not be confused with gamma benzene hexachloride ($C_6 H_6 Cl_6$), the insecticide used for the treatment of scabies and pediculosis.[61] Although diabetes mellitus is present in 25% to 50% of patients with porphyria cutanea tarda, the reason for this high association is unknown.

The exact genetic and enzymatic defect in porphyria cutanea tarda remains unknown. Basically a disease of the liver, it has been associated with specific enzyme deficiencies (uro- and coprodecarboxylase). The primary cutaneous lesion of porphyria cutanea tarda is a photosensitivity to the uroporphyrin deposited in the skin. Light in the 400 nm range is necessary for production of cutaneous lesions. Skin lesions in this disease consist of vesicles or blisters on light-exposed cutaneous surfaces, especially the dorsal aspect of the hands (Fig 11–5). Other features include increased fragility of the skin, with erosions and ulcerations as a result of relatively minor trauma, and hypertrichosis and melanosis of the face that appear to be related to sun exposure.

Blisters seen in association with this disorder vary markedly in size from 1 mm to 2 to 3 cm across, with small blisters often being overlooked. They are most commonly filled by clear or slightly turbid liquid, soon rupture, turn into erosions, and become infected. On healing, the blister sites may scar or evolve into milia (rounded, yellowish, or pale-colored intraepidermal inclusions 1 to 2 mm or more in diameter).

DIAGNOSIS.—Confirmation of the clinical diagnosis of porphyria cutanea tarda can be made by increased levels of uroporphyrin, slightly elevated fecal coproporphyrin and protoporphyrin, and positive fluorescence of the

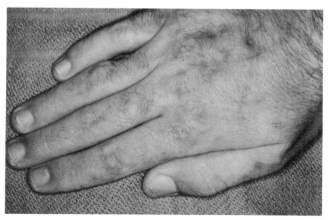

Fig 11–5.—Vesicles, erosions and ulcerations on the dorsal aspect of the hand following sunlight exposure in a patient with porphyria cutaneous tarda. (Department of Dermatology, Yale University School of Medicine).

patient's urine with a Wood's light. Skin biopsy of vesicular lesions shows subepidermal bullae with dermal papillae rising irregularly from the floor of the bulla into its cavity. Immunofluorescent studies show deposition of IgG and, less commonly, IgM or complement around the upper dermal vessels and at the dermoepidermal junction. Electron microscopic examination reveals reduplication of the basal lamina of the upper dermal vessels and dermoepidermal junction, suggesting repeated injury to the endothelial and basal cells.[47] Since similar observations can be made in other forms of porphyria, none of the above findings is pathognomonic of PCT.

TREATMENT.—Treatment is dependent upon the elimination of alcohol, estrogen, or iron ingestion, the avoidance of exposure to environmental toxins and phlebotomy, with the number and frequency of phlebotomies dependent upon clinical response, hemoglobin levels, and urinary porphyrin levels. Low-dose chloroquine therapy has also been recommended as an effective treatment. The therapeutic effect proposed for chloroquine in this disorder appears to be related to chloroquine destruction of hepatocyte mitochondria and the formation of a water-soluble complex with porphyrin that can be excreted by the kidneys.[63]

Porphyria Variegata

Porphyria variegata (congenital cutaneous hepatic porphyria) is an autosomal dominant disorder that represents a combination of acute intermittent porphyria (AIP) and porphyria cutanea tarda (PCT). This disease, not

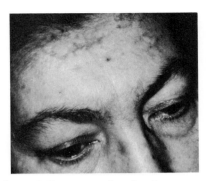

Fig 11–6.—Hyperpigmentation, a weather-beaten appearance and excessive furrowing of the forehead in porphyria variegata. (From Hurwitz S.: *Clinical Pediatric Dermatology.* W.B. Saunders Co., Philadelphia, 1981. Used by permission.)

seen in young children, has its onset after puberty and generally appears in the fourth to fifth decades of life. Clinical features include sun sensitivity in adult life, with vesicles or blisters on light-exposed surfaces, hyperpigmentation, a weather-beaten or waxy complexion with excessive furrowing of the forehead (cutis rhomboidalis frontalis), scars on the back of the neck and frontal hair margin, milia, and scleroderma-like plaques (Fig 11–6).[63, 64] The urinary findings overlap those of both AIP and PCT. Treatment consists of avoidance of hepatoxic agents and sun exposure, repeated phlebotomies, and low-dose chloroquine therapy.

REFERENCES

1. Ramsay C.A.: Photosensitivity in children, in Rasmussen J.E. (Guest Editor), *Symposium on Pediatric Dermatology II, Pediatric Clinics of North America,* W.B. Saunders Co., Philadelphia, 1983, pp. 687–699.
2. Epstein J.H.: Photoallergy. A review. *Arch. Dermatol.* 106:741–778, 1972.
3. Reed W.B., Landing B., Sugarman G., et al.: Xeroderma pigmentosum. Clinical and laboratory investigation of its basic defect. *J.A.M.A.* 207:2073–2079, 1969.
4. Robbins J.H., Kraemer K.H., Lutzner M.A., et al.: Xeroderma pigmentosum—an inherited disease with sun sensitivity, multiple cutaneous neoplasms, and abnormal DNA repair. *Ann. Int. Med.* 80:221–248, 1974.
5. Cleaver J.E.: DNA damage and repair in light-sensitive human skin disease. *J. Invest. Dermatol.* 54:181–195, 1970.
6. Rook A.: Genetics in dermatology, in Rook A., Wilkinson, D.S., Ebling F.J.G. (eds.): *Textbook of Dermatology, ed. 2.* Blackwell Scientific Publications, Oxford, 1972, pp. 91–126.
7. Reed W.B., Sugarman G.I., Mathis R.A.: DeSanctis-Cacchione syndrome. A case report with autopsy findings. *Arch. Dermatol.* 113:1561–1563, 1977.
8. Ramsay C.A., Coltart T.M., Blunt C., et al.: Prenatal diagnosis of xeroderma

pigmentosum: report of first successful case. *J. Invest. Dermatol.* 63:392–396, 1974.

9. Ramsay C.A., Giannelli F.: The erythemal action spectrum and deoxyribonucleic acid repair synthesis in xeroderma pigmentosum. *Brit. J. Derm.* 92:49–56, 1975.

10. Epstein E.H., Jr., Burk P., Cohen I.K., et al.: Dermatome shaving in the treatment of xeroderma pigmentosum. *Arch. Dermatol.* 105:589–590, 1972.

11. Editorial comment in Malkinson F.D., Pearson R.S.: *The Year Book of Dermatology, 1975.* Year Book Medical Publishers, Inc., Chicago, 1975, p. 180.

12. Bloom D.: Congenital telangiectatic erythema resembling lupus erythematosus in dwarfs. *Am. J. Dis. Child.* 88:754–758, 1954.

13. Dicken C.H., Dewald G., Gordon H.: Sister chromatid exchanges in Bloom's syndrome. *Arch. Derm.* 114:755–760, 1978.

14. Hutteroth T.H., Litwin S.D., German J.: Abnormal immune responses of Bloom's syndrome lymphocytes in vitro. *J. Clin. Invest.* 56:1–7, 1975.

15. Weemaes C.M.R., Bakkerson A.J.M., ter Haar B.G.A., et al.: Immune responses in four patients with Bloom syndrome. *Clin. Immunol. Immunopath.* 12:12–19, 1979.

16. Silver H.K.: Rothmund-Thomson syndrome: an oculocutaneous disorder. *Am. J. Dis. Child.* 111:182–190, 1966.

17. Gilchrest B.A.: Premature aging syndromes affecting the skin, in Blandau R.J. (Editor), *Morphogenesis and Malformation of the Skin.* Alan R. Liss, Inc., New York, 1981, pp. 227–241.

18. Kraus B.S., Gottlieb M.A., Meliton H.R.: The dentition in Rothmund's syndrome. *J. Am. Dent. Assoc.* 81:894–915, 1970.

19. Cockayne E.A.: Case reports: Dwarfism with retinal atrophy and deafness. *Arch. Dis. Child.* 11:1–8, 1936.

20. Cockayne E.A.: Case reports: dwarfism with retinal atrophy and deafness. *Arch. Dis. Child.* 21:52–54, 1946.

21. MacDonald E.B., Fitch K.D., Lewis I.C.: Cockayne's syndrome. *Pediatrics* 25:997–1007, 1960.

22. Scrivastava R.N., Gupta P.C., Mayekar G., et al.: Cockayne's syndrome in two sisters. *Acta Pediatr. Scand.* 63:461–464, 1974.

23. Moosa A., Dubowitz V.: Peripheral neuropathy in Cockayne's syndrome. *Arch. Dis. Child.* 45:674–677, 1970.

24. Higginbottom M.C., Griswold W.R., Jones K.C., et al.: The Cockayne syndrome: an evaluation of hypertension and studies of renal pathology. *Pediatrics* 64:929–933, 1979.

25. Kraemer K.H., Coon H.G., Petinga R.A., et al.: Genetic heterogeneity in xeroderma pigmentosum: complementation groups and their relationship to DNA repair rate. *Proc. Natl. Acad. Sci.* 72:59, 1975.

26. Ohno T., Hirooka M.: Renal lesions in Cockayne's syndrome. *Tohoku J. Exp. Med.* 89:151–161, 1966.

27. Coles W.H.: Ocular manifestations of Cockayne's syndrome. *Am. J. Ophthal.* 67:762–764, 1969.

28. Andrews A.D., Barrett S.F., Yoder F.W., et al.: Cockayne's syndrome fibroblasts have increased sensitivity to ultraviolet light but normal rates of unscheduled DNA synthesis. *J. Invest. Dermatol.* 70:237–239, 1978.

29. Schmickel R.D., Chu E.H.Y., Trosko J.E., et al.: Cockayne syndrome: a cellular sensitivity to ultraviolet light. *Pediatrics* 60:135–139, 1977.

30. Baron D.N., Dent C.E., Harris H., et al.: Hereditary pellagra-like skin rash with temporary cerebellary ataxia, constant renal aminoaciduria and other bizarre chemical features. *Lancet* 2:421–428, 1956.
31. Dent C.E.: Hartnup disease: An inborn error of metabolism. *Arch. Dis. Child.* 32:363–372, 1957.
32. Srikantia S.G., Vankatachalam P.S., Reddy V.: Clinical and biochemical features of a case of Hartnup disease. *Br. Med. J.* 1:282–285, 2964.
33. Jepson J.B.: Hartnup disease, in Stanbury J.B., Wyngaarden J.B., Fredrickson D.S.: *The Metabolic Basis of Inherited Disease, ed. 2.* McGraw-Hill Book Company, New York, 1966, pp. 1283–1299.
34. Fischer E., Jung E.G.: Photosensitivity and the genodermatoses, in Rook A.J., Maibach H.I. (eds.): *Seminars in Dermatology.* Thieme Stratton, Inc., New York, 1:169–174, 1982.
35. Baron B.N., Dent C.E., Harris H., et al.: Hereditary pellagra-like skin rash with temporary cerebellar ataxia, constant renal aminoaciduria and other bizarre biochemical features. *Lancet* 2:421–428, 1956.
36. Freedberg I.M.: Hartnup disease, in Demis D.J., Dobson R.C., McGuire J.: *Clinical Dermatology, ed. 10.* Harper & Row, Philadelphia, 1983, 12-8:1–2.
37. Wilcken B., Brown D.A.: Natural history of Hartnup disease. *Arch. Dis. Child.* 52:38–40, 1977.
38. Honeycut W.M., Huldin B.H.: Reactions to isoniazid. *Arch. Dermatol.* 88:190–194, 1963.
39. Cohen L.K., George W., Smith R.: Isoniazid-induced acne and pellagra. *Arch. Dermatol.* 109:377–381, 1974.
40. Stratigos J.D., Katsambas A.: Pellagra: a still existing disease. *Br. J. Dermatol.* 96:99–106, 1977.
41. Behar M., Viteri F., Bressani R., et al.: Principles of treatment and prevention of severe protein malnutrition in children (Kwashiorkor). *Ann. N.Y. Acad. Sci.* 69:954–968, 1958.
42. Trowell H.C., Davies J.P.N., Dean R.F.A.: *Kwashiorkor.* London, Arnold & Co., 1954.
43. Williams C.D.: Council on foods and nutrition. Kwashiorkor. *J.A.M.A.* 153:1280–1285, 1953.
44. Levere R.D., Kappas A.: The porphyric diseases of man. *Hospital Practice* 5:61–73, 1970.
45. Konrad K., Hönigsmann H., Gschnait F., et al.: Mouse model for protophyria II. Cellular and subcellular events in the photosensitivity flare of the skin. *J. Invest. Dermatol.* 65:300–310, 1975.
46. Poh-Fitzpatrick M.B.: Erythropoietic porphyrias: current mechanistic, diagnostic, and therapeutic considerations. *Semin. Hematol.* 14:211–219, 1977.
47. Epstein J.H., Tuffanelli D.L., Epstein W.L.: Cutaneous changes in the porphyrias. *Arch. Dermatol.* 107:689–698, 1973.
48. Nordlund J.J. Klaus S.N., Mathews-Roth M.M., et al.: New therapy for polymorphous light eruptions. *Arch. Dermatol.* 108:710–712, 1973.
49. Magnus I.A.: The porphyrias. *Seminars in Dermatology,* 1:197–210, 1982.
50. Bickers D.R.: Porphyrias, in Callen J.P. (Ed.): *Cutaneous Aspects of Internal Disease,* Year Book Medical Publishers, Inc., Chicago, 1981, pp. 549–567.
51. Klatzkin G., Bloomer J.R.: Birefringence of hepatic pigment deposits in erythropoietic protoporphyria: specificity and sensitivity of polarization microscopy in the identification of hepatic protoporphyrin deposits. *Gastroenterology* 67:295–302, 1974.

52. Bloomer J.R., Phillips N.J., Davidson D.C., et al.: Hepatic disease in erythropoietic protoporphyria. *Am. J. Med.* 58:869–882, 1975.
53. DeLeo V.A., Mathews-Roth M., Poh-Fitzpatrick M., et al.: Erythropoietic porphyria. Ten years' experience. *Am. J. Med.* 60:8–22, 1976.
54. Cripps D.J., Scheuer P.J.: Hepatobiliary changes in erythropoietic protoporphyria. *Arch. Path.* 80:500–508, 1965.
55. Cripps D.J., Gilbert L.A., Goldfarb S.S.: Erythropoietic protoporphyria: juvenile protoporphyrin hepatopathy cirrhosis and death. *J. Pediatr.* 91:744–748, 1977.
56. Poh-Fitzpatrick M.B., Piomelli S., Young P., et al.: Rapid quantitative assay for erythrocyte porphyrins: rapid quantitative microfluorometric assay applicable for diagnosis of erythropoietic protoporphyria. *Arch. Dermatol.* 110:225–230, 1974.
57. Zaynoun S.T., Hunter J.A.A., Darby F.J., et al.: The treatment of erythropoietic protoporphyria: experience with beta-carotene. *Br. J. Dermatol.* 97:663–668, 1977.
58. Mathews-Roth M.M., Patach M.A., Fitzpatrick T.B., et al.: Beta-carotene, an oral photoprotective agent in erythropoietic protoporphyria. *J.A.M.A.* 228:1004–1008, 1974.
59. Corbett M.F., Herxheimer A., Magnus, I.A., et al.: The long term treatment with betacarotene in erythropoietic protoporphyria: a controlled trial. *Brit. J. Derm.* 97:655–668, 1977.
60. Kasky A.: Porphyria cutanea tarda in a two-year-old girl. *Br. J. Dermatol.* 90:213–216, 1974.
61. Cam C., Nigogosyan G.: Acquired toxie porphyria cutanea tarda due to hexachlorobenzene. *J.A.M.A.* 183:89–91, 1963.
62. Beeaff D.: Porphyria. *Dermatology* 1:15–27, 1978.
63. Mustajoki P.: Variegate porphyria. *Q. J. Med.* 49:191–203, 1980.
64. Kramer S.: Porphyria variegate. *Clin. Haematol.* 9:303–322, 1980.

12 / The Reticuloendothelial Disorders

THE RETICULOENDOTHELIAL SYSTEM is a term used to designate a group of cells located in the dermis of the skin, endothelial cells of connective tissue, the reticulum of lymph nodes, the spleen, phagocytic monocytes in the peripheral blood and phagocytic cells of the connective tissue. These cells are frequently altered by infection, foreign body reactions, allergic or metabolic conditions and neoplastic disorders. In this chapter the term will be utilized to categorize disorders designated as the histiocytic diseases (Letterer-Siwe disease, Hand-Schüller-Christian disease, and eosinophilic granuloma), malignant histiocytosis, juvenile xanthogranuloma and xanthoma disseminatum, the various forms of mastocytosis, sarcoidosis, and mycosis fungoides (a malignant reticuloendotheliosis seen primarily in adults but also occasionally seen in children).

Histiocytosis X

Histiocytosis X is a term originated by Lichtenstein in 1953 to identify three clinical entities of unknown etiology characterized by histiocyte proliferation.[1] This classification includes Letterer-Siwe disease, Hand-Schüller-Christian disease, and eosinophilic granuloma. Each of these disorders presents a distinct clinical picture with overlapping transitional stages suggesting that they are all variants of the same basic disease process.

Numerous etiologies have been proposed for this group of disorders. These include a disturbance of intracellular lipid metabolism, a reactive histiocytocytic response to an infectious process, and a neoplastic disorder of histiocytes. Since data are insufficient to support any of these theories, the true pathogenesis remains obscure. Proof of unity of the three syndromes, however, is recognized by their histologic similarity and electron microscopic demonstration of Langerhans granules in the cytoplasm of histiocytes in all three syndromes. Recent studies of Letterer-Siwe disease in uniovular twins, reports of familial incidence, and cases of consanguinity suggest a hereditary influence, perhaps an autosomal recessive gene with reduced penetrance.[2]

Letterer-Siwe Disease

Letterer-Siwe disease is seen at the severe fulminating end of the histiocytosis spectrum, as the acute disseminated form of the disease. It usually occurs during the first year of life and is almost exclusively limited to children up to three years of age. In virtually all patients with Letterer-Siwe disease, skin markers may represent the first recognizable sign of the disorder. The infant may appear healthy for many months before fever, anemia, thrombocytopenia, adenopathy, hepatosplenomegaly, or skeletal tumors become apparent (Table 12–1).

CLINICAL FEATURES.—Cutaneous involvement, seen in 80% of cases, is usually part of the initial presentation of this disease. The skin eruption presents in several forms. It frequently begins with a scaly, erythematous seborrhea-like eruption on the scalp, behind the ears, and in the axillary, inguinal or perineal areas (Figs 12–1, 12–2, 12–3).[3] On close inspection, the presence of basic lesions of histiocytosis (reddish-brown or purpuric papules) may identify the disorder (Fig 12–4). In infants, vesicular or crusted papules may predominate (Fig 12–5). Purpuric nodules on the palms and soles of infants appear to be a particularly bad prognostic sign. Buccal and gingival ulcerations, chronic otitis media, and ulceration of the postauricular, inguinal, or perineal regions also represent important diagnostic clues (Fig 12–3). When the diagnosis is indeterminant, the character and distribution of lesions should suggest the true nature of the eruption. Diagnosis, then, can be confirmed easily by skin biopsy.[2]

This disease was considered an invariably fatal disorder until 1951 when Aronson reported the first incidence of recovery.[4] Since then, additional long-term survivals have been reported. Careful clinical reviews have shown that prognosis is related to age of onset, duration of symptoms, and the degree of systemic involvement. Benign and purely cutaneous forms, although rare, have been reported.[5–9] The absence of thrombocytopenia and a lack of extensive visceral involvement favor a good prognosis.

The highest mortality is seen in patients under the age of 6 months,

TABLE 12–1.—LETTERER-SIWE DISEASE

1. Usually in first year of life (almost exclusively in children up to age 3)
2. Not necessarily uniformly fatal
3. Cutaneous features
   a. Scaly erythematous seborrhea-like rash
   b. Petechiae, purpuric papules and nodules
   c. Vesicles as crusted papules may predominate in infants.
4. Other features: fever, anemia, thrombocytopenia, adenopathy, hepatosplenomegaly

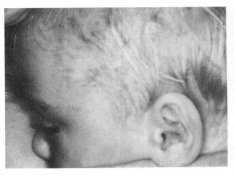
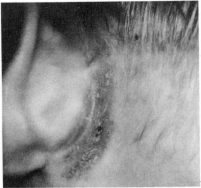

Fig 12–1 (left).—Histiocytosis X. Scaly, erythematous seborrhea-like eruption on the scalp of a 14-month-old infant with Letterer-Siwe disease.

Fig 12–2 (right).—Letterer-Siwe disease. Scaly erythematous seborrhea-like eruption with purpuric papules in the postauricular area of a 14-month-old infant.

particularly those with widespread systemic involvement. Purpura of the palms, a finding seldom seen in other skin disease, early age of onset, and lung involvement appear to be signs of a particularly poor prognosis. Death, when it occurs, may be caused by pulmonary, hepatic, or splenic involvement and frequently is attributed to hemorrhage, anemia, or infection. Despite reports of long standing that Letterer-Siwe disease bears a

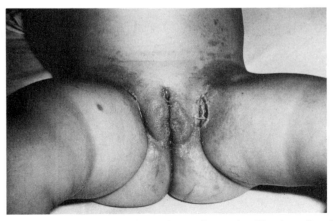

Fig 12–3.—Histiocytosis X (Letterer-Siwe disease) with ulceration in the inguinal region. (From Braverman I.M.: *Skin Signs of Systemic Disease.* W.B. Saunders Co., Philadelphia, 1970. Used by permission.)

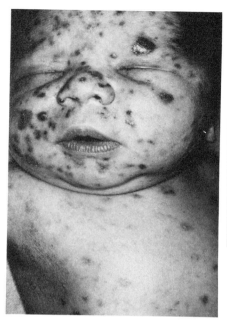 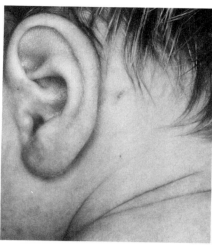

Fig 12–4 (left).—Reddish-brown purpuric papules and nodules on the face and chest of a newborn with congenital Letterer-Siwe disease.

Fig 12–5 (right).—Crusted vesicular lesion in the postauricular area of a 1-month-old infant with congenital Letterer-Siwe disease.

poor prognosis, the disease course fluctuates and spontaneous remissions have been documented. Although Letterer-Siwe disease often implies a fatal outcome, therapy is often beneficial, spontaneous remissions have occurred, and at times the illness may evolve into a more chronic phase of histiocytosis X such as Hand-Schüller-Christian disease.[2]

Hand-Schüller-Christian Disease

This is the variant of histiocytosis generally seen in children between 2 and 6 years of age (Table 12–2). Classically this syndrome consists of a triad of osteolytic defects, diabetes insipidus, and exophthalmos. The bony lesions are invariably present; only 50% of patients, however, have diabetes insipidus, and a mere 10% demonstrate exophthalmos. Chronic otitis media secondary to histiocytic infiltration of the mastoid is common. Histiocytic proliferation may also cause necrosis, ulcerations, and small tumors of the gums and oral mucous membranes. Roentgenograms of the skull often reveal sharply defined areas of osseous rarefaction, termed "geographic

TABLE 12–2.—HAND-SCHÜLLER-CHRISTIAN DISEASE

1. Generally in children 2 to 6 years of age
2. A triad of osteolytic defects, diabetes mellitus and exophthalmos
3. Other features: chronic otitis media, necrosis, ulcerations and small tumors of gums and oral mucous membranes, and pulmonary involvement (in 30%)
4. Cutaneous lesion (in 30% to 50%)
   a. Similar to Letterer-Siwe disease (coalescing scaling or crusted brown to flesh-colored papules)
   b. Purpura less common
   c. Lesions less vivid and less destructive

skull," or erosions of the tooth-bearing portion of the mandible, with loosening or extrusion of the teeth. The lungs and pleura represent a major cause of disability and are affected in 30% of patients, with death resulting from pulmonary fibrosis, associated ventricular hypertrophy, and right-sided heart failure.

Skin lesions, seen in 30% to 50% of patients, are similar to those of the Letterer-Siwe syndrome, except that in Hand-Schüller-Christian disease purpura is less common and the skin lesions are neither as vivid nor as destructive. The skin lesions consist of coalescing, scaling or crusted, brown to flesh-colored papules. Occasionally, lesions of long duration develop a shiny yellowish hue. As in Letterer-Siwe disease, granulomatous infiltrates with ulceration are also found in the axillary or anogenital areas.

Eosinophilic Granuloma

Eosinophilic granuloma represents the third and most benign form of histiocytosis. Usually seen in children over age 6 and young adults, the onset is insidious (Table 12–3). The patient is generally symptom-free until headaches, localized pain, tenderness, or swelling of soft tissues suggest

TABLE 12–3.—EOSINOPHILIC GRANULOMA

1. Least severe of histiocytosis X group
2. Usually in children over 6 years and adults
3. Clinical features
   a. Headaches, localized pain, tenderness or swelling of soft tissues suggest the diagnosis
   b. Single or multiple skeletal lesions
   c. Cutaneous lesions (rare, but identical to L-S or H-S-C disease)
      (1) Reddish-brown papules or nodules in retroauricular and perineal areas
      (2) Ulcerated granulomatous lesions of buccal mucous membranes, inguinal, perineal or vulvar areas

the diagnosis. In children, eosinophilic granuloma often represents an early or transitional form of Letterer-Siwe or Hand-Schüller-Christian disease. The disorder may present as single or multiple skeletal lesions and often goes undetected until a spontaneous fracture or an incidental roentgenographic examination suggests the diagnosis. Although the course is usually benign, 10% of patients manifest multifocal disease within six months,[10] and it usually represents a benign yet chronic illness.

Skin lesions are rare, but may be identical to those seen in Letterer-Siwe or Hand-Schüller-Christian disease. Again they may consist of crusting of the scalp (suggesting seborrheic dermatitis); reddish-brown papules or nodules in the retroauricular and perineal areas; or ulcerated granulomatous lesions of the buccal mucous membranes, inguinal, perineal or vulvar regions. The course is characteristically chronic, with a strong tendency to spontaneous remission. Diabetes insipidus, pulmonary lesions, and Langerhans granules have been reported, adding to the evidence that all three forms of histiocytosis are caused by a common disease process.

TREATMENT.—Therapeutic regimens for histiocytosis X vary widely, and since the disease is of variable activity, evaluation of therapy is often difficult. In general, patients with diffuse systemic disease of the reticulohistiocytic system suffer impaired immunity, and subsequently, diminished resistance to infection. Blood transfusions and antibiotics may improve the long-term outlook for such patients, in particular for those with anemia, leukopenia, or thrombocytopenia.

Immunosuppressive drugs currently offer the greatest hope for survival. Simultaneous combination of drugs has been most effective. This suggests that aggressive combination regimens with good symptomatic care may achieve further long-term remissions, and possibly eventual cure. In general, patients with Hand-Schüller-Christian disease and eosinophilic granuloma are more responsive to therapy than patients with Letterer-Siwe disease. Radiation therapy, particularly when initiated early in the course of the disease, is very effective for localized skeletal lesions. Diabetes insipidus is controllable with vasopressin (Pitressin) by injection or nasal insufflation. X-ray therapy or curettage is effective for bone lesions of eosinophilic granuloma.

Histiocytosis, although still a potentially fatal disorder, particularly in young children, can be diagnosed early by characteristic cutaneous manifestations. These skin signs may appear alone or in combination with systemic symptoms. Although the disease reputedly has a poor prognostic outlook, it often presents in much less severe form, so that prognosis is frequently more optimistic than the literature suggests. Vigorous therapeutic approaches, with a combination of steroids, immunosuppressive drugs, and general supportive measures, appear to offer the greatest hope for survival. With accumulation of data, the fatalistic approach to the disease must be reassessed. Aggressive chemotherapy and good supportive care may allow children not only hope for long-term remission but, perhaps, even eventual complete cure.[11-15]

Xanthoma Disseminatum

Xanthoma disseminatum is a rare, benign, histiocytic proliferative disorder of unknown cause characterized by disseminated xanthomatosis in predominantly young male adults. Although it may merely represent a variant of Hand-Schüller-Christian disease, various differences suggest that it may warrant separate consideration. In 30% of cases, the disorder begins before the age of 15 (Table 12–4). Lesions consist of closely set, round to oval, yellowish-orange or yellowish-brown to mahogany-brown or purple papules, nodules, and plaques that are present mainly on the face, flexor surfaces of the neck, antecubital fossae, periumbilical area, perineum, and genitalia. Xanthomatous deposits have been observed in the mouth and upper respiratory tract (epiglottis, larynx, and trachea in 40% of cases), occasionally leading to respiratory difficulty.[16]

Diabetes insipidus is present in 40% of cases. Although the cutaneous lesions are similar in xanthoma disseminatum and Hand-Schüller-Christian disease and both diseases share the fairly common occurrence of diabetes insipidus, the question as to whether xanthoma disseminatum is a form fruste of Hand-Schüller-Christian disease remains controversial.

The distribution of lesions, their histologic features, and the usual lack of disturbed lipid metabolism help establish the diagnosis. Histologic examination of lesions shows a mixture of xanthoma cells, numerous Touton giant cells, and an inflammatory infiltrate. In early lesions, however, lipidization of histiocytes and the formation of foam cells occurs, and the more typical histopathologic features of the disorder become apparent.

TABLE 12–4.—XANTHOMA DISSEMINATUM

---

1. Usually a disorder of young male adults (30% start before the age of 15 years)
2. A benign disorder (possibly a variant of H-S-C disease)
3. Cutaneous lesions
   a. Closely set round to oval yellowish-brown to purple papules, nodules and plaques
   b. Usually on face, flexor surface of neck, antecubital fossae, periumbilical area, perineum and genitalia
4. Other features
   a. Xanthomatous deposits in mouth and upper respiratory tract may lead to respiratory difficulty
   b. Diabetes insipidus in 40%

Except for severe laryngeal involvement occasionally necessitating tracheostomy, the disease tends to run a chronic but benign course and the lesions have been seen to regress spontaneously. If diabetes insipidus occurs, it is usually mild and may be transient, so that continued therapy with vasopressin injections (Pitressin) becomes unnecessary.

Malignant Histiocytosis

Malignant histiocytosis, originally described in 1939 as histiocytic medullary reticulosis, is a rare histiocytic proliferative disorder that often has an acute onset, severe malaise, and used to progress on to a fatal course within a few months[17-20] (Table 12–5). Clinical features include fever, wasting, generalized lymphadenopathy, hepatosplenomegaly, jaundice, pancytopenia, cutaneous purpura, and papules and nodules that often undergo ulceration. Although involvement of the skin or subcutaneous tissues has been estimated to occur in about 10% of cases,[18] in children the incidence appears to be somewhat higher.[19]

Cutaneous lesions consist of papules, nodules or plaques that undergo ulceration. The cutaneous infiltrate, usually located in the middle to lower portion of the dermis and in the subcutaneous fat, consists of atypical as well as normal histiocytes with acute and chronic inflammation and focal areas of necrosis. The atypical histiocytes are characterized by large, hyperchromatic, pleomorphic, nuclei with coarse clumped chromatin, nuclear debris, fragments of leukocytes in their cytoplasm[20] and one or more small nucleoli adjacent to a prominent nuclear membrane. Erythrophagocytosis (a hallmark of malignant histiocytosis) may occasionally be seen.[21]

Although previously considered an invariable fatal disease with death occurring within weeks or months after the onset of symptoms, some reports have shown that patients may occasionally respond to chemotherapy with survivals of six or more years.[19]

Juvenile Xanthogranuloma

Juvenile xanthogranuloma (JXG), a designation that is replacing the term nevoxanthoendothelioma, represents a benign, self-limiting disease of in-

TABLE 12–5.—MALIGNANT HISTIOCYTOSIS

1. Acute onset, malaise, fever, wasting, generalized lymphadenopathy, hepatosplenomegaly, pancytopenia
2. Affects children as well as adults
3. Cutaneous features (in 10%): papules, nodules or plaques that undergo ulceration
4. Previously invariably fatal within weeks or months, but survivals up to six years or more with chemotherapy

fants and children characterized by a cutaneous infiltrate. Since histiocytes represent the basic cell, and internal lesions similar to those seen in Hand-Schüller-Christian disease occasionally occur, many authors consider juvenile xanthogranuloma to be an abortive cutaneous form of histiocytosis.[20] The lesions have no relationship to nevi, and endothelial cells are not responsible for the histogenesis of this disorder. Accordingly, the earlier term, nevoxanthoendothelioma (a misnomer), has been replaced by the name juvenile xanthogranuloma (Table 12–6).

JXG represents a benign, self-limiting disorder of childhood characterized by solitary or multiple yellow to reddish-brown papules and nodules of the face, scalp, neck, and proximal portions of the extremities or trunk (Fig 12–6). Lesions also occur on mucous membranes or at mucocutaneous junctions (the mouth, vaginal orifice, and perineal area). Typically the lesions are present at birth (20%) or during the first six to nine months of life. The lesions run a benign course, often increasing in number until about 1 to 1½ years of age, and then involute spontaneously. There may be as few as one or two lesions or as many as several hundred. They may range in diameter from several millimeters to one centimeter and frequently have a discrete, firm or rubbery consistency.

About 90% of patients with this disorder have a self-limiting cutaneous disease. Juvenile xanthogranuloma was regarded as a lesion limited to the skin until 1949, when Blank reported a lesion of the iris in a 4-month-old infant with this condition.[22] Lesions also may occur in the lung, pericardium, meninges, liver, spleen, and testes. Patients with pulmonary involvement often show spontaneous regression of lesions. Ocular tumors of the iris or epibulbar area, however, are the most frequent internal complications and often require therapy if extensive glaucoma, hemorrhage, or blindness is to be avoided. Once the proper diagnosis has been established, therapy of ocular lesions includes radiation and topical or systemic steroids; skin lesions, however, involute spontaneously and require no treatment.

TABLE 12–6.—Juvenile Xanthogranuloma
(Nevoxanthoendothelioma)

1. 0.5 to 1 cm yellow to reddish-brown papules and nodules (solitary or multiple)
   a. Usually on face, scalp, neck or proximal extremities
   b. Occasionally in mouth, vaginal orifice, or perineal area
2. 90% are self-limiting purely cutaneous lesions
3. Occasionally may affect the lungs, pericardium, meninges, spleen, liver, testes or eyes
4. Possible association of leukemia in patients with a combination of neurofibromatosis and juvenile xanthogranuloma

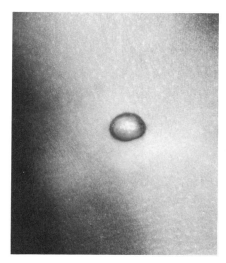

Fig 12–6.—Firm yellow to reddish-brown nodular lesion on the right thigh of an 8-month-old girl with juvenile xanthogranuloma (nevoxanthoendothelioma).

There have been patients with a combination of juvenile xanthogranuloma and neurofibromatosis who developed chronic myelogenous leukemia or acute monomyelocytic leukemia. Patients with this combination should be checked periodically for the possibility of an associated leukemia.[23]

Mastocytosis

Mastocytosis is a term used to describe a group of clinical disorders characterized by the accumulation of mast cells in the skin and at times, generally in adults, other organs of the body. It may appear at any time from birth to middle age; approximately three quarters of all cases develop during infancy or early childhood (generally before the age of 2), and most of the remaining 25% of cases begin at or after puberty (usually between the ages of 15 and 40).[24-26] The etiology is unknown. Reports of mastocytosis in twins, siblings, and families suggest an inherited basis for this disorder. Further studies of genetic pedigrees, however, are required to clarify the possible role of inheritance in patients with this disorder.[27-29]

The clinical spectrum of mastocytosis includes: (1) single or multiple small cutaneous nodules (solitary mastocytoma) (Fig 12–7); (2) a cutaneous form characterized by multiple hyperpigmented macules or papules (urticaria pigmentosa) (Figs 12–8, 12–9); (3) a diffuse form in which virtually all of the skin is infiltrated with mast cells (diffuse cutaneous mastocytosis) (Figs 12–10, 12–11); (4) unusual telangiectases of the trunk and extremities usually seen in adults and rarely in children (telangiectasia macularis eruptiva perstans); (5) systemic mastocytosis, a condition in which mast cell pro-

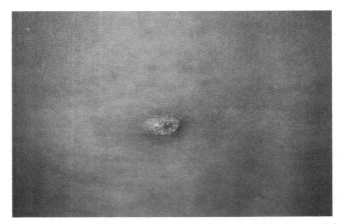

Fig 12–7.—Solitary bullous mastocytoma. A flesh-colored to reddish-brown nodular aggregation of mast cells on the back of a 6-month-old infant. Stroking or gentle rubbing of such lesions causes localized erythema, urticarial wheals and, at times, blisters in this variant of mastocytosis.

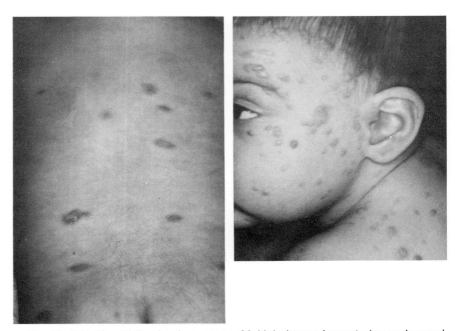

Fig 12–8 (left).—Urticaria pigmentosa. Multiple hyperpigmented macules and nodules on the back of a 5-year-old girl with mastocytosis.

Fig 12–9 (right).—Bullous urticaria pigmentosa in a 6-year-old boy. Vesicles and bullae are prominent features of this form of mast cell disease.

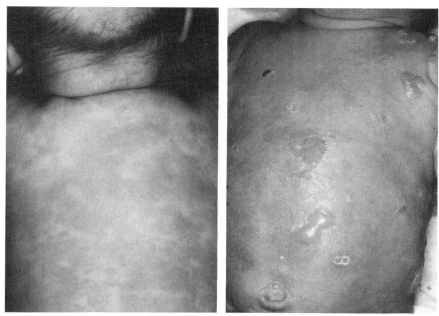

Fig 12–10 (left).—Diffuse cutaneous erythrodermic mastocytosis in a 5-month-old infant.
Fig 12–11 (right).—Bullous mastocytosis. Diffuse cutaneous erythrodermic mastocytosis with extensive bulla formation.

liferation occurs in various organ systems (the skin, liver, spleen, lymph nodes, lungs, bones, and gastrointestinal tract); and (6) a rare malignant form of mast cell leukemia seen primarily in adults and rarely in children (Table 12–7).

The classification of the forms of mastocytosis, often confusing because of their varied manifestations, can be simplified by separation into child-hood and adult varieties. In children the disorder appears in three forms: (1) individual lesions (solitary mastocytosis); (2) a generalized form termed urticaria pigmentosa; and (3) a relatively rare variant (diffuse cutaneous mastocytosis). All three of these childhood forms may display vesicular or bullous variants. Seen primarily in children under 2, they may be termed bullous mastocytoma, bullous urticaria pigmentosa, or bullous mastocytosis. Although the cause of vesiculation in this age group remains unknown, it is presumably related to a histamine-induced transudate in a group susceptible to vesicle formation by insecure attachments of the epidermis to the underlying dermis.[30]

The prognosis and course of mastocytosis depends on the clinical presen-

TABLE 12–7.—CLINICAL SPECTRUM OF
MASTOCYTOSIS*

1. Solitary mastocytoma
2. Urticaria pigmentosa
3. Diffuse cutaneous mastocytosis
4. Telangiectasia macularis eruptiva perstans (usually in adults, rare in children)
5. Systemic mastocytosis
   a. Seen in adults
   b. Asymptomatic systemic involvement of a limited degree may occur in urticaria pigmentosa of childhood, but it is uncommon
6. Mast cell leukemia (primarily in adults; rare in childhood)

*Childhood forms of mastocytosis include solitary mastocytoma, urticaria pigmentosa and diffuse cutaneous mastocytosis. All three may display vesicular or bullous variations.

tation and its age of onset. In general, children have a better prognosis than adults (in children under 10, it is almost always a purely cutaneous disease that resolves spontaneously). In adults, however, the skin lesions seldom disappear, and 30% to 55% of patients have evidence of systemic involvement.[24, 25]

The diagnosis of cutaneous mastocytosis is aided by Darier's sign. This finding, a hallmark of the disorder, is seen in 90% of patients with cutaneous mastocytosis and consists of localized erythema and urticarial wheals that develop after gentle mechanical irritation, such as might be induced by a tongue blade or the blunt end of a pen or pencil. Erythema and urtication, apparently the result of liberation of histamine by mast cells, usually develop within a few minutes and may persist from 30 minutes to several hours. The degranulation of mast cells seems to be correlated with an increased production of cyclic adenosine monophosphate and prostaglandin D_2, with histamine, heparin, and prostaglandin D_2 being responsible for many of the systemic features seen in patients with this disorder.[31–33]

Solitary Mastocytosis

The terms *solitary mastocytosis* and *solitary mastocytoma* are used to designate patients with one or more isolated or individual lesions, a variant estimated to occur in 10% to 15% of all cases of mastocytosis.[34] Lesions usually appear at birth or in infancy, increase somewhat in size for several months, and eventually regress spontaneously, usually within several years. In most patients with this form of mastocytosis, lesions are solitary. Many children, however, may develop as many as three or four individual lesions (in one instance, a 4-month-old male infant had nine solitary mastocytomas,[35] and a few patients with solitary mastocytosis have been reported to progress to a generalized form of urticaria pigmentosa).[36]

CLINICAL MANIFESTATIONS.—Solitary mastocytomas may occur on any part of the body but are noted most frequently on the arms (especially near the wrists), the neck, and trunk. Clinically they are seen as slightly elevated flesh-colored to light-brown or tan plaques or nodules. Occasionally they may display a yellowish or pink hue. Lesions are usually round or oval and measure 1 to 5 cm in diameter. They may have a thick or rubbery quality with a smooth or pebbly peau d'orange (orange peel-like) consistency. Darier's sign is positive, and stroking or rubbing the lesions may at times produce symptoms of flushing or colic.

Infant skin is more likely to respond to various noxious stimuli by forming blisters. Accordingly, bullous lesions are seen as common variants of this disorder. When present in association with solitary lesions of mastocytosis, this disorder (frequently misdiagnosed as bullous impetigo) is termed bullous mastocytoma (Fig 12–7). This tendency toward vesiculation and bulla formation usually disappears in one to three years.

Solitary mastocytomas have the most favorable prognosis of all cutaneous forms of mastocytosis. Symptoms, when present, are usually mild, and spontaneous resolution within several years is the rule (almost always before age 10). Parents should be advised that symptoms, if present, usually abate after one or two years (even before the lesions disappear) and that surgical excision, except in cases that are symptomatic and troublesome, is generally unnecessary.

Urticaria Pigmentosa

Urticaria pigmentosa, seen in about two-thirds of patients with cutaneous mastocytosis, is the most common manifestation of the mastocytosis syndrome.[24] Primarily a disease of children, the disorder may be present at birth, with the majority of cases originating during the first three to nine months of life. In a study of 139 patients with urticaria pigmentosa, 86% had the onset of their disorder before 15 years of age; the remaining had their onset between ages 15 and 40.[37]

CLINICAL MANIFESTATIONS.—The cutaneous lesions of urticaria pigmentosa generally appear as multiple reddish-brown (occasionally yellowish-brown) hyperpigmented macules, papules, or nodular lesions that urticate in a characteristic manner when traumatized (Darier's sign) (Fig 12–8). When the normal-appearing skin also urticates, it usually does so to a lesser extent. Dermographism of the apparently uninvolved skin has occurred in one-third to one-half of all patients with urticaria pigmentosa. This finding, when present, appears to be due to an increase in mast cells throughout the dermis of otherwise apparently normal skin.[24]

Lesions of urticaria pigmentosa may occur anywhere on the body but generally involve the trunk, often in a symmetrical fashion. In later stages, lesions may spread to the extremities and the neck. Involvement of the scalp, face, palms, and soles, although occasionally present, is infrequent and uncommon; a few cases have been reported in which lesions were present in the buccal, palatal, or pharyngeal mucosa, or on the anal mucous membrane.

Individual lesions are usually round or oval, vary in size from one millimeter to several centimeters in diameter, and are larger in children than in adults. Pigmentation, particularly in older lesions, is common. The reason for increased pigmentation of lesions is unknown. Increased levels of tyrosinase due to reduction of tyrosine inhibitor by the release of mucopolysaccharides from the mast cells has been suggested as the cause of this phenomenon. This hypothesis, however, remains unsubstantiated and requires further investigation and corroboration.[24]

Vesicles or bullae occasionally occur as prominent features of urticaria pigmentosa of childhood. Although the mechanism of vesiculation is unknown, this appears to be related to the release of histamine and the fact that infantile skin blisters more easily than adult skin. When bullae are present in addition to pigmented skin lesions, the disease is termed bullous urticaria pigmentosa[30] (Fig 12–9).

Telangiectasia macularis eruptiva perstans (TMEP) is a variant generally seen in patients with the adult form of urticaria pigmentosa. This variant, uncommon in childhood, has been reported in children with this disorder.[24] Patients with TMEP have an extensive eruption of small, persistent, brownish-red hyperpigmented telangiectatic macules on the trunk and extremities with little or no tendency toward urtication. This uncommon disorder is thought by some to be related to frequent dilatation of blood vessels by repeated release of histamine, and although this concept remains unsubstantiated, it has been suggested that patients with TMEP may have an increased incidence of peptic ulcer.[25]

PROGNOSIS.—When seen in children under age 10, urticaria pigmentosa has an excellent prognosis and is almost always a cutaneous disorder that tends toward spontaneous remission; in about one-half of the cases in which the disorder has its onset in infancy or early childhood, the lesions disappear by adolescence, and another 25% will have partial resolution of lesions by adulthood.[38, 39] Although systemic involvement has been reported in children with urticaria pigmentosa, a review of childhood cases having widespread and occasionally fatal extracutaneous mast cell infiltrates (liver, spleen, lymph nodes, and bone marrow) found these cases to be diffuse cutaneous or erythrodermic forms of mastocytosis rather than true urticaria pigmentosa.[38] When urticaria pigmentosa has its onset in later childhood (beyond the age of 10 years) the outlook is less favorable with regard to disappearance of cutaneous lesions,[38, 39] and the majority of patients with associated systemic disease occur in this group. Although it is impossible to accurately estimate what proportion of patients are likely to develop a systemic form of the disease, systemic involvement seems to occur in approximately 10% to 15% (generally adults) of all patients with mastocytosis.[24]

When systemic mastocytosis occurs, almost any organ or tissue of the body may be affected. The most frequently involved organs are the bones, liver, spleen, lymph nodes, and peripheral blood. Mast cell accumulations, however, have also been found in the lung, kidney, gastrointestinal tract, skeletal muscle, myocardium, pericardium, omentum, and other tissues. Hepatomegaly, present in 10% to 15% of patients, and splenomegaly (usually seen in association with hepatic enlargement) seem to occur in an equal percentage of patients. Although an incidence as high as 30% had been reported for bone involvement (either localized or diffuse areas of osteoporosis or osteosclerosis) in patients with systemic disease, 10% or 15% is a more realistic figure for this association.[24]

Since systemic involvement occurs in 10% to 30% of patients with urticaria pigmentosa whose skin lesions appear after the age of 10 years, all patients with late-onset or adult forms of this disorder should be carefully evaluated.[39] Although the measurement of urinary histamine excretion may be of indirect help in the diagnosis of systemic mastocytosis, further experience is required to substantiate the value of this laboratory study.[25] Symptoms of the mastocytosis syndrome may include intense pruritus, urticaria, headache, flushing, tachycardia, gastrointestinal symptoms, nonspecific abnormalities of blood clotting, hypotension, and syncope. Patients with bone involvement may have bone pain. Hemorrhagic diatheses, although rare, may be related to hepatosplenic involvement, heparin liberation, or to the infrequent association of mastocytosis with mast cell leukemia or lymphoma.[32]

The development of leukemia or a related malignant condition affecting tissues of the reticuloendothelial system is the main hazard in adult patients with mastocytosis. The presence of mast cells in the peripheral blood of patients with mastocytosis is a grave prognostic sign. A 5-year-old child with urticaria pigmentosa and acute lymphoblastic leukemia was reported in 1973. Although perhaps coincidental, this report raises the question as to whether this association was more than just a chance occurrence.[40]

Diffuse Cutaneous and Erythrodermic Mastocytosis

Diffuse cutaneous mastocytosis is a rare form of childhood mastocytosis that bears little clinical resemblance to urticaria pigmentosa. In this disorder, large areas of the dermis are infiltrated with mast cells, and the skin develops a thickened boggy, doughy, and at times lichenified appearance. The cutaneous surface may be smooth, or it may contain numerous minute papules that give it a scotch-grained, leather-like appearance, frequently with a yellow carotenemia-like tint or a diffusely reddened appearance (diffuse erythrodermic mastocytosis). In some cases, diffuse cutaneous mastocytosis may be accompanied by multiple cutaneous mastocytomas[41] and extensive bullous eruptions (Figs 12–10, 12–11). In the latter variant (bullous mastocytosis), the prognosis seems to be related to the age of onset of bullous lesions. When bullae develop early in the neonatal period, the prognosis is more guarded and systemic involvement frequently occurs.[42] With delayed onset of blisters, however, extracutaneous manifestations appear to bear less significance and the prognosis is more favorable.[30]

The diffuse cutaneous forms of mastocytosis may present symptoms of intense generalized pruritus, flushing, temperature elevation, vomiting, diarrhea, abdominal pain, and acute respiratory distress, with wheezing, cyanosis, apnea, and, at times, severe shock-like states. In a review of eight infants with this variant, two died; five of the remaining six had mast cell infiltration of the reticuloendothelial system; and one had gastrointestinal involvement, an increased number of mast cells in the bone marrow, and mast cells in the peripheral blood.[43]

DIAGNOSIS.—Typical cases of cutaneous mastocytosis generally present little diagnostic problem to the physician familiar with this disorder. Urtication following the mechanical irritation of lesions (Darier's sign) is highly diagnostic and will frequently help to confirm the true nature of the disease. Atypical and more unusual forms of cutaneous mastocytosis, however, are more difficult to diagnose and require a high index of suspicion on the part of the clinician.

When the diagnosis is indeterminate, cutaneous biopsy can help confirm the true nature of the disorder. Since loss of granules may occur owing to handling of lesions during biopsy, the injection of local anesthetic too close to lesions or biopsy of a lesion that had previously been urticated makes histopathologic identification of mast cells difficult. Specimens should be handled gently and removed whenever possible without previous urtication, and avoidance of local anesthetic infiltration into the area of the biopsy site may be necessary to establish the proper histopathologic diagnosis.

All forms of mastocytosis are characterized by abnormal accumulation of mast cells. In the macular and papular type of lesions, there is generally a sparse mast cell infiltrate in the upper dermis, usually with a perivascular and periappendageal distribution. A scarcity of mast cells in some sections may make histologic confirmation difficult, and at times the true nature of the disorder may be established only after performing repeated biopsies.

Cutaneous biopsies of juvenile forms of urticaria pigmentosa are characterized by dense aggregates of mast cells in the subpapillary layers and midcutis. The cells may have a peculiar arrangement, being packed into tumor-like clumps or arranged in strands or columns of varying width. The dense packing of mast cells may cause them to appear cuboidal, polyhedric, or flattened, thus resembling fibroblasts with spindle-shaped nuclei. Nodular lesions and isolated mastocytomas tend to have massive mast cell infiltrates throughout the entire corium, and the skin of patients with diffuse cutaneous mastocytosis has a band-like infiltrate of mast cells close to the epidermis. Mast cells are characterized by the presence of metachromatic granules in their cytoplasm. Although these granules are not often visible on routine stains, they can generally be visualized after staining with Giemsa, azure A, methylene-blue or toluidine-blue stains.

TREATMENT.—There is no satisfactory treatment for mastocytosis. Children with diffuse cutaneous mastocytosis and those with onset after the age of 10 years should be observed closely and screened for possible involvement of other organs. Proper screening in such cases includes frequent examination of blood smears, thrombocyte, bleeding, and coagulation time studies, and, if indicated by history, gastrointestinal survey and bone scans. Patients with all forms of this disorder should avoid aspirin, codeine, opiates, procaine, alcohol, polymyxin B, hot baths, and vigorous rubbing after showering or bathing in an effort to minimize the release of histamine. Hydroxyzine (Atarax or Vistaril) or various antihistamines may be helpful in the relief of pruritus and may modify flushing or other symptoms associated with the mastocytosis syndrome. Cyproheptadine (Periactin) has the advantage of both antihistamine and antiserotonin activity. For some, it is the drug of choice for the management of symptoms associated with this disorder. Inhibition of the enzyme histidine decarboxylase thus far has been ineffective for the relief of symptoms of mast cell disease. Oral cromolyn sodium (disodium cromoglycate) in dosages of 10 to 20 mg four times a day has been reported to be helpful in infants with gastrointestinal involvement, in infants with blistering and urticaria associated with bullous and diffuse cutaneous forms of mastocytosis, and in adults with systemic involvement.[44, 45] Recent reports suggest the use of cimetidine and chlorpheniramine for the treatment of the systemic manifestations of mastocytosis.[46] Other authorities recommend oral psoralen followed by long-wave ultraviolet light (PUVA) for the treatment of some individuals with urticaria pigmentosa.[47] Evaluation of these modalities, however, remain inconclusive and require further investigative studies.

Sarcoidosis

Sarcoidosis is a systemic granulomatous disorder of unknown etiology with widespread manifestations predominantly affecting the lungs, eyes, skin and reticuloendothelial system. Rarely seen in children, the greatest incidence of this disorder is in patients between 20 and 40 years of age. Although the youngest reported patient was a 2-month-old infant, of the relatively few childhood cases in the literature, most have occurred in the preadolescent or adolescent age group (between 9 and 15 years of age)[48] (Table 12–8).

The disease occurs in blacks, mongoloids, and Caucasians and appears to be most common among Scandinavians, American blacks, and Caucasians of the southeastern United States. There have been few case reports involving Caucasian children of Northern European ancestry and the disorder is rarely seen in African blacks. Most children with sarcoidosis in the United States have been black, from the "sarcoid belt" of the southeastern states, and symptomatic with a high incidence of reticuloendothelial involvement, hyperglobulinemia, and hypercalcemia.[44–48]

The etiology of sarcoidosis is unknown. Although many agents (mycobacteria, fungal, viral and bacterial) have been postulated to be involved in its pathogenesis, little evidence exists to favor any one etiologic agent. The cause appears to be the end result of multiple factors with an abnormal host response, delayed hypersensitivity and abnormal immunoregulation all contributing to the clinical features of affected individuals.

TABLE 12–8.—SARCOIDOSIS

---

1. A systemic granulomatous disorder of unknown etiology (an abnormal host response with delayed hypersensitivity and abnormal immunoregulation?)
2. Relatively uncommon in children (most cases in the United States are in blacks from the southeastern United States)
3. Skin lesions (in up to 50%), lungs (50%), ocular lesions (25%), splenomegaly (17%), osseous lesions (12%), cranial nerve paresis (5%), hilar lymphadenopathy (70%), peripheral lymphadenopathy (30%), hepatomegaly (20%)
4. Cutaneous lesions
   a. Soft, red to yellowish-brown or violaceous flat-topped papules
   b. Nodules or infiltrated plaques
   c. Subcutaneous tumors
   d. Scaly erythematous patches
5. Serum angiotensin-converting enzyme (SACE) levels (often of diagnostic value in adults but less significant in children)

CLINICAL MANIFESTATIONS.—The signs and symptoms of sarcoidosis are due primarily to local tissue infiltration and injury from pressure and displacement by sarcoidal lesions. The skin, lungs, eyes, liver, spleen, lymph nodes, bones, muscles, nervous system, and exocrine glands may be involved, with clinical manifestations of the disorder dependent upon the organ or system involved and its degree of involvement.[49]

Arthralgias, low-grade fever, and abdominal pain are the most frequent symptoms in children with sarcoidosis.[44] Pulmonary involvement, the earliest and most frequently seen symptom in adults, also occurs in most childhood forms of this disorder. Pulmonary symptoms are usually mild and often consist of a dry hacking cough, with or without mild to moderate dyspnea. The most common roentgenographic finding in children is that of bilateral hilar lymph node enlargement, with or without detectable lung changes.[49, 50] Ocular involvement, too, is extremely common in children. Uveitis and iritis constitute the most frequently observed lesions, but keratitis, retinitis, glaucoma, and involvement of the eyelids and lacrimal glands may also occur. Although examination of the world literature suggests that eye lesions in children are not usually severe, involvement of the eye, with resultant partial or total blindness, occurs in a relatively high percentage of children with sarcoidosis.[48, 51]

Facial nerve paralysis and central nervous system involvement, although common in adults, are rare in children. Osseous involvement is also rarely seen in children. When present, however, the metacarpals, metatarsals, and phalanges are the bones most frequently affected. Uveoparotid fever (a combination of uveitis, parotitis, and Bell's palsy) and Sjögren's syndrome without arthritis (keratoconjunctivitis sicca and enlargement of the parotid and lacrimal glands), though often seen in adults, are quite rare in children. Parotid gland enlargement and peripheral adenopathy are commonly seen in children. Hepatic and splenic involvement, though clinically uncommon, are frequently seen at necropsy.

CUTANEOUS FEATURES.—Although the incidence of skin lesions noted in patients with sarcoidosis depends upon the observer and therefore varies in different series, of the 113 children with sarcoidosis reviewed by McGovern and Merritt, 57 patients (50%) were noted to have skin lesions.[49] Cutaneous lesions can arise anywhere on the body, and although they do not have a pathognomonic clinical morphology, they exhibit highly characteristic features that should strongly suggest the presence of the disease. In children under the age of 6, the disorder characteristically involves the skin, eyes and synovial tissues in a chronic progressive course.[52–54]

Cutaneous lesions of sarcoidosis include papules, nodules, infiltrated plaques, subcutaneous tumors, and scaly erythematous patches with little or no palpable infiltration, with the latter often leaving pitted scars in children less than six years of age.[54] The most common lesions are soft, red to yellowish-brown or violaceous flat-topped papules, with a predilection for the face. Although the extremities, neck, and trunk may be affected, an annular configuration of these lesions around the nares, lips, and eyelids is highly characteristic of this disorder. Frequently these lesions will present a waxy or translucent appearance. Occasionally the mucous membranes may be involved as well. If the cutaneous lesions are pressed out with a glass slide (diascopy), a characteristic yellowish-brown or "apple-jelly" color may be demonstrated.

Other forms of sarcoidosis in the skin have received special designations. One of these is *lupus pernio*, a variant in which soft infiltrated violaceous plaques are located on the nose, cheeks, ears, forehead, dorsa of the hands, fingers, or toes. *Angiolupoid* is a term used to describe purplish infiltrated plaques or nodules, particularly on or around the nose, with a characteristic telangiectatic vascular component. *Erythrodermic sarcoidosis* is a term used to describe a rare variant of this disorder. Characterized by extensive, sharply demarcated, brownish-red scaly patches with little or no palpable infiltration, these lesions often involute spontaneously. Another form of skin involvement is a nodular vasculitis with a granulomatous infiltrate largely confined to the subcutaneous tissue. This variant has been termed the *Darier-Roussy* type of sarcoidosis. These skin-colored or violaceous, round or oval, deep-seated nodules appear primarily on the trunk and legs, usually without subjective symptoms.

Erythema nodosum, occasionally seen in association with sarcoidosis, is a striking but not diagnostic finding; it represents a hypersensitivity phenomenon and is not specific for this disorder.

DIAGNOSIS.—There is no single fully reliable test for sarcoidosis. Since the clinical picture may be mimicked by other diseases, histologic proof in the form of either a biopsy or a positive *Kveim* test is advisable. The Kveim test consists of intradermal injection of a 10% suspension of human sarcoidal tissue in normal saline. During the following weeks a small papule may develop at the site of injection. Biopsy of the papule four to six weeks after the injection reveals specific distinctive sarcoidal granulomas. In general, the frequency of a positive response to the Kveim test is greatest in early cases of sarcoidosis. Because of loss of reactivity as the disease progresses, this test has been found to have prognostic as well as diagnostic value. However, since reliable Kveim antigen is difficult to obtain, this test frequently has more of a theoretical than a practical application. Tuberculin, histoplasmin, coccidioidin, and cat-scratch antigen tests also should be performed, as these conditions may closely resemble sarcoidosis in children. The diagnosis often is hindered by a lack of the classic laboratory findings of hyperglobulinemia, hypercalcemia, leukopenia, and eosinophilia. Although occasionally found, they rarely prove to be reliable diagnostic features of this disorder in childhood.[49]

It has recently been demonstrated that 50% to 60% of patients with active sarcoidosis have elevated serum levels of angiotensin-converting enzyme (ACE).[55-60] In a study of 21 children with sarcoidosis, 80% had elevation of serum ACE levels. In this study the levels were significantly higher than those in adults with similar type disease. It has been suggested that this is a very sensitive indicator of disease activity, especially in individuals with pulmonary sarcoidosis. However, ACE levels are often elevated in normal individuals under the age of 20 and are frequently normal when the sarcoidosis is limited to the skin.[59] In patients where the serum angiotensin converting enzyme does not decrease following adequate steroid therapy, it may indicate progressive disease with a relatively poor prognosis.[56, 60]

TREATMENT.—The natural course of sarcoidosis in childhood is insidious, follows a smoldering course, and often regresses completely after many years. Mortality is reported to be about 5%, and tuberculosis has been estimated to occur in 10% of children with sarcoidosis.[52]

Since the etiology is unknown, specific therapy is not available. Corticosteroids, however, can suppress the acute manifestation of sarcoidosis. Because of the well-known hazards of prolonged systemic corticosteroid therapy, the indications for treatment are determined by the specific organ system involved and the severity of the involvement. Corticosteroids should be used in patients with hypercalcemia, ocular involvement, severe or debilitating lung disease, or lung disease that is progressing rapidly, and for the management of ocular sarcoidosis. In ocular sarcoidosis, corticosteroid ophthalmic preparations may be utilized in conjunction with the systemic therapy. In children the dose of prednisone is 1 mg/kg of body weight, with gradual reduction to the lowest dosage that will suppress the symptoms and signs of the disorder. The course of treatment is usually about six months, but the duration is determined by the response to therapy and the type or severity of involvement.

Mycosis Fungoides

Mycosis fungoides is a chronic, often fatal disease of the lymphoreticular system whose initial clinical manifestations appear in the skin, often remaining there for years before terminating as a malignant lymphoma with lymph node and visceral involvement. Generally seen in patients in the fifth to seventh decades of life, it has also been seen in children and early adulthood[61] (Table 12–9). The etiology of mucosis fungoides remains unknown with current hypotheses suggesting a viral origin,[62] chronic antigenic stimulation in which epidermally located antigens act as stimulants

TABLE 12–9.—MYCOSIS FUNGOIDES

---

1 Generally seen in fifth to seventh decades of life (only occasionally in children and early adulthood)
2. Etiology unknown (? chronic antigenic stimulation in skin)
3. Cutaneous lesions
    a. Erythematous (premycotic) stage
    b. Plaque (mycotic) stage
    c. Tumor stage
4. Poor prognosis (50% mortality within 2–4 years of onset of tumor stage)

---

for blast formation of T cells, or a malignant lymphoma in which the mycosis cell (a T lymphocyte) represents the neoplastic cell.[63–65]

CUTANEOUS MANIFESTATIONS.—Clinically as well as histologically, in typical cases mycosis fungoides can be divided into erythematous, plaque and tumor stages. In affected individuals, the disorder may begin with any of the stages, only one or two phases may be noted, and in some instances lesions of all three stages may be present at the same time.

The erythematous (premycotic) stage is characterized by pruritus and flat erythematous, eczematous or psoriasiform lesions. Most lesions of this premycotic stage are asymptomatic or pruritic, macular, dull pink, and round or oval with poorly formed scale.

In the plaque (mycotic) phase the premycotic lesions become infiltrated, well-demarcated and appear as red, reddish-brown to purple slightly indurated plaques. Central clearing often develops and the lesions may assume serpiginous, arciform, horseshoe or other bizarre shapes. In many instances, the entire integument may become infiltrated producing a thickened red hide with or without scaling, islands of normal skin often remaining for a time before the universal erythroderma becomes complete.[66] Although extensive exfoliative erythroderma may occur in patients with atopic, contact or seborrheic dermatitis, psoriasis or pityriasis rubra pilaris, patients with de novo onset of generalized erythroderma and no evidence for drug eruption may have an associated malignancy such as mycosis fungoides.

In the third (tumor) stage multiple round, dome- or irregularly shaped raised tumors may appear (Fig 12–12). These are flesh-colored or smooth brown to bluish-red lesions covered with a thin stretched, atrophic-appearing epidermis, with or without telangiectasia. Lesions often undergo necrosis or ulceration and, at times, may disappear spontaneously. Once the development of tumors, lymphadenopathy, or cutaneous ulceration occur during the course of the disease, the prognosis is extremely poor, and 50% of patients die in 2½ to 4 years (0.1 to 48.3 years, with an average of 6 years).[67]

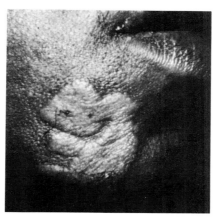

Fig 12–12.—An irregularly shaped nodular tumor on the face of a 10-year-old black male with mycosis fungoides. (Courtesy of Dr. Emily Omura, Birmingham, Alabama.)

OTHER CLINICAL FEATURES.—A disorder termed *parapsoriasis en plaque* has been defined as both a benign and a premalignant form. Those in the premalignant variety may be characterized by round or oval yellowish to red smooth or slightly scaly plaques 2 to 4 cm in diameter which occur chiefly on the trunk and thighs. In patients where parapsoriasis en plaque progresses to mycosis fungoides, the skin assumes a dusky reddish brown hue upon which numerous telangiectatic vessels involve the entire skin, poikilodermatous lesions become atrophic with a folded wrinkled telangiectatic surface, mild scaling, and hyper- and hypopigmentation, and eventually plaque-like infiltration and ulcerations develop. *Alopecia mucinosa* (follicular mucinosis) has also been shown to be a feature of mycosis fungoides and, on occasion, malignant lymphoma in adults. However, in the majority of cases (children and adults under the age of 40) it is a totally benign condition not associated with mycosis fungoides.

About 15% of patients with mycosis fungoides develop generalized or universal redness and scaling of the skin with weeping, crusting, fissuring, and some degree of hyperpigmentation. Pruritus usually is severe and excoriations are prominent. Some patients are simply red with little alteration of the epidermis *(l'homme rouge)*; thickening of the palms and soles (keratoderma palmaris et plantaris) and alopecia of the scalp are often seen, and tumors may develop late in the course. The term *Sézary syndrome* has been used for this condition. Although this syndrome was first believed to be an independent entity, available evidence now indicates that, with few exceptions, it represents a manifestation of mycosis fungoides.[66]

DIAGNOSIS.—In the premycotic stage, mycosis fungoides may be extremely difficult to diagnose. Pruritus with or without skin lesions may be the only finding. Skin lesions are usually nondescript and eczematous in nature, frequently suggesting a diagnosis of psoriasis, parapsoriasis, eczema, seborrheic dermatitis, or neurodermatitis. The histology of the lesion is usually not helpful at this stage.

When clinical infiltration is noted, however, histopathologic examination of lesions usually exhibit histologic changes consistent with this disorder. The histopathology varies with the stage of the disease. A great multiplicity of cell types with pleomorphism of the histiocytes, immature and atypical reticulum cells, scattered mycotic figures, a patchy infiltrate in the lower dermis, and the presence of Pautrier microabscesses in the epidermis help establish the diagnosis of mycosis fungoides.

TREATMENT.—Since most patients live for many years before mycosis fungoides becomes life-threatening, early stages of the disease may be treated conservatively with topical and systemic antipruritics and topical corticosteroids. For those with more advanced disease, localized x-ray therapy,[68] PUVA therapy,[69] electron beam, topically applied nitrogen mustard (Mustargen),[70] and systemic chemotherapy are frequently necessary. Patients with mycosis fungoides who go on to die from the disorder usually do so because of infection or as the result of systemic dissemination of the disease. Many deaths, however, are unexplained and seem to occur following years of unsuccessful stressful struggle with the disorder.[71]

REFERENCES

1. Lichtenstein L.: Histiocytosis X: integration of eosinophilic granuloma of bone, "Letterer-Siwe disease", and "Schüller-Christian disease" as related manifestations of a single nosological entity. *Arch. Pathol.* 56:84–102, 1953.
2. Hurwitz S.: Histiocytosis in children. *Mod. Prob. Paediat.* 17:204–210, 1975.
3. Lipman M.B., Berry R.S., Peltzik R.L., et al.: Letterer-Siwe disease presenting as seborrheic dermatitis. *Cutis* 22:303–306, 1978.
4. Aronson R.P.: Streptomycin in Letterer-Siwe disease. *Am. J. Dis. Child.* 117:236–238, 1969.
5. Esterly N.B., Swick H.M.: Cutaneous Letterer-Siwe disease. *Am. J. Dis. Child.* 117:236–238, 1969.
6. Freeman S.: A benign form of Letterer-Siwe disease. *Aust. J. Dermatol.* 12:165–171, 1971.
7. Bierman H.R.: Apparent cure of Letterer-Siwe disease. *J.A.M.A.* 196:368–370, 1966.
8. Bonifazi E., Caputo R., Ceci A., et al.: Congenital self-healing histiocytosis. *Arch. Dermatol.* 118:267–272, 1982.
9. Hashimoto K., Griffin D., Koshsabi M.: Self-healing reticulohistiocytosis: a clinical, histologic, and ultrastructural study of the fourth case in the literature. *Cancer* 49:331–337, 1982.

10. Fox J.L., Berman B.: T6-antigen-bearing cells in eosinophilic granuloma of bone. *J.A.M.A.* 249:3071–3072, 1983.
11. Doede K.G., Rappaport H.: Long-term survival of patients with acute differentiated histiocytosis (Letterer-Siwe disease). *Cancer* 20:1782–1795, 1967.
12. Starling K.A., Donaldson M.H., Haggard M.E., et al.: Therapy of histiocytosis X with vincristine, vinblastine, and cyclophosphamide—the Southwest Cancer Chemotherapy Study Group. *Am. J. Dis. Child.* 123:105–110, 1972.
13. Lahey M.E.: Histiocytosis X: Comparison of three treatment regimens. *J. Pediatr.* 87:179–183, 1975.
14. Lahey M.E.: Histiocytosis X: Analysis of prognostic factors. *J. Pediatr.* 87:184–188, 1975.
15. Zachariae H.: Histiocytosis X in two infants—treated with topical nitrogen mustard. *Br. J. Dermatol.* 100:433–438, 1979.
16. Mishkel M.A., Cockshott W.P., Nazir D.J., et al.: Xanthoma disseminatum: clinical, metabolic, pathologic and radiologic aspects. *Arch. Dermatol.* 113:1094–1100, 1977.
17. Scott R.B., Robb-Smith A.H.T.: Histiocytic medullary reticulosis. *Lancet* 2:194–198, 1939.
18. Abele D.C., Griffin T.B.: Histiocytic medullary reticulosis. *Arch. Dermatol.* 106:319–329, 1972.
19. Zucker J.M., Cailleaux J.M., Vanel D., et al.: Malignant histiocytosis in childhood. *Cancer* 45:2821–2829, 1980.
20. Lever W.F., Schaumburg-Lever G.: Lipidoses, lymphoma and leukemia, in *Histopathology of the Skin*, ed. 6. J.B. Lippincott Co., Philadelphia, 1983, pp. 383–406, 726–761.
21. Morgan N.E., Fretzin D.F.: Cutaneous manifestations of malignant histiocytosis, in American Society of Dermatology abstracts. *Arch. Dermatol.* 115:1348, 1979.
22. Blank H., Eglick P.G., Beerman H.: Nevoxanthoendothelioma with ocular involvement. *Pediatrics* 4:349–354, 1949.
23. Royer P., Blondet C., Guihard J.: Xantholeucémie du nourisson et neurofibromatose de Recklinghausen. *Ann. Pediatr.* 5:260, 1958.
24. Sagher R., Even-Paz Z.: *Mastocytosis and the Mast Cell.* Year Book Medical Publishers, Inc., Chicago, 1967.
25. Demis D.J.: The mastocytosis syndrome: clinical and biological studies. *Ann. Int. Med.* 59:194–206, 1963.
26. Schachner L., Press S.: Vesicular, bullous and pustular disorders in infancy and childhood, in Rasmussen J.E. (Guest Editor): *Symposium on Pediatric Dermatology II, Pediatric Clinics of North America.* W.B. Saunders Co., Philadelphia, 1983, Vol. 30, No. 4, pp. 609–620.
27. Selmanowitz V.J., Orentreich N.O., Tiagco C.C., et al.: Uniovular twins discordant for cutaneous mastocytosis. *Arch. Dermatol.* 102:34–41, 1970.
28. Selmanowitz V.J., Orentreich N.O.: Mastocytosis: a clinical genetic evaluation. *J. Hered.* 61:91–94, 1970.
29. Klaber M., Pegum J.S.: Diffuse cutaneous mastocytosis in mother and daughter. *Proc. R. Soc. Med.* 69:16–18, 1976.
30. Orkin M., Good R.A., Clawson C.C., et al.: Bullous mastocytosis. *Arch. Dermatol.* 101:547–564, 1970.
31. Soter N.A., Austen K.F.: The diversity of mast cell derived mediators. impli-

cations for acute, subacute, and chronic cutaneous inflammatory disorders. *J. Invest. Dermatol.* 67:313–319, 1976.

32. Guillet G., Dore N., Melville J.: Heparin liberation in urticaria pigmentosa. *Arch. Dermatol.* 118:532–533, 1982.

33. Roberts L.J., Sweetman B.J., Lewis R.A., et al.: Increased production of prostaglandin D_2 in patients with systemic mastocytosis. *N. Engl. J. Med.* 303:1400–1404, 1980.

34. Johnson W.C., Helwig E.B.: Solitary mastocytosis (urticaria pigmentosa). *Arch. Dermatol.* 84:806–815, 1961.

35. Burkhart C.G.: Letters to the editors: Benign mastocytomas. *Arch. Dermatol.* 118:449–450, 1982.

36. Lantis S.H., Koblenzer P.H.: Solitary mast cell tumor: progression to disseminated urticaria pigmentosa in a negro infant. *Arch. Dermatol.* 99:60–63, 1969.

37. Hurwitz S.: Mastocytosis, in Hurwitz S.: *Clinical Pediatric Dermatology*, W.B. Saunders Publishing Co., Philadelphia, 1981, pp. 435–440.

38. Klaus S.N., Winkelmann R.K.: Course of urticaria pigmentosa in children. *Arch. Dermatol.* 86:116–119, 1962.

39. Caplan R.M.: Urticaria pigmentosa and systemic mastocytosis. *J.A.M.A.* 194:1077–1080, 1965.

40. Fromer J.L., Jaffe N., and Paed D.: Urticaria pigmentosa and acute lymphoblastic leukemia. *Arch. Dermatol.* 107:283–284, 1973.

41. Willemze R., Ruiter J., Scheffer E., et al.: Diffuse cutaneous mastocytosis with multiple cutaneous mastocytomas. *Br. J. Dermatol.* 102:601–607, 1980.

42. Harrison P.V., Cook L.J., Lake H.J., et al.: Diffuse cutaneous mastocytosis: a report of neonatal onset. *Acta Derm. Vener.* 59:541–543, 1979.

43. Burgoon C.F., Graham J.H., McCafree D.L.: Mast cell disease: a cutaneous variant with multisystem involvement. *Arch. Dermatol.* 98:590–605, 1968.

44. Soter N.A., Austen K.F., Wasserman S.I.: Oral disodium cromoglycate in the treatment of systemic mastocytosis. *N. Engl. J. Med.* 301:465–469, 1979.

45. Czarnetzki B.M., Behrendt H.: Urticaria pigmentosa: clinical picture and response to oral disodium cromoglycate. *Br. J. Dermatol.* 105:563–567, 1981.

46. Gerrard J.W., Chieu K.O.: Urticaria pigmentosa: treatment with cimetidine and chlorpheniramine. *J. Pediatr.* 94:843–845, 1979.

47. Christophers E., Hanigsmann H., Wolf K., et al.: PUVA-treatment of urticaria pigmentosa. *Br. J. Dermatol.* 98:701–702, 1978.

48. Kendig E.L.: Medical progress. Sarcoidosis among children—a review. *J. Pediatr.* 61:229–278, 1962.

49. McGovern J.P., Merritt D.H.: Sarcoidosis in childhood. *Advances in Pediatrics, Vol. 8.* Year Book Medical Publishers, Chicago, 1957, pp. 97–135.

50. Beier R.F., Lahey M.D.: Sarcoidosis among children in Utah and Idaho. *J. Pediatr.* 65:350–359, 1964.

51. Schmitt E., Appelman H., Threatt B.: Sarcoidosis in children. *Radiology* 106:621–625, 1973.

52. Kendig E.L., Jr., Brummer D.L.: The prognosis of sarcoidosis in children. *Chest* 70:351–353, 1976.

53. Siltzbach L.E., Greenberg G.M.: Childhood sarcoidosis—a study of 18 patients. *N. Engl. J. Med.* 279:1239–1245, 1968.

54. Rasmussen J.E.: Sarcoidosis in young children. *J. Am. Acad. Derm.* 5:556–570, 1981.

55. Lieberman J.: Elevation of angiotensin-converting enzyme (ACE) in sarcoidosis. *Am. J. Med.* 59:365–372, 1975.
56. Silverstein E., Friedland J., Lyons H.A.: Serum angiotensin converting enzyme in sarcoidosis: clinical significance. *Isr. J. Med. Sci.* 13–II: 1001–1006, 1977.
57. DeRemee R.A., Rohrbach M.S.: Serum angiotensin-converting enzyme activity and evaluating the clinical course of sarcoidosis. *Ann. Int. Med.* 92:361–365, 1980.
58. Studdy P., Bird R., Geraint James, G.: Serum angiotensin-converting enzyme (SACE) in sarcoidosis and other granulomatous disorders. *Lancet* 2:II: 1331–1334, 1978.
59. Rodriguez G., Shin B.C., Abernathy R.S., et al.: Serum angiotensin-converting enzyme activity in normal children and in those with sarcoidosis. *J. Pediatr.* 99:68–72, 1981.
60. Schultz T., Miller W.C., Bedrossain C.W.M.: Clinical application of measurement of angiotensin-converting enzyme. *J.A.M.A.* 242:439–441, 1979.
61. Taniguchi S., Horio T., Komura J.: Mycosis fungoides in the tumor stage treated by PUVA: a successful trial in a 12-year-old girl. *Dermatologica* 160:409–413, 1980.
62. Poliesz B.J., Ruscetti F.W., Gadzar A.F., et al.: Detection and isolation of type C retrovirus particles from fresh and cultured lymphocytes of a patient with cutaneous T-cell lymphoma. *Proc. Nat'l. Acad. Sci.* 77:7415–7419, 1980.
63. Greene M.H., Dalager N.A., Lanberg S.I., et al.: Mycosis fungoides: epidemiological observations. *Cancer Treat. Rep.* 63:597–606, 1979.
64. Tan R.S.H., Butterworth C.M., McLaughlin H., et al.: Mycosis fungoides—a disease of antigen persistence. *Br. J. Dermatol.* 91:607–616, 1974.
65. Rowden G., Lewis M.G.: Comment. Langerhan cells: involvement in the pathogenesis of mycosis fungoides. *Br. J. Dermatol.* 95:665–672, 1976.
66. Braverman I.M.: Lymphomas and allied disorders, in Braverman I.M.: *Skin Signs of Systemic Diseases*, ed. 2. W.B. Saunders Co., Philadelphia, 1981, pp. 109–178.
67. Epstein E.H., Jr., Levin D.L., Croft J.D., Jr., et al.: Mycosis fungoides. Survival, prognostic features, response to therapy, and autopsy findings. *Medicine* 51:61–72, 1972.
68. Hoppe R.T., Fuks Z., Bagshaw M.A.: The rationale for curative radiotherapy in mycosis fungoides. *Int. J. Radiat. Oncol. Biol. Phys.* 2:843–851, 1977.
69. Roenigk H.H.: Photochemotherapy for mycosis fungoides. *Arch. Dermatol.* 113:1047–1051, 1977.
70. Vanderheid E.C., Van Scott E.J., Johnson W.C., et al.: Topical chemotherapy and immunotherapy of mycosis fungoides. *Arch. Dermatol.* 113:454–462, 1977.
71. Lynch P.J.: Mycosis fungoides and Sézary syndrome, in Callen J.P.: *Cutaneous Aspects of Internal Disease.* Year Book Medical Publishers, Inc., Chicago, 1981, pp. 257–273.

Subject Index

A

Abdomen
  in epidermolysis bullosa, recessive
    dystrophic, 264
  in epidermolysis bullosa, recessive
    dystrophic in newborn, 261
  pain (*see* Pain, abdomen)
Abscess (*see* Microabscess)
Acetylcholine, 5
Acetylsalicylic acid: in juvenile
    rheumatoid arthritis, 146
Achilles tendon: rupture in
    alkaptonuria, 190
Acne
  steroid, in Cushing's syndrome, 177
  vulgaris in adrenogenital syndrome,
    178–179
Acoustic neuroma, 220
Acrocyanosis, 2, 7
Acrodermatitis enteropathica, 250–253
  clinical manifestations, 251–253
  course of, 252
  diagnosis, 253
  etiology, 250
  inheritance pattern of, 250
  pathogenesis, 250
  periorificial lesions in, 251, 252
  secondary infection in, 250, 252
  treatment, 253
  zinc in (*see* Zinc)
Acrodermatitis, papular (*see* Gianotti-
    Crosti syndrome)
Acrogeria: elastosis perforans
    serpiginosa in, 113
Acromegaly: in adult in
    hyperpituitarism, 179
Acrosclerosis, 137, 138
ACTH-stimulating test, 176
Actinic damage: chronic, at early age,
    313
Addisonian hyperpigmentation, 177
Addisonian pigmentation: in
    hyperthyroidism, 164

Addison's disease, 174–176
  clinical manifestations, 175–176
  diagnosis, 176
    differential, 194
  etiologic factors, 174
  hyperpigmentation in, 175
  hypoparathyroidism and, 172
  neurofibromatosis and, 226
  treatment, 176
Adenocarcinoma: in ataxia
    telangiectasia, 305
Adenoma
  functional, in hyperthyroidism, 163
  sebaceum, 227, 229
    discussion of term, 228
    in sclerosis, tuberous, 232
    treatment for cosmetic reasons,
      232
Adenomatosis, endocrine (*see* Multiple
    endocrine adenomatosis
    syndromes)
Adenopathy
  cervical, in Kawasaki disease, 47
  in Letterer-Siwe disease, 337
  in sarcoidosis, 355
Adrenal disorders, 174–179
Adrenogenital syndrome, 178–179
  clinical manifestations, 178–179
  congenital, 179
  diagnosis, 179
  treatment, 179
Agenesis: of thyroid, 157
Aging, premature
  in Cockayne syndrome, 319
  of skin, 312
  in xeroderma pigmentosum,
    314
Albinism, partial
  tuberous sclerosis and, 229, 231
  in Waardenburg syndrome, 239
Albright's syndrome, 222
  café au lait spots in, 223
  lesions resembling coast of Maine in,
    223

Alcohol: home-brewed, and porphyria cutanea tarda, 330
Alcoholic cirrhosis: and porphyria cutanea tarda, 330
Alcoholism: chronic, and acrodermatitis enteropathica, 351
Alezzandrini syndrome, 240
   relationship to Vogt-Koyanagi-Harada syndrome, 240
Alkaline phosphatase: low in hypothyroidism, 161
Alkaptonuria, 190, 193–195
   in Addison's disease, 176
   clinical manifestations, 193–194
   diagnosis, 194
   systemic manifestations, 194
   treatment, 195
Allergens
   contact, 3
   inhalant, 3
Allergic granulomatosis, 42–45
Allodermanyssus sanguineus, 82
Allopurinol: in Lesch-Nyhan syndrome, 198
Alopecia
   in acrodermatitis enteropathica, 250, 251
   areata, in hyperthyroidism, 164
   in biotin deficiency, 199, 200
   in incontinentia pigmenti, 236
   in lupus erythematosus, 120, 122, 124
   in mixed connective tissue disease, 149
   mucinosa in mycosis fungoides, 359
   in mycosis fungoides, 359
   in Rothmund-Thomson syndrome, 317
   in Vogt-Koyanagi-Harada syndrome, 239, 240
Alpha-L-fucosidase: deficiency in fucosidosis, 297
Alpha-lipoproteins, 203
Amino acid chromatography: in homocystinuria, 193
Aminoaciduria
   in Hartnup disease, 319, 320
   in hepatolenticular degeneration, 190
Amniocentesis: in xeroderma pigmentosum, 315

Amphotericin: in candidiasis, systemic, 86
Ampicillin in infectious mononucleosis, 79
   rashes after, 80–81
Amyloidosis: in familial Mediterranean fever, 275, 276
Anal mucosa: in dyskeratosis congenita, 270
Anaphylactoid purpura (*see* Henoch-Schönlein purpura)
Anemia
   in dyskeratosis congenita, 272
   Fanconi's, in dyskeratosis congenita, 271
   hemolytic, in erythropoietic porphyria, 325, 327
   in Letterer-Siwe disease, 337
   pernicious, and hypoparathyroidism, 172
   recalcitrant, in junctional epidermolysis bullosa, 260
Aneurysms
   arteriovenous, in Klippel-Trenaunay-Parkes-Weber syndrome, 290
   of circle of Willis, congenital, elastosis perforans serpiginosa in, 113
Angiitis: diffuse, in lupus erythematosus, 123
Angiitis, leukocytoclastic, 35
   palpable purpura as hallmark of, 36
Angioedema, 2
Angiofibroma
   on nose and cheek, 229
   tuberous sclerosis and, 228
Angiography
   coronary, abnormalities in Kawasaki disease, 51
   of spine in Cobb syndrome, 294
Angioid streaks: in pseudoxanthoma elasticum, 111
Angiokeratoma, 294–299
   circumscriptum, 294
   in Cobb syndrome, 294
   corporis diffusum, 294–297
      afflicted women, discussion of, 296
      cataracts with spoke-like appearance in, 296
      clinical features, 295–296

Angiokeratoma *(cont.)*
diagnosis, 296
heterozygous females in, 295
metabolic defect in, 295
prenatal diagnosis, 296
treatment, 296–297
disseminated, on hip and thigh in
fucosidosis, 297
of Fordyce, 294
in fucosidosis, 297
of Mibelli, 294
multiple, 294
of scrotum, 294
solitary, 294
of vulva, 294
Angiolipoma
in Cobb syndrome, 294
Angiolupoid, 356
Angioma
in epidermal nevus syndrome, 244
of gastrointestinal tract, in blue
rubber-bleb nevus syndrome,
291
Angiomatosis
encephalofacial *(see* Sturge-Weber
syndrome)
encephalotrigeminal *(see* Sturge-
Weber syndrome)
meningeal, in Sturge-Weber
syndrome, 287
Angioneurotic edema, hereditary, 9–11
clinical manifestations, 10
diagnosis, 10–11
treatment, 11
Angiosarcoma: in Maffucci's syndrome,
291
Angiotensin-converting enzyme: levels
in sarcoidosis, 354, 357
Ankle
edema in angiokeratoma corporis
diffusum, 296
in Mediterranean fever, familial, 277
Anomalies
in basal cell nevus syndrome, 242,
243
in hypomelanosis of Ito, 237–238
in incontinentia pigmenti, 236
Anorexia: in kwaskiorkor, 324
Antibiotics
in eosinophilic granuloma, 341

in erythema chronicum migrans, 72
in Lyme disease, 75
prophylactic, in epidermolysis
bullosa, 266
in pyoderma gangrenosum, 273
Antibody(ies)
anti-DNA, 124
antigluten, 254
anti-nDNA, 126
antinuclear, 126, 150
antithyroid, 157
heterophile, studies in infectious
mononucleosis, 79
Anticoagulants: in Henoch-Schönlein
purpura, 39
Anti-DNA antibody, 124
Antigen(s)
Australian, 77
extractable nuclear, 148, 150
hepatitis B surface, 76
histocompatibility, 129
HLA, and Vogt-Koyanagi-Harada
syndrome, 240
Antigluten antibodies, 254
Antihistamines, 4
in mastocytosis, 353
in Stevens-Johnson syndrome, 25
in urticaria, 3
Antimalarials: in lupus erythematosus,
127
Anti-nDNA antibodies, 126
Antinicotinic substance ingestion: and
pellagra, 321
Antinuclear antibody, 126, 150
Antithyroid antibodies, 157
Antithyroid medication, 158
in hyperthyroidism, 165
Aortic
stenosis, calcific, in alkaptonuria, 190
valve disease in mucolipidosis III,
216
Apathy: in Kwashiorkor, 324
Aplasia: cutis congenita, 301
Arachnodactyly: in homocystinuria,
190, 192
Arcus
cornea, 208
hyperlipoproteinemia and, type II,
208
juvenilis, 208

lipoides, 208
Argon laser: in Sturge-Weber
    syndrome, 289
Argyria: differential diagnosis, 194
Arm: in incontinentia pigmenti, 234
Armenian disease (*see* Mediterranean
    fever, familial)
Arteries
    calcification, 170
    coronary, disease in angiokeratoma
        corporis diffusum, 296
Arteriovenous
    aneurysm, in Klippel-Trenaunay-
        Parkes-Weber syndrome, 290
    fistula, pulmonary, in hereditary
        hemorrhagic telangiectasia, 302
    shunts, and diffuse neonatal
        hemangiomatosis, 293
Arteritis: coronary, 57
Arthralgia
    in Kawasaki disease, 47, 52
    lupus erythematosus and, 120, 124
    in mixed connective tissue disease,
        149
    in sarcoidosis, 355
Arthritis
    in alkaptonuria, 190
    complicating alkaptonuria, 194
    in Henoch-Schönlein purpura, 38
    of interphalangeal joints, in
        angiokeratoma corporis
        diffusum, 296
    in Kawasaki disease, 47, 52
    lupus erythematosus and, 120
    Lyme, 73
    in Mediterranean fever, familial,
        276
    in mixed connective tissue disease,
        149
    rheumatoid (*see* Rheumatoid
        arthritis)
Arthus-like response, 40
Ascorbic acid
    in Ehlers-Danlos syndrome, 101
    in tyrosinemia, in newborn, 200
Aspirin: in familial Mediterranean
    fever, 275
Atabrine: bluish pigmentation after,
    194
Atarax: in mastocytosis, 353

Ataxia
    cerebellar, in Hartnup disease, 320
    in Cockayne syndrome, 318
Ataxia telangiectasia, 303–305
    cause, 304
    clinical manifestations, 304–305
    diagnosis, 305
        rapid test for, 305
    malignancy in, high incidence, 304
    prenatal diagnosis, 305
    treatment, 305
Atheromatous vascular disease: in
    Cockayne syndrome, 318, 319
Atherosclerosis
    coronary, and tendinous xanthoma,
        206
    of vessels, and hyperlipoproteinemia,
        type III, 208
Atopic dermatitis: in hyperthyroidism,
    164
Atresia: pyloric, in epidermolysis
    bullosa, 261
Atrial myxoma: in NAME syndrome,
    242
Atrioventricular block: congenital, 130
Atrophy
    in Bloom syndrome, 315
    in dyskeratosis congenita, 270
    in epidermolysis bullosa,
        generalized, 260
    of lingual papillae in biotin
        deficiency, 199
    in lupus erythematosus, 121, 122
    optic, in Cockayne syndrome, 319
    in pellagra, 322
    retina in Cockayne syndrome, 318,
        319
    in Rothmund-Thomson syndrome,
        317
    of scars in epidermolysis bullosa, 261
    skin
        in Cockayne syndrome, 319
        in dermatomyositis, 134
    of spinal muscle in ataxia
        telangiectasia, 305
Auditory impairment: in Vogt-
    Koyanagi-Harada syndrome,
    240
Austin type: of leukodystrophy, 216
Australian antigen, 77

Autoimmune disorder
  congenital hypoparathyroidism as,
    172
  Vogt-Koyanagi-Harada syndrome as,
    239
Autoimmunity: and Addison's disease,
    174
Autonomic nervous system: in
    neurofibromatosis, 226
Avidin: and biotin deficiency, 199
Axillae: in alkaptonuria, 190
Azotemia: in angiokeratoma corporis
    diffusum, 296
Azure lunulae: in hepatolenticular
    degeneration, 190, 195

B

Back
  mast cells on, in mastocytosis, 346
  urticaria pigmentosa of, in
    mastocytosis, 346
Bacterial chrondritis: in Addison's
    disease, 176
Bantus: porphyria cutanea tarda of, 330
Bart syndrome, 265
Basal cell epithelioma, 242
Basal cell nevus syndrome, 242–243
  clinical manifestations, 242–243
  comedonal lesions in, 243
  diagnosis, 243
  endocrine findings in, 243
  neurologic abnormalities in, 243
  neurologic anomalies in, 242, 243
  ophthalmic anomalies in, 242, 243
  treatment, 243
Beau's lines, 50
  in hypoparathyroidism, 172
Bed rest: in lupus erythematosus, 128
Beer: home-brewed, and porphyria
    cutanea tarda, 330
Behcet syndrome, 57–60
  aphthous lesions of, 58
  clinical manifestations, 58–60
  diagnosis, 60
  etiology, 58
  treatment, 60
Bell's palsy: in Lyme disease, 73
Benzoyl peroxide: in necrobiosis
    lipoidica diabeticorum, 182

Berry aneurysms: of circle of Willis,
    elastosis perforans serpiginosa
    in, 113
Beta-carotene
  in erythropoietic porphyria, 328
  in erythropoietic protoporphyria, 329
Beta galactosidase deficiency: in GM_1
    gangliosidosis, 216
Beta-lipoproteins, 203
Biopsy
  cutaneous punch, in toxic epidermal
    necrolysis, 28
  liver, in erythropoietic
    protoporphyria, 328
  rectal, in familial Mediterranean
    fever, 276
  in rickettsial disease, 83
  of skin, in mastocytosis, diffuse
    cutaneous, 352–353
  in staphylococcal scalded skin
    syndrome, 68
Biotin-binding capacity, 199
Biotin deficiency, 198–203
  diagnosis, 199–200
  juvenile form, 199, 200
  in newborn, 199, 200
  treatment, 200
Biotin-deficient parenteral therapy,
    199
Biting: compulsive self-destructive, in
    Lesch-Nyhan syndrome, 198
"Black tongue:" in pellagra, 323
Bleeding (see Hemorrhage)
Blepharitis: in dyskeratosis congenita,
    271
Blindness: in sarcoidosis, 355
Blisters: in porphyria cutanea tarda,
    330
Bloch-Sulzberger syndrome (see
    Incontinentia pigmenti)
Block
  atrioventricular, congenital, 130
  heart, congenital, 128
Blood
  eosinophilia, 141
  fresh whole, in purpura fulminans,
    307
  transfusion (see Transfusion)
Bloodhound-like appearance: in cutis
    laxa, 108, 109

Bloom syndrome, 315–316
  clinical manifestations, 315–316
  diagnosis, 316
  as recessive disorder, 315
  treatment, 316
Blue nevi: in LAMB syndrome, 242
Blue rubber-bleb nevus syndrome, 291–292
Blue sclerae
  in Ehlers-Danlos syndrome, 100, 105
  in Marfan's syndrome, 105
  in osteogenesis imperfecta, 104, 105
  in pseudoxanthoma elasticum, 112
Body segment ratio: increase in upper to lower, in hypothyrodism, 160
Bone
  cysts in basal cell nevus syndrome, 243
  development defects in Rothmund-Thomson syndrome, 317
  disappearing, 293
  disease, lysosomal, and fucosidosis, 298
  fragility, in erythropoietic porphyria, 327
  hypertrophy in Klippel-Trenaunay-Parkes-Weber syndrome, 290
  imaging in screening for mastocytosis, 353
  involvement in urticaria pigmentosa, 351
  malformations in basal cell nevus syndrome, 242
  necrosis, ischemic, 124
  skull, in Cockayne syndrome, 319
  vanishing bone disease, 293
Bougienage
  in dyskeratosis congenita, 272
  in epidermolysis bullosa, 267
Brain calcification: sclerotic, in tuberous sclerosis, 232
Breast milk: and zinc, 251
Brockenheimer's syndrome, 300
Bruch's membrane, 111
Bruisability: excessive, in Kwashiorkor, 324
Buccal mucosae: in angiokeratoma corporis diffusum, 295
"Buffalo hump:" in Cushing's syndrome, 177

Bürger-Grütz disease (see Hyperlipoproteinemia, type I)
Butterfly rash: in lupus erythematosus, 120, 124
"Buttonholing:" in neurofibroma, 224
Bypass: intestine, causing acrodermatitis enteropathica, 251

C

Café au lait spots
  in ataxia telangiectasia, 304
  in basal cell nevus syndrome, 243
  in Bloom syndrome, 315
  in epidermal nevus syndrome, 244
  in neurofibromatosis, 220, 221–223
    freckle-like, 223
  in sclerosis, tuberous, 227, 229
Calcification
  in Addison's disease, 176
  of arteries, 170
  of brain, in tuberous sclerosis, 232
  fat, subcutaneous, 170
  intracranial, in Cockayne syndrome, 318
  leg, in alkaptonuria, 194
  muscle, 170
  in scleroderma, 138
  in sclerosis, systemic, 137
  skin, 170
    metastatic, 170
  in Sturge-Weber syndrome, 289
Calcinosis
  in Addison's disease, 176
  in dermatomyositis, 134
  in scleroderma, systemic, 139
  skin, and dermatomyositis, 132
Calcitonin
  in hyperparathyroidism, 171
  in hyperthyroidism, 169
  in osteogenesis imperfecta, 106
Calcium
  deposits, ectopic, in basal cell nevus syndrome, 243
  extrusion in hyperparathyroidism, 170
Cancer
  in ataxia telangiectasia, high incidence, 304

Cancer (*cont.*)
   dermatomyositis and, 132, 133
   dyskeratosis congenita and, 270
   lymphoreticular, in ataxia
      telangiectasia, 303, 305
   in Peutz-Jeghers syndrome, 268
   skin
      in epidermolysis bullosa, 271
      in dyskeratosis congenita, 271
      in xeroderma pigmentosum, 314
   Sweet's syndrome and, 40
   thyroid, in hyperthyroidism, 163
Candida albicans: in acrodermatitis
      enteropathica, 252
Candidiasis
   chronic mucocutaneous, 87
      treatment, 88
   hypoparathyroidism and, 172
   mucocutaneous, in
      hypoparathyroidism, 172
   oral, in hypoparathyroidism, 173
Candidiasis, systemic, 85–88
   diagnosis, 86
   treatment, 86–88
Carcinoma
   with degeneration in Gardner's
      syndrome, 275
   epidermoid, in dyskeratosis
      congenita, 271
   epidermolysis bullosa and, 267
   nevoid basal cell carcinoma
      syndrome (*see* Basal cell nevus
      syndrome)
   in Peutz-Jeghers syndrome, 269
   Sweet's syndrome and, 41
   thyroid carcinoma syndrome,
      medullary, 166
   thyroid, medullary, 167
   in hyperthyroidism, 169
Cardiomyopathy: and dermatomyositis,
      136
Carditis: in Kawasaki disease, 47
Carotenemia: and hypopituitarism, 180
Carpal tunnel syndrome, 141
Cartilage: pigmentary changes in
      alkaptonuria, 193
Casal's necklace: in pellagra, 322
CAT scan: in tuberous sclerosis, 232
Cat scratch fever: in erythema
      nodosum, 18

Cataracts
   in angiokeratoma corporis diffusum,
      296
   in basal cell nevus syndrome, 243
   in Cockayne syndrome, 318, 319
   juvenile, in Rothmund-Thomson
      syndrome, 317
   in Rothmund-Thomson syndrome,
      317
"C" cells, 167
Celiac
   disease, 251, 254
   sprue, 254
Cell(s)
   basal (*see* Basal cell)
   "C," 167
   "gargoyle," in Hurler syndrome, 212
   giant (*see* Giant cell)
   mast (*see* Mast cell)
   -mediated immunity, and candidiasis,
      172
   mulberry, in angiokeratoma corporis
      diffusum, 296
   mycosis, 358
   Schwann, 223
Cellulitis-like lesions: in familial
      Mediterranean fever, 276
Central nervous system
   degeneration in hepatolenticular
      degeneration, 195
   dysfunction in hypomelanosis of Ito,
      237
   in epidermal nevus syndrome, 244
   in fucosidosis, 298
   in Henoch-Schönlein purpura, 38
   in incontinentia pigmenti, 236
   in Kawasaki disease, 51, 52
   in nevus unius lateris, 245
   in sclerosis, tuberous, 231
   involvement
      in Behcet's syndrome, 59
      in sarcoidosis, 355
Ceramidetrihexoside, 294, 295
Cerebellar ataxia
   in ataxia telangiectasia, 303
   in Hartnup disease, 320
Cerebral
   cortex in Sturge-Weber syndrome,
      287
   manifestations of Lesch-Nyhan

syndrome, 198
palsy, spastic, in Lesch-Nyhan
    syndrome, 198
Cerebrovascular accidents
in angiokeratoma corporis diffusum,
    296
in homocystinuria, 190, 192
livedo reticularis and, 299
susceptibility to, in angiokeratoma
    corporis diffusum, 296
Ceruloplasmin: and copper increase,
    195
C_1-esterase inhibitor, 9
"Charlie Chaplin-like" gait: in
    homocystinuria, 190, 192
Cheeks
angiofibroma on, 229
in Cushing's syndrome, 177
in dermatomyositis, 132
puffiness in hypothyroidism, 160
sagging, in cutis laxa, 109
telangiectasia on, in Bloom
    syndrome, 316
Cheilitis: angular, in pellagra, 323
Chelating agents: in hepatolenticular
    degeneration, 195
Chemotaxis defect: in acrodermatitis
    enteropathica, 252
Chemotherapy: systemic, in mycosis
    fungoides, 360
Cherry red spot-myoclonus syndrome,
    215
Chest
in ataxia telangiectasia, 303
deformities in homocystinuria, 192
in Letterer-Siwe disease, in
    newborn, 339
nevus unius lateris of, in boy, 245
Chickenpox: in purpura fulminans, 306
Chilblains, 123
Chloramphenicol: in Q fever, 83
Chloroquine, 6
bluish pigmentation after, 194
in porphyria
    cutanea tarda, 331
    variegata, 332
Cholecystitis, 38
in erythropoietic protoporphyria, 328
Cholelithiasis: in erythropoietic
    protoporphyria, 328

Cholesterol
in hyperlipoproteinemia, type II, 207
in hypothyroidism, 161
metabolism derangement in type II
    hyperlipoproteinemia, 207
Cholinergic urticaria, 4
treatment, 5
Chondritis: bacterial, in Addison's
    disease, 176
Chondrosarcoma: in Maffucci's
    syndrome, 291
Choreoathetosis
in ataxia telangiectasia, 304
in Lesch-Nyhan syndrome, 198
Chromatography: amino acid, in
    homocystinuria, 193
Churg-Strauss syndrome, 42, 44
etiology, 44
respiratory symptoms, 44
skin lesions of, 44
Chylomicrons
in hyperlipoproteinemia, type I, 206
lipoprotein, 203
Cimetidine, 4
in mastocytosis, 353
Cirrhosis
alcoholic, and porphyria cutanea
    tarda, 330
in hepatolenticular degeneration, 195
Claw hand: in Hurler syndrome, 211,
    213
Clinodactyly: in Bloom syndrome, 315
Clothing: staining of, in alkaptonuria,
    190, 194
Clotrimazole: in candidiasis, systemic,
    86
Coagulation, disseminated intravascular
    (*See also* Purpura, fulminans)
in Kasabach-Merritt syndrome, 287
in rickettsial disease, 85
in toxic shock syndrome, 69
Coagulopathy: consumptive, 306
Cobb syndrome, 294
Coccidioidomycosis: in erythema
    nodosum, 18
Cockayne syndrome, 318–319
clinical manifestations, 318–319
diagnosis, 319
    prenatal, 319
quick bird-like movements in, 318

Cockayne syndrome *(cont.)*
  treatment, 319
Coffee-colored skin: in Kwashiorkor,
    324
Colchicine
  in Behcet's syndrome, 60
  in Mediterranean fever, familial, 275,
    277
Cold
  intolerance to, in hypothyroidism,
    158, 160
  livedo reticularis and, 299
  urticaria, 4, 6–7
Colitis: ulcerative, in erythema
    nodosum, 18
Collagen
  disorders, 96–108
  in epidermolysis bullosa, recessive
    dystrophic, 262
  type I, synthesis abnormality, 104
  vascular disorders, 119–156
Collagenase: in recessive dystrophic
    epidermolysis bullosa, 262
Colon: transplant in epidermolysis
    bullosa, 267
Complement
  first component, 9
  fixation test, 82
    in Q fever, 82
    in rickettsial disease, 83
  immunofluorescence and dermatitis
    herpetiformis, 255
Computed tomography: in tuberous
    sclerosis, 232
Conjunctiva
  in ataxia telangiectasia, 303
  hyperemia in toxic shock syndrome,
    69
  in Kawasaki disease, 47, 48
  neuroma of, 168
  vessels of, tortuosity in
    angiokeratoma corporis
    diffusum, 296
Conjunctivitis
  in dyskeratosis congenita, 271
  in porphyria, erythropoietic, 325–327
  in xeroderma pigmentosum, 314
Connective tissue
  disease, 96–118
  disease, mixed, 138, 145, 148–151

clinical manifestations, 149–150
diagnosis, 150
differences between adult and
  childhood forms, 150
mucosal dryness in, 149
overlapping features with other
  diseases, 150
prognosis, 150, 151
treatment, 151
disease, undifferentiated, maternal,
  neonatal lupus erythematosus
  after, 128
Contractures
  in alkaptonuria, 190
  of joints in Cockayne syndrome, 319
Convulsions: in tuberous sclerosis, 231
Copper
  excessive tissue accumulation, in
    hepatolenticular degeneration,
    195
  increase, and ceruloplasmin, 195
  in Menkes' kinky hair syndrome, 196
  storage disease in Menkes' kinky hair
    syndrome, 196
Cornea
  arcus, 208
  clouding
    in GM_1 gangliosidosis, 216
    in Hurler syndrome, 211
    in mucolipidosis III, 216
  opacities
    in angiokeratoma corporis
      diffusum, 295, 296
    in xeroderma pigmentosum, 314
Coronary
  angiography, abnormalities in
    Kawasaki disease, 51
  arteritis, 57
  artery disease, in angiokeratoma
    corporis diffusum, 296
  atherosclerosis and tendinous
    xanthoma, 206
  occlusion in homocystinuria,
    192–193
  thrombosis, and Kawasaki disease, 47
Corticosteroids
  (See also Steroids)
  in dermatomyositis, 136
  in granuloma annulare, 185
  in Henoch-Schönlein purpura, 39

in Kasabach-Merritt syndrome, 287
in lupus erythematosus, 128
  complications of, 128
in periarteritis nodosa, adult, 57
in rheumatoid arthritis, juvenile, 146
in sarcoidosis, 357
in scleroderma, 140
systemic
  in Behcet's syndrome, 60
  in Churg-Strauss syndrome, 44
  in Cushing's syndrome, 177
  in fasciitis, eosinophilic, 141, 142
  in hemangioma, cavernous, 286
  in hemangiomatosis, diffuse
    neonatal, 293
  Sjögren's syndrome, 148
  in Stevens-Johnson syndrome, 26
  in Sweet's syndrome, 41
  Wegener's granulomatosis and, 43
topical, in lupus erythematosus, 127
Counseling (*see* Genetic counseling)
Covermark; in Sturge-Weber
    syndrome, 289
Coxiella burnetti, 82
"Cretinism," 158
Crithiden luciliae immunofluorescent
    technique, 126
Cromolyn sodium: in mastocytosis, 353
Crowe's sign: in neurofibromatosis,
    221, 223
CRST syndrome, 139
Cryoglobulinemia, 7
  livedo reticularis in, 122, 299
Cryptorchidism: in Bloom syndrome,
    315
Curettage: for bone lesions in
    eosinophilic granuloma, 341
Cushingoid syndrome, 176
Cushing's disease, 176
Cushing's syndrome, 176–178
  adrenogenital syndrome and, 178
  clinical manifestations, 176–177
  diagnosis, 177
  endogenous, 176
  exogenous, 176
  striae in, 177
  treatment, 178
Cutaneous (*see* Skin)
Cuticular
  erythema in dermatomyositis, 133

telangiectasia (*see* Telangiectasia,
    cuticular)
Cutis
  aplasia cutis congenita, 301
  hyperelastica (*see* Ehlers-Danlos
    syndrome)
  laxa, 108–110
    bloodhound-like appearance in,
      108, 109
    clinical manifestations, 108–110
    diagnosis, 110
    elastosis perforans serpiginosa in,
      113
    pathogenesis, 108
    treatment, 110
  marmorata, livid mottling of skin in,
    299
  marmorata telangiectatica congenita,
    299–301
    etiology, 300
    in Riley-Smith syndrome, 293
  rhomboidalis frontalis, and porphyria
    variegata, 332
  verticis gyrata in hyperpituitarism,
    180
Cyanide nitroprusside test: in
    homocystinuria, 190, 193
Cyclophosphamide: in Wegener's
    granulomatosis, 43
Cyproheptadine, 7
  in mastocytosis, 353
Cyst
  bone, in basal cell nevus syndrome,
    243
  epidermal
    in Gardner's syndrome, 274
    of limbs, in basal cell nevus
      syndrome, 243
  jaw, odontogenic, in basal cell nevus
    syndrome, 242
  in sclerosis, tuberous, 232
Cystathionine synthetase
  absence or deficiency in
    homocystinuria, 192
  defect in homocystinuria, 190
Cytotoxic agents
  in Churg-Strauss syndrome, 44
  in dermatomyositis, 136
  in Henoch-Schönlein purpura, 39
  Wegner's granulomatosis and, 43

D

Dapsone
  in dermatitis herpetiformis, 255, 256
  in pyoderma gangrenosum, 273
  side effects of, 256
Darier's sign
  in mastocytosis, 348
    solitary, 349
  in urticaria pigmentosa, 349
Deafness
  in Alezzandrini syndrome, 240
  in Cockayne syndrome, 318, 319
  in multiple lentigines syndrome, 240
  neural, congenital, in Waardenburg
    syndrome, 239
  in neurofibromatosis, 225
  in Vogt-Koyanagi-Harada syndrome,
    239
Dejection: in Kwashiorkor, 324
Dementia: in pellagra, 321
Dental
  (See also Teeth)
  anomalies
    in hypomelanosis of Ito, 238
    in incontinentia pigmenti, 236
  defects
    in Bloom syndrome, 315
    in dyskeratosis congenita, 271
    in Rothmund-Thomson syndrome,
      317–318
  enamel in epidermolysis bullosa,
    junctional, 260
  hygiene in epidermolysis bullosa, 268
  malformations in epidermolysis
    bullosa, recessive dystrophic,
    261
  manifestations of incontinentia
    pigmenti, 234
Dentition
  defective in hypothyroidism, 158
  delayed in hypothyroidism, 158
Deoxyribonucleic acid (see DNA)
Depigmentation
  in epidermolysis bullosa, dominant
    dystrophic, 263
  of hair in Kwashiorkor, 324
  in xeroderma pigmentosum, 314
Dermabrasion: and dominant
    dystrophic epidermolysis
    bullosa, 263

Dermacenter
  andersonii, 83
  variabilis, 83
Dermal deposition: of pigment in
    alkaptonuria, 193
Dermal-epidermal junction: and
    dermatitis herpetiformis, 255
Dermal hypoplasia (see Focal dermal
    hypoplasia)
Dermatitis
  atopic, in hyperthyroidism, 164
  in biotin deficiency, 199
  eczematoid, in phenylketonuria, 189,
    190
  exfoliative, in hypoparathyroidism,
    172
  herpetiformis, 253–257
    cause of, 254
    clinical manifestations, 254–255
    diagnosis, 255
    treatment, 255–257
  infectious eczematoid, in chronic
    granulomatous disease of
    childhood, 89
  in pellagra, 321
  periorificial, in biotin deficiency, 200
  scaly, in biotin deficiency, 199
Dermatomyositis, 131–136, 138
  cheeks in, 132
  clinical manifestations, 132–135
  contrasted with mixed connective
    tissue disease, 148–149
  course, 135
    different in children than in adults,
      133
  diagnosis, 135
    criteria for, 135
  etiology, 131–132
  eyelids in, 132
  genetic predisposition, 132
  interphalangeal joints in, 133
  mucous membranes in, 134
  shoulder in, 133
  Sjögren's syndrome and, 146
  in telangiectasia, cuticular, 123
  treatment, 135–136
Dermatosis
  bullous, in diabetes, 183, 184
  febrile neutrophilic (see Sweet's
    syndrome)
Dermis: fibroma in neurofibroma, 223

Dermographism, 4
in urticaria pigmentosa, 349
Dermopathy, diabetic, 182–183
diagnosis, 183
pathogenesis, 183
treatment, 183
DeSanctis-Cacchione syndrome, 313
Desquamation: in Kwashiorkor, 324
deToni-Fanconi syndrome: and tyrosine
metabolism disorders, 201
Development retardation: in
homocystinuria, 192
Dexamethasone suppression test: in
adrenogenital syndrome, 179
Dextran: in purpura fulminans, 307
Diabetes insipidus
eosinophilic granuloma and, 341
vasopressin for, 341
in Hand-Schüller-Christian disease,
339
in xanthoma disseminatum, 342, 343
Diabetes mellitus
in Addison's disease, 176
in Cushing's syndrome, 177
dermatosis in, bullous, 183, 184
dermopathy of (see Dermopathy,
diabetic)
disorders associated with, 181–185
granuloma annulare in, 183–185
in Hand-Schüller-Christian disease,
340
latent, 184
porphyria cutanea tarda and, 330
xanthoma and, 205
Diaper
crystals resembling sand in, in
Lesch-Nyhan syndrome, 197
orange uric acid crystals in, in Lesch-
Nyhan syndrome, 198
urine-moistened, dark brown stains
on, in alkaptonuria, 193
Diarrhea
in acrodermatitis enteropathica, 251
in Kawasaki disease, 47
in pellagra, 321
Diascopy, 356
Diatheses: hemorrhagic, in urticaria
pigmentosa, 351
Diet
fat-free, in familial Mediterranean
fever, 275, 277

gluten-free, in dermatitis
herpetiformis, 254, 255, 256
low fat, in hyperlipoproteinemia,
type I, 207
zinc deficient, and acrodermatitis
enteropathica, 251
DiGeorge syndrome
hypothyroidism and, 172, 173
thymic transplant in, 174
Diiodohydroxyquin: in acrodermatitis
enteropathica, 253
Dilantin: in epidermolysis bullosa, 267
Diphenylhydantoin
in angiokeratoma corporis diffusum,
296
in epidermolysis bullosa, 267
Disodium cromoglycate: in
mastocytosis, 353
Diuretics: in hypercalcemia, 171
DL-alpha tocopherol: in epidermolysis
bullosa, 266
DNA
cross-links defect, and dyskeratosis
congenita, 272
photosensitivity as a decrease in
ability to repair, 312
tests for excision repair of in
fibroblasts, in xeroderma
pigmentosum, 313
Down's syndrome: elastosis perforans
serpiginosa in, 113
Drooling: in acrodermatitis
enteropathica, 252
Drug(s)
antithyroid (see Antithyroid
medications)
hypersensitivity to, 3, 26
reactions in erythema nodosum, 18
Duhring's disease (see Dermatitis,
herpetiformis)
Dwarfism: in Cockayne syndrome,
318
Dysacousia: in Vogt-Koyanagi-Harada
syndrome, 239
Dyschondroplasia: with hemangiomata,
291
Dyschromia: in Kwashiorkor, 324
Dysgenesis of thyroid, 157
hypothyroidism due to, 158
Dysgerminoma: ovarian, in ataxia
telangiectasia, 305

Dyskeratosis congenita, 270–272
  clinical manifestations, 270–272
  diagnosis, 272
  histopathology in, 272
  infection in, 272
  treatment, 272
Dysostosis multiplex
  GM$_1$ gangliosidosis and, 216
  in mucolipidosis II, 215
Dysphagia, 139
  in epidermolysis bullosa, recessive
    dystrophic, 267
Dysplasia: polyostotic fibrous, with
    sexual precocity, in girls, 223
Dystopia canthorum
  in basal cell nevus syndrome, 243
  in Waardenburg syndrome, 239
Dystrophic Epidermolysis Bullosa
    Research Association, 268
Dystrophy
  in epidermolysis bullosa (see under
    Epidermolysis bullosa)
  nail
    in acrodermatitis enteropathica,
      250
    in candidiasis, 87
    in dyskeratosis congenita, 270, 272
    in epidermolysis bullosa,
      generalized atrophic, 260
    in incontinentia pigmenti, 236

E

Ears
  in Addison's disease, 176
  "alabaster"-like, in hypothyroidism,
    158
  in alkaptonuria, 190, 194
  in ataxia telangiectasia, 303
  large, in Cockayne syndrome, 319
  protruding, with "Mickey Mouse"-
    like appearance in Cockayne
    syndrome, 318
  of werewolves, 327
EB (see Epidermolysis bullosa)
Ecchymoses
  in Cushing's syndrome, 177
  in hypothyroidism, 162
Echocardiography: in Kawasaki disease,
    53

Ectasias: in Klippel-Trenaunay-Parkes-
    Weber syndrome, 290
Ectodermal defects: in
    hypoparathyroidism, 172
Ectopia lentis: in homocystinuria, 190,
    192, 193
Ectropion
  in dyskeratosis congenita, 271
  in xeroderma pigmentosum, 314
Edema
  in angiokeratoma corporis diffusum,
    296
  angioneurotic (see Angioneurotic
    edema)
  in dermatomyositis, 132
  of eyelid in infectious mononucleosis,
    79
  in Kwashiorkor, 324
  of palms in toxic shock syndrome, 70
  periorbital, in dermatomyositis, 134
  Quincke's, 2
  in rickettsial disease, 83
  subcutaneous, in toxic shock
    syndrome, 69
Ehlers-Danlos syndrome, 96–101
  arthrochalasis type, 100
  benign familial hypermobile type, 98
  blue sclerae in, 105
  clinical manifestations, 96–98
  contrasted with cutis laxa, 110
  diagnosis, 100
  fibronectin type, 100
  gravis type, 98
  maternal, 100
  mitis form, 98
  ocular type, 100
  periodontal type, 100
  Sack type, 99
  treatment, 100–101
  type I, 98
  type II, 98
  type III, 98
  type IV, 99
    elastosis perforans serpiginosa in,
      113
  type V, 99
  type VI, 100
  type VII, 100
  type VIII, 100
  type IX, 100
  type X, 100

Elastin disorders, 108–115
Elastolysis, generalized (*see* Cutis, laxa)
Elastosis perforans serpiginosa, 99, 107,
    113–115
  clinical manifestations, 113–114
  diagnosis, 114–115
  penicillamine and, 195
  penicillamine-induced, 114
  treatment, 115
Electrocardiography
  abnormalities in Kawasaki disease, 51
  conduction defects in multiple
    lentigines syndrome, 240
Electroencephalography: in Sturge-
    Weber syndrome, 288
Electron beam: in mycosis fungoides,
    360
Electron microscopy
  in epidermolysis bullosa
    recessive dystrophic, 261
    simplex, 257
  in incontinentia pigmenti, 235
  in sclerosis, tuberous, 231
Emotional lability: in Hartnup disease,
    320
Enamel: dental, in junctional
    epidermolysis bullosa, 260
Encephalofacial angiomatosis (*see*
    Sturge-Weber syndrome)
Encephalotrigeminal angiomatosis (*see*
    Sturge-Weber syndrome)
Endocrine
  adenomatosis (*see* Multiple endocrine
    adenomatosis syndrome)
  disorders, 157–188
    in multiple lentigines syndrome,
      241
    in neurofibromatosis, 226
  features, of basal cell nevus
    syndrome, 242
  neoplasia (*see* Multiple endocrine
    neoplasia)
Endocrinopathy: and chronic
    mucocutaneous candidiasis, 87
Endonuclease, 312
Endotoxin: in toxic shock syndrome, 68
Enteritis: regional, and acrodermatitis
    enteropathica, 251
Enteropathy, gluten-sensitive, 254
  celiac type, 254
    immunologic process of dermatitis

herpetiformis related to, 255
Enterotoxin E: in toxic shock
    syndrome, 68
Enzymatic defect: in hypothyroidism,
    157
Enzyme
  angiotensin-converting, levels in
    sarcoidosis, 354
  temperature-sensitive cytolytic, in
    epidermolysis bullosa simplex,
    257–259
Eosinophilia, 142
  blood, 141
  in fasciitis, eosinophilic, 140–141
  in incontinentia pigmenti, 234
Eosinophilic
  fasciitis (*see* Fasciitis, eosinophilic)
  granuloma (*see* Granuloma,
    eosinophilic)
EP (*see* Porphyria, erythropoietic)
Ephelides: in NAME syndrome, 242
Epidermal nevus syndrome, 244–245
  bilateral nevi in, 244
  diagnosis, 244–245
  histopathologic features, 244
  treatment, 245
Epidermis
  cysts of limbs in basal cell nevus
    syndrome, 243
  necrolysis (*see* Toxic epidermal
    necrolysis)
  normal, in neurofibromatosis, 222
Epidermolysis bullosa, 257–268
  acquired, 265–266
    diagnosis of, 265–267
  acquisita (*see* acquired *above*)
  benign, 260
  dermolytic (*see* dystrophic *below*)
  Dowling-Meara, 259–260
  dystrophic, 257, 260–264
    differentiating dominant from
      recessive forms, 262
    dominant, 262–264
    dominant, albopapuloid form, 263,
      264
    dominant, milia in, 263
    recessive, 260–262
    recessive, pathogenesis, 262
    recessive, prenatal diagnosis, 262
    recessive, secondary infection in,
      261

Epidermolysis bullosa *(cont.)*
  generalized atrophic, 260
  hereditary, classification of, 258
  Herlitz variant, 260
  herpetiformis, 259–260
  junctional, 257, 260
  nondystrophic *(see* simplex *below)*
  nursing care in, 268
  prevalence, 257
  simplex, 257–259
    blisters after trauma, 259
    generalized, 257–259
    localized, 259
    localized, pathophysiology of, 259
    Ogna variant, 260
  treatment, 266–268
  Weber-Cockayne, 259
Epilepsy: in tuberous sclerosis, 232
Epinephrine, 4
Epiphyses: femoral, in hypothyroidism, 158
Epistaxis
  in angiokeratoma corporis diffusum, 295
  in telangiectasia, hereditary
      hemorrhagic, 301
    recurrent epistaxis, 302
Epithelioma: basal cell, 242
EPP *(see* Protoporphyria,
      erythropoietic)
Epstein-Barr virus, 78
Errors: of metabolism, 189–219
Erysipelas-like lesions: in familial
      Mediterranean fever, 276, 277
Erythema
  annular, 11–17
  annulare centrifugum, 11, 16–17
    diagnosis, 17
    differentiated from erythema
        chronicum migrans, 15
    etiology, 16
    treatment, 17
  in Bloom syndrome, 315, 316
  bulbar, in toxic shock syndrome, 70
  chronicum migrans, 11, 14–15, 73
    in Lyme disease, 72
    with tick bite, 72
  contusiformis, 19
  cuticular, in dermatomyositis, 133
  of face, in lupus erythematosus,
      neonatal, 129

  of forehead, in lupus erythematosus,
      neonatal, 130
  heliotrope, in dermatomyositis, 132,
      134
  of interphalangeal joints in
      dermatomyositis, 133
  marginatum, 11, 12–14
  in mixed connective tissue disease,
      149
  multiforme, 2, 19–23
    bullous *(see* Stevens-Johnson
        syndrome)
    classification, 21
    clinical manifestations, 20–23
    contrasted with Henoch-Schönlein
        purpura, 36
    generalized loss of epidermis in,
        20
    herpes simplex as etiologic factor
        in, 23
    major *(see* Stevens-Johnson
        disease)
    minor, 20
    pathogenesis, 20
  nodosum, 17–19
    clinical manifestations, 18–19
    diagnosis, 19
    etiologic causes, 17
    in sarcoidosis, 356
    treatment, 19
  of palms and fingers in lupus
      erythematosus, 123
  periungual, in mixed connective
      tissue disease, 149
  rash in Kawasaki disease, 47
  of scalp in neonatal lupus
      erythematosus, 130
  telangiectatic, congenital *(see* Bloom
      syndrome)
  in xeroderma pigmentosum, 312, 313
Erythematous blotches: in
      homocystinuria, 192
Erythrocyte fluorescence: in
      erythropoietic protoporphyria,
      329
Erythroderma: in mycosis fungoides,
      358
Erythrodermic *(see* Mastocytosis,
      erythrodermic)
Erythrophagocytosis: in malignant
      histiocytosis, 343

Esophagus
dysfunction, and scleroderma, 139
motility disturbances in mixed
connective tissue disease, 149
webs and strictures in epidermolysis
bullosa, 261
Estrogen therapy: precipitating
porphyria cutanea tarda, 330
Ethacrynic acid: in hypercalcemia, 171
Exanthem
in infectious mononucleosis, 79
in Kawasaki disease, 48–49
Exfoliation, 65
Exophthalmos
in Hand-Schüller-Christian disease,
339, 340
hyperthyroidism and, 163, 165
Exotoxin: in toxic shock syndrome, 68
Extremities
bowed, in homocystinuria, 192
epidermal cysts of, in basal cell
nevus syndrome, 243
erythematous blotches, in
homocystinuria, 192
hypertrophy in Klippel-Trenaunay-
Parkes-Weber syndrome, 290
in Kawasaki disease, 49–50
long, disproportionately, in Cockayne
syndrome, 318
long slender, in multiple mucosal
neuroma syndrome, 168
lower
calcifications, subcutaneous, in
alkaptonuria, 194
in cutis marmorata telangiectatica
congenita, 301
in epidermolysis bullosa, dominant
dystrophic, 263
erythematous scaly eruptions in
pellagra, 322
in Henoch-Schönlein purpura, 37
hyperpigmentation in
hepatolenticular degeneration,
190
purpura fulminans with Rocky
Mountain spotted fever, 306
in sclerosis, tuberous, 230
upper, in incontinentia pigmenti, 234
Eye
abnormality
in Hartnup disease, 320

in tyrosinemia II, 202
anomalies in epidermal nevus
syndrome, 244
in ataxia telangiectasia, 303
changes in pseudoxanthoma
elasticum, 111
disturbances in hypomelanosis of Ito,
237
hypertelorism in multiple lentigines
syndrome, 240
in incontinentia pigmenti, 236
lens (see Lens)
lesions in Behcet's syndrome, 59
manifestations of incontinentia
pigmenti, 234
puffiness in hypothyroidism, 160
in sarcoidosis, 355
in Sjögren's syndrome, 147
tumors in juvenile xanthogranuloma,
344
Eyebrows
confluent, in Waardenburg
syndrome, 239
sparse in hypoparathyroidism, 172
tangled, in Menkes' kinky hair
syndrome, 196
Eyelids
in ataxia telangiectasia, 303
cavernous hemangioma of, 285
complication rate of, 286
in dermatomyositis, 132
edema
in hyperpituitarism, 180
in infectious mononucleosis, 79
heliotrope rash, in mixed connective
tissue disease, 149
neuroma of, 168
strawberry hemangioma of, 284
of werewolves, 327

F

Fabry syndrome (see Angiokeratoma,
corporis diffusum)
Face
coarse
in Hunter syndrome, 212
in Menkes' kinky hair syndrome,
197
erythema
in Bloom syndrome, 315, 316

Face (*cont.*)
  in butterfly distribution in
    Cockayne syndrome, 319
  in lupus erythematosus, neonatal,
    129
  erythematous eruptions in pellagra,
    322
  flushing in hyperthyroidism, 164
  in Gionotti-Crosti syndrome, 77
  in Letterer-Siwe disease, in
    newborn, 339
  in lupus erythematosus, 120, 121
    neonatal, 130
  milia on, in basal cell nevus
    syndrome, 243
  pallid in Menkes' kinky hair
    syndrome, 196
  papillomatous lesions in xeroderma
    pigmentosum, 314
  in scleroderma, 139
  skin, widepored, 192
  tumor in mycosis fungoides, 359
  verrucous lesions in xeroderma
    pigmentosum, 314
Facies
  "bird-like," 319
    in Cockayne syndrome, 318
  coarse
    in fucosidosis, 298
    in Menkes' kinky hair syndrome,
      196
  in cutis laxa, 109
  dull expressionless, in
    hypothyroidism, 160, 162
  "moon," in Cushing's syndrome, 176,
    177
  puffy myxedematous, in
    hypothyroidism, 158
  in Rothmund-Thomson syndrome,
    317
  in sclerosis, systemic, 137
  widepored, in homocystinuria, 190
Factor: Hageman, 9
Failure to thrive: and acrodermatitis
    enteropathica, 251
Fanconi's anemia: in dyskeratosis
    congenita, 271
Fasciitis: diffuse, 141
Fasciitis, eosinophilic, 140–142
  clinical manifestations, 141

  cobblestone appearance in, 141
  diagnosis, 141–142
  etiology, 141
  histopathologic examination in, 142
  male preponderance in, 141
  pathogenesis, 141
  treatment, 142
Fat
  -free diet in familial Mediterranean
    fever, 275, 277
  subcutaneous
    calcification, 170
    loss in Cockayne syndrome, 319
Fatigue: in lupus erythematosus, 127
Febrile neutrophilic dermatosis (*see*
    Sweet's syndrome)
Feet
  in diabetes, 184
  eruptions in epidermolysis bullosa,
    259
  hemangiomatosis of, diffuse neonatal,
    292
  in Kawasaki disease, 47, 50
  large, in Cockayne syndrome, 318,
    319
  in Mediterranean fever, familial, 277
  puffy, in hypothyroidism, 162
  in purpura fulminans with Rocky
    Mountain spotted fever, 306
  "rocker-bottom"
    in homocystinuria, 190
    in phenylketonuria, 192
Femur: epiphyses in hypothyroidism,
    158
Ferric chloride test: in
    phenylketonuria, 190, 191
Ferric ferricyanide reduction: in
    alkaptonuria, 190
Ferrochelatase deficiency: in
    erythropoietic protoporphyria,
    328
Fetus: protein for, 304
Fever
  cat scratch, in erythema nodosum, 18
  in Kawasaki disease, 47
  in Letterer-Siwe disease, 337
  low-grade, in sarcoidosis, 355
  Mediterranean (*see* Mediterranean
    fever)
  Q, 81, 82–83

rheumatic (*see* Rheumatic fever)
Rocky Mountain spotted (*see* Rocky
  Mountain spotted fever)
scarlet, staphylococcal, 68
typhus (*see* Typhus fever)
uveoparotid, in sarcoidosis, 355
Fibroma
  angiofibroma (*see* Angiofibroma)
  in basal cell nevus syndrome, 243
  dermal, in neurofibroma, 223
  gingival, and tuberous sclerosis, 227,
    228
  periungual, and tuberous sclerosis,
    227, 228
  sclerosis and, tuberous, 228
  subungual, and tuberous sclerosis,
    228
Fibrosis: in Addison's disease, 176
Finger(s)
  clubbing, drumstick-like, in
    hyperthyroidism, 165
  in Hunter syndrome, 212
  hyperextensibility in Ehlers-Danlos
    syndrome, 98
  in Kawasaki disease, 51
  in lupus erythematosus, 123
  mitten-like deformities in
    epidermolysis bullosa, recessive
    dystrophic, 261
  in mixed connective tissue disease,
    149
  spindling in juvenile rheumatoid
    arthritis, 142, 145
Fingernails
  in alkaptonuria, 194
  loss in erythropoietic porphyria,
    327
Fingertip
  blistering in epidermolysis bullosa,
    junctional, 260
  erosions of, in tyrosinemia II, 202
  in Kawasaki disease, 47
  ulcer, in dermatomyositis, 134
Fistula: pulmonary arteriovenous, in
    hemorrhagic telangiectasia, 302
Flea
  -borne typhus fever, 81–82
  rat, 82
Floppy mitral valve syndrome, 98, 100,
  106

Flucytosine: in candidiasis, systemic,
  86
Fluorescence
  of erythrocytes in erythropoietic
    protoporphyria, 329
  of urine in porphyria cutanea tarda,
    331
Focal dermal hypoplasia, 103–104
  clinical manifestation, 103–104
  diagnosis, 104
    differential, 104
  "lobster-claw" deformities in, 103
  treatment, 104
Foods: hypersensitivity to, 3
Foot (*see* Feet)
Fordyce angiokeratoma, 294
Forehead
  furrowing in porphyria variegata, 332
  in lupus erythematosus, neonatal,
    130
Forelock: white, in Waardenburg
    syndrome, 239
Freckle
  -like café au lait spots in
    neurofibromatosis, 223
  white, in tuberous sclerosis, 231
Freckling
  axillary, in neurofibromatosis, 221,
    223, 226
  in xeroderma pigmentosum, 312–313
Frontal bossing: in basal cell nevus
    syndrome, 243
Frostbite: in Addison's disease, 176
Fucosidosis, 294, 297–299
  clinical features, 297–298
  diagnosis, 298–299
  treatment, 299
  type III, 298
  variants of, 298
Fumarylacetoacetate (FAA) hydrolase
    deficiency: in tyrosinemia I, 201
Fungal infection
  in Cushing's syndrome, 177
  in erythema nodosum, 18
Furosemide: in hypercalcemia, 171

G

Gait
  "Charlie Chaplin-like," in

Gait (*cont.*)
  homocystinuria, 190, 192
  unsteady in Hartnup disease, 320
Gallbladder hydrops: in Kawasaki
    disease, 53
Gamma globulin: 7S, in
    hyperthyroidism, 164
Ganglioneuromatosis: intestinal, in
    multiple endocrine adenomatosis
    syndromes, 167
Gangliosidosis (*see* GM$_1$ gangliosidosis)
Gardner's syndrome, 274–275
  clinical manifestations, 274–275
  diagnosis, 275
  treatment, 275
"Gargoyle cells:" in Hunter syndrome,
    212
Gastroesophageal reflux, 139
Gastrointestinal
  complaints in Behcet's syndrome, 59
  disturbances in scleroderma, 139
  hemorrhage (*see* Hemorrhage,
    gastrointestinal)
  infection in Bloom syndrome, 316
  involvement
    in mastocytosis, 352
    in toxic shock syndrome, 69
  polyposis in Peutz-Jeghers syndrome,
    268
  polyps in Peutz-Jeghers syndrome,
    269
  survey in screening for mastocytosis,
    353
  tract
    angioma in blue rubber-bleb nevus
      syndrome, 291
    in neurofibromatosis, 226
    skin and, 250–282
Gaucher disease, 211
Genetic abnormalities: risk associated
    with transmitting, 266
Genetic counseling
  in granulomatous disease of
    childhood, chronic, 89
  in incontinentia pigmenti, 236, 237
  in neurofibromatosis, 227
  in sclerosis, tuberous, 232
  in xeroderma pigmentosum, 314–315
Genetic pedigrees: in mastocytosis, 345
Genetics
  of acrodermatitis enteropathica, 250

  in dermatitis herpetiformis, 254
  of epidermolysis bullosa simplex, 260
  of incontinentia pigmenti, 233
  in lupus erythematosus, neonatal,
    129
Genital ulcer: in Behcet's syndrome, 59
Genitalia
  abnormalities in multiple lentigines
    syndrome, 240
  in alkaptonuria, 190
Gianotti-Crosti syndrome, 75–78
  clinical manifestations, 76–78
  diagnosis, 78
  face in, 77
  histologic features, 78
  treatment, 78
Giant cell
  granulomatosis (*see* Wegener's
    granulomatosis)
  Touton, in xanthoma disseminatum,
    342
Giant pigment granules: in
    neurofibromatosis, 222, 226
Giant urticaria, 2
Gigantism: in hyperpituitarism,
    179–180
Gingiva
  fibroma, 227
    in tuberous sclerosis, 228
  in Hand-Schüller-Christian disease,
    339
  tumors in Hand-Schüller-Christian
    disease, 340
  ulcer in Letterer-Siwe disease, 337
Glaucoma
  in Marfan syndrome, 193
  in Sturge-Weber syndrome, 287, 288
Glioma
  in ataxia telangiectasia, 305
  of optic nerve in neurofibromatosis,
    225
  in sclerosis, tuberous, 232
Glossitis: in biotin deficiency, 199
Glucocorticosteroids: in neonatal lupus
    erythematosus, 131
Glucose-6-phosphate dehydrogenase
    deficiency: screening test for,
    256
Glucose tolerance test: abnormalities in
    necrobiosis lipoidica
    diabeticorum, 181

Glutamic pyruvic transaminase: and
epidermolysis bullosa simplex,
260
Gluten
dietary, 254
-free diet in dermatitis herpetiformis,
254, 255, 256
-sensitive (see Enteropathy, gluten-
sensitive)
Glycolipids: in fucosidosis, 297
GM$_1$ gangliosidosis, 216
beta galactosidase deficiency causing,
216
cherry red macules in, 216
Goiter
diffuse toxic, 163
endemic, 157–158
Gold therapy; in juvenile rheumatoid
arthritis, 146
Goltz syndrome (see Focal dermal
hypoplasia)
Gorham's syndrome, 293
Gorlin syndrome (see Basal cell nevus
syndrome)
Gottron's papules: in dermatomyositis,
132, 133, 134
Graft-vs.-host reaction, 26
Granuloma
annulare
cause, 184
corticosteroids in, 185
diabetes and, 183–185
rheumatoid nodules in, 184
subcutaneous forms, 184
eosinophilic, 340–342
curettage in, 341
treatment, 341–342
ulcer in, 340
Granulomatosis
allergic, 42–45
giant cell (see Wegener's
granulomatosis)
lymphomatoid, 42, 44–45
contrasted with Wegener's
granulomatosis, 44–45
Wegener's (see Wegener's
granulomatosis)
Granulomatous disease of childhood,
chronic, 88–89
clinical manifestations, 88–89
diagnosis, 89

fatal, 88
treatment, 89
Graves' disease, 163
in hyperthyroidism, 165
Grönglad-Strandberg syndrome, 112
Growth
impairment in Kwashiorkor, 324
retardation
in acrodermatitis enteropathica,
252
in Bloom syndrome, 315
in Cockayne syndrome, 318, 319
in epidermolysis bullosa,
junctional, 260
in fucosidosis, 298
in Kwashiorkor, 324
in multiple lentigines syndrome,
240
in porphyria, erythropoietic, 327
in xeroderma pigmentosum, 313
Gums (see Gingiva)
Günther's disease (see Porphyria,
erythropoietic)
Guthrie test: in phenylketonuria, 190,
191

H

Hageman factor, 9
Hair
abnormalities in Kwashiorkor, 324
anomalies in hypomelanosis of Ito,
238
body
loss in angiokeratoma corporis
diffusum, 296
loss in hypopituitarism, 180
in candidiasis, 172
coarse, in hypothyroidism, 158, 160,
162
color in acrodermatitis enteropathica,
252
depigmentation in Kwashiorkor, 324
in dyskeratosis congenita, 271
friable, in homocystinuria, 190, 192
greying, premature, in Rothmund-
Thomson syndrome, 317
lanugo, in Cushing's syndrome, 177
loss
in candidiasis, chronic
mucocutaneous, 87

Hair (cont.)
  premature, in Rothmund-Thomson
    syndrome, 317
  premature development in
    adrenogenital syndrome, 179
  of scalp, graying in ataxia
    telangiectasia, 304
  in Sjögren's syndrome, 147
  sparse
    in Cockayne syndrome, 319
    in hypoparathyroidism, 172
  steel wool, in Menkes' kinky hair
    syndrome, 196, 197
  straw color, in Kwashiorkor, 324
  thinning and loss, in
    hypoparathyroidism, 172
Hamartoma
  of iris, 220
  renal, in tuberous sclerosis, 232
  in tuberous sclerosis, 228
Hand
  claw, in Hurler syndrome, 211, 213
  eruptions in epidermolysis bullosa,
    259
  hyperpigmentation in Addison's
    disease, 175
  in Kawasaki disease, 47, 50
  large, in Cockayne syndrome, 318,
    319
  puffy, in hypothyroidism, 162
  swollen, in mixed connective tissue
    disease, 150
Hand-Schüller-Christian disease, 336,
    339–340
  granulomatous infiltrates with ulcer
    in, 340
  xanthoma and, 205
HANE (see Angioneurotic edema,
    hereditary)
Hartnup disease, 319–321
  clinical manifestations, 320
  diagnosis, 321
  infections in, intercurrent, 320
  neurologic abnormalities in, 319
  treatment, 321
Hashimoto's (see Thyroiditis,
    Hashimoto's)
Headache: in eosinophilic granuloma,
    340
Healing: in Cushing's syndrome, 177

Hearing impairment: in Vogt-Koyanagi-
    Harada syndrome, 240
Heart
  abnormalities
    in Lyme disease, 74
    in multiple lentigines syndrome,
      241
  anomalies in incontinentia pigmenti,
    236
  block, congenital, 128
  changes in pseudoxanthoma
    elasticum, 112
  complications in lupus
    erythematosus, 124
  disease
    alkaptonuria complicating, 194
    ischemic, with type II
      hyperlipoproteinemia, 207
  evaluation in LAMB syndrome,
    242
  failure, in hemangiomatosis, diffuse
    neonatal, 292
  involvement
    in lupus erythematosus, neonatal,
      130
    in mixed connective tissue disease,
      150
  manifestations in incontinentia
    pigmenti, 234
  system in epidermal nevus
    syndrome, 244
Heat: intolerance in hyperthyroidism,
    164
Heliotrope
  eruption on shoulder in
    dermatomyositis, 133
  erythema in dermatomyositis, 134
  patches on face in dermatomyositis,
    132
  rash over eyelids in mixed
    connective tissue disease, 149
Hemangioma
  capillary, 283
  cavernous, 283, 285–286
    in blue rubber-bleb nevus
      syndrome, 291
    in Cobb syndrome, 294
  of eyelid, 285
  of eyelid, complication rate in, 286
  of foot, 292

of Klippel-Trenaunay-Parkes-
Weber syndrome, 290
in Maffucci's syndrome, 291
with thrombocytopenia, 286
treatment, 285
with dyschondroplasia, 291
liver, 293
in Maffucci's syndrome, 291
origin of, 283
skin, 283–286
strawberry, 283–284
of eyelid, 284
resolution of, 284
Hemangiomatosis
benign neonatal, 292
diffuse neonatal, 292–293
of foot, 292
multinodular, 292
Hematemesis: in Peutz-Jeghers
syndrome, 269
Hematuria: in Lesch-Nyhan syndrome,
197
Hemihypertrophy
in epidermal nevus syndrome, 244
in nevi achromicus, 239
Hemiplegia: in Sturge-Weber
syndrome, 287, 288
Hemochromatosis: differential
diagnosis, 194
Hemoglobinuria: dark urine in, 194
Hemolytic anemia: in erythropoietic
porphyria, 325, 327
Hemoptysis: in angiokeratoma corporis
diffusum, 295
Hemorrhage
gastrointestinal
in hemangiomatosis, diffuse
neonatal, 292
in telangiectasia, hereditary
hemorrhagic, 301
of scrotum in Henoch-Schönlein
purpura, 38
in telangiectasia, hereditary
hemorrhagic, 302
of testes in Henoch-Schönlein
purpura, 38
in toxic shock syndrome, 70
Hemorrhagic
diatheses, in urticaria pigmentosa,
351

infarction, and purpura fulminans,
307
telangiectasia (see Telangiectasia,
hereditary hemorrhagic)
Henoch-Schönlein purpura, 35–39
arthritic symptoms, 38
clinical manifestations, 35–37
contrasted with Wegener's
granulomatosis, 43
diagnosis, 39
etiologic factor, 35
gastrointestinal symptoms, 38
lower extremities in, 37
prognosis, 39
systemic manifestations, 37–39
treatment, 39
Heparin: in purpura fulminans,
307
Hepatic
(See also Liver)
porphyria, 329–332
congenital cutaneous, 331
Hepatitis
B surface antigen, 76
in Gianotti-Crosti syndrome, 75, 77
icteric, in infectious mononucleosis,
79
in Kawasaki disease, 52
in Q fever, 82
serum, 3
Hepatobiliary disease: and Sjögren's
syndrome, 146
Hepatolenticular degeneration, 190,
195
clinical features, 195
treatment, 195
Hepatomegaly
in Gianotti-Crosti syndrome, 76, 77
urticaria pigmentosa and, 351
Hepatosplenomegaly
in infectious mononucleosis, 79
in Letterer-Siwe disease, 337
Herpes simplex: and etiologic factor in
erythema multiforme, 23
Heterochromia iridis, 237
in Waardenburg syndrome, 239
Heterophile antibody studies: in
infectious mononucleosis, 79–80
Hexachlorobenzene: porphyria cutanea
tarda after, 330

Hip: disseminated angiokeratoma in
    fucosidosis, 297
Hirsutism
    in adrenogenital syndrome, 178, 179
    in ataxia telangiectasia, 304
    in hyperpituitarism, 180
Histamine: in urticaria pigmentosa, 351
Histiocytosis
    malignant, 343
    X, 336
        classification, 336
        etiology, numerous, 336
        hereditary influence in, 336
        ulcer in inguinal region in, 338
Histocompatibility antigens, 129
Histoplasmosis: in erythema nodosum,
    18
HLA
    antigen and Vogt-Koyanagi-Harada
        syndrome, 240
    -B8 and dermatitis herpetiformis, 254
    -DRW3 in dermatitis herpetiformis,
        254
Holocarboxylase synthetase: activity
    deficiency and biotin deficiency,
    199
Homocystine: increased urinary
    excretion of, in homocystinuria,
    192
Homocystinuria, 190, 192–193
    clinical features, 192–193
    diagnosis, 193
    treatment, 193
Homogentisic acid defect: in
    alkaptonuria, 190, 193, 194
Hormone(s)
    melanocyte-stimulating (see MSH)
    TSH in hyperthyroidism, 164
    hypersecretion, 163
Hunter syndrome, 211, 213
    (See also Mucopolysaccharidosis II)
    facial features in, coarse, 212
    fingers in, 212
    nodules in reticular pattern on
        shoulder in, 214
    papules of, flesh-colored, 214
    pathognomonic lesions in, 213
    shoulder in, 214
Hurler syndrome, 211–212
    claw hand in, 212

diagnosis, 211–212
distinguished from mucolipidosis II,
    216
features of, 211
prenatal diagnosis, 212
Scheie syndrome as variant of,
    212–213
Hyalinosis cutis et mucosae (see Lipoid
    proteinosis)
Hyaluronic acid: in Marfan syndrome,
    106
Hydrops: of gallbladder in Kawasaki
    disease, 53
p-Hydroxyphenyl-pyruvate oxidase
    deficiency: and neonatal
    tyrosinemia, 200
Hydroxyzine
    in mastocytosis, 353
    in urticaria, 3
Hyperbetalipoproteinemia, familial (see
    Hyperlipoproteinemia, types III
    and IV)
Hypercalcemia: secondary, 170
Hypercalcinosis: and hyperthyroidism,
    169
Hypercholesterolemia, familial (see
    Hyperlipoproteinemia, type II)
Hyperchylomicronemia: familial,
    208–209
Hyperemia
    conjunctival, in toxic shock
        syndrome, 69
    in toxic shock syndrome, 70
    of mucous membranes, 71
Hypereosinophilic syndrome, 28–30
    clinical manifestations, 28–30
    diagnosis, 30
    pathogenesis, 28
    treatment, 30
Hyperextensibility: of joints in Ehlers-
    Danlos syndrome, 97–98
Hypergammaglobulinemia, 141, 142
    in fasciitis, eosinophilic, 141
Hyperhidrosis
    in dyskeratosis congenita, 270
    in epidermolysis bullosa simplex,
        localized, 259
    in scleroderma, 138
Hyperkeratosis
    in dermatomyositis, 134

with erosions
  in tyrosine metabolism disorders, 201
  in tyrosinemia II, 201
palmoplantar, in dyskeratosis congenita, 270
of palms and soles in epidermolysis bullosa, 260
  generalized atrophic, 260
in xeroderma pigmentosum, 314
Hyperlipemia: in hyperlipoproteinemia, type I, 206
Hyperlipidemia, 203
  familial, 205
  type II, 205
  type III, 205
Hyperlipoproteinemia, 203
  classification, 206–209
  type I, 205, 206–207
    abdominal pain in, 206
    chylomicrons in, 206
  type II, 205, 207–208
    cholesterol levels in, 207
    cholesterol metabolism derangement in, 207
  type III, 205, 208
    electrophoresis showing broad beta band in, 208
    lipoprotein clearance disturbance in, 208
  type IV, 205, 208
    abdominal pain in, 208
    lipemia retinalis in, 208
  type V, 205, 208–209
Hyperparathyroidism, 170–171
  clinical manifestations, 170
  diagnosis, 171
  secondary to chronic renal failure, 170
  treatment, 171
Hyperpigmentation
  Addisonian, 177
  in ataxia telangiectasia, 304
  in dermatitis herpetiformis, 254–255
  in dermatomyositis, 134
  in epidermolysis bullosa, dominant dystrophic, 263
  freckled, in xeroderma pigmentosum, 313, 314
  of hands, in Addison's disease, 175

in hepatolenticular degeneration, 195
in hyperparathyroidism, 170
in hyperpituitarism, 180
in hypoparathyroidism, 172
of legs in hepatolenticular degeneration, 190
melanin, in Addison's disease, 174
in mixed connective tissue disease, 149
of mucous membranes of mouth in Addison's disease, 175
in mycosis fungoides, 359
in porphyria
  erythropoietic, 327
  variegata, 332
reticulated, in dyskeratosis congenita, 270
in Rothmund-Thomson syndrome, 317
in scleroderma, 138
in sclerosis, tuberous, etiology, 230
Hyperpituitarism, 179–180
  diagnosis, 180
Hyperplasia: parathyroid, 169
Hyperprebetalipoproteinemia (*see* Hyperlipoproteinemia, types III and V)
Hypersensitivity
  to drugs, 26
  syndromes, 1–34
Hypersplenism: in erythropoietic protoporphyria, 328
Hypertelorism
  in hypoparathyroidism, 173
  in hypothyroidism, 158, 159
  in multiple lentigines syndrome, 240
Hypertension
  in angiokeratoma corporis diffusum, 296
  in Cockayne syndrome, 318
  in Cushing's syndrome, 176, 177
Hyperthyroidism, 163–166
  in Addison's disease, 176
  in children, causes, 163
  clinical features, 164
  clinical manifestations, 163–165
  diagnosis, 165, 169
  of newborn, 163
    transient, 163
  thyroidectomy in, 166

Hyperthyroidism *(cont.)*
  treatment, 165, 169
Hypertrichosis
  in dermatomyositis, 134
  in hypothyroidism, 162
    acquired, 161
    porphyria cutanea tarda and, 330
  in porphyria, erythropoietic, 325
Hypertriglyceridemia: and xanthoma,
  205
Hypertrophy
  of bone in Klippel-Trenaunay-Parkes-
    Weber syndrome, 290
  in epidermolysis bullosa, dominant
    dystrophic, 263
  of extremities in Klippel-Trenaunay-
    Parkes-Weber syndrome, 290
  soft tissue, in Klippel-Trenaunay-
    Parkes-Weber syndrome, 290
Hyperuricemia: in Lesch-Nyhan
  syndrome, 197, 198
Hypocomplementemia, 122
Hypogonadism
  in basal cell nevus syndrome, 243
  in Rothmund-Thomson syndrome,
    317
Hypohidrosis: in angiokeratoma
  corporis diffusum, 296
Hypomelanosis of Ito, 235, 237–238
  diagnosis, 238
  genetic pattern in, 237
  histologic examination in, 237
  internal manifestations, 235, 237
  neurologic assessment in, 238
  treatment, 238
Hyponatremia: in rickettsial disease, 85
Hypoparathyroidism, 171–174
  clinical manifestations, 172–173
  congenital, 172
  maculopapular eruptions in, 173
  parathyroid removal and, 172
  surgical injury and, 172
  treatment, 173–174
Hypopigmentation
  ash-leaf-shaped, in tuberous
    sclerosis, 230
  in ataxia telangiectasia, 304
  in dermatomyositis, 134
  in dyskeratosis congenita, 270
  in epidermal nevus syndrome, 244

  of macules in tuberous sclerosis,
    227–233
  in mixed connective tissue disease,
    149
  in mycosis fungoides, 359
  in nevus achromicus, 238
  in phenylketonuria, 189
  in Rothmund-Thomson syndrome,
    317
  of scars in dermatitis herpetiformis,
    255
  in scleroderma, 138
  in sclerosis, tuberous, 231
    etiology, 230
  in vitiligo, 231
Hypopigmented atrophic plaques: in
  lupus erythematosus, neonatal,
  129
Hypopituitarism, 180
Hypoplasia
  focal dermal (*see* Focal dermal
    hypoplasia)
  of ovaries in multiple lentigines
    syndrome, 241
Hypoproteinemia: in Kwashiorkor, 324
Hypotension
  postural, in toxic shock syndrome, 70
  in toxic shock syndrome, 69
Hypothenar eminence: in juvenile
  rheumatoid arthritis, 144
Hypothermia: in Menkes' kinky hair
  syndrome, 196
Hypothyroidism, 157–163
  acquired, 157, 159–163
    clinical features, 162–163
    clinical manifestations, 159–163
    delayed development in, 162
    Hashimoto's thyroiditis causing,
     158
    placid disposition in, 162
    sallow appearance in, 162
    treatment, 161–163
  in children
    etiology, 158
    iodine therapy of, radioactive, 158
    maternal causes, 158
  clinical manifestations, 158
  congenital, 157–158
    cause, 158
    clinical features of, 159

diagnosis, 158–159, 161
screening of newborn for, 159
after thyroidectomy, 172
Hypotrichosis: in Rothmund-Thomson syndrome, 317
Hypoxanthineguanine phosphoribosyl transferase: and Lesch-Nyhan syndrome, 197
Hypsarrhythmia: in tuberous sclerosis, 231

I

Ichthyosis hystrix, 244
Ig (see Immunoglobulin)
Ileitis: regional, in erythema nodosum, 18
Imaging: bone, for mastocytosis screening, 353
Immune complexes: IgA circulating, 254
Immunity: cell-mediated, in candidiasis, 172
Immunodeficiency: combined, in ataxia telangiectasia, 303, 305
Immunofluorescence
complement, and dermatitis herpetiformis, 255
in lupus erythematosus, 126
in mixed connective tissue disease, 150
Immunofluorescent staining: in rickettsial disease, 83
Immunofluorescent studies
in lupus erythematosus, neonatal, 131
in porphyria cutanea tarda, 331
Immunofluorescent technique: with Crithiden luciliae, 126
Immunofluorescent tests
in Q fever, 82
in rickettsialpox, 82
Immunoglobulin
A
deposition in dermatitis herpetiformis, 254
in dermatitis herpetiformis, 255
immune complexes, circulating, 254
G cryoprecipitates, 73

M cryoprecipitates, 73
reduction of, in Bloom syndrome, 316
Immunologic deficiency: and candidiasis, chronic mucocutaneous, 87
Immunosuppression
in eosinophilic granuloma, 341
livedo reticularis after, 122
in lupus erythematosus, 128
in mixed connective tissue disease, 151
in periarteritis nodosa, adult, 57
in pyoderma gangrenosum, 273–274
in Sjögren's syndrome, 148
Impetigo: bullous, 65, 66
Incontinentia pigmenti, 233–237
achromians (see Hypomelanosis of Ito)
arm lesions in, 234
bullae of, 234
Chinese-figure-like patches in, 235
clinical manifestations, 233–236
depigmented lesions in, 235
diagnosis, 236
genetics of, 233
histopathologic examination in, 236
mutation in, 233
phase 1, 234
phase 2, 234
phase 3, 235
phase 4, 235–236
pigmentary incontinence in, 235
pigmentary state begins, 235
systemic manifestations, 234, 236
treatment, 237
vesicles of, 234
Infarction
hemorrhagic, and purpura fulminans, 307
splenic, in type I hyperlipoproteinemia, 207
Infection, 65–95
hypersensitivity to, 3
Infectious mononucleosis, 78–81
ampicillin in, rashes after, 80–81
clinical manifestations, 79
diagnosis, 79–80
treatment, 80–81

Inguinal region: ulcer in, in
    histiocytosis X, 338
Inheritance (*see* Genetics)
Insect bites: hypersensitivity to, 3
Intellectual deficits: in ataxia
    telangiectasia, 305
Intellectual development: delay in
    phenylketonuria, 189
Intellectual function: after
    phenylketonuria treatment, 191
Interphalangeal joints
    arthritis of, in angiokeratoma corporis
        diffusum, 296
    in dermatomyositis, 133
Intestine
    bypass causing acrodermatitis
        enteropathica, 251
    ganglioneuromatosis in multiple
        endocrine adenomatosis
        syndromes, 167
    perforation in Henoch-Schönlein
        purpura, 38
    polyposis, in Gardner's syndrome,
        274
    polyps (*see* Polyps, intestinal)
    small, studies for dermatitis
        herpetiformis, 256
Intoxication: vitamin D, hypercalcemia
    secondary to, 170
Intracranial calcification: in Cockayne
    syndrome, 318
Intralesional injection: of systemic
    corticosteroids in cavernous
    hemangioma, 286
Intussusception, 38
    in Peutz-Jeghers syndrome, 269
Involuntary movements: in Lesh-Nyhan
    syndrome, 198
Iodine: maternal, during pregnancy,
    157
Iridocyclitis: in juvenile rheumatoid
    arthritis, 146
Iris
    hamartoma of, 220
    neurofibroma on, 225
    in xanthogranuloma, juvenile, 344
Iritis: in sarcoidosis, 355
Ischemic
    heart disease, in type II
        hyperlipoproteinemia, 207

necrosis of bone, 124
Ixodes dammini, 14, 72

J

Jaundice: in toxic shock syndrome, 69
Jaw
    cysts, odontogenic, in basal cell
        nevus syndrome, 242
    lantern, in hyperpituitarism, 180
Job syndrome, 89–90
    clinical manifestations, 89–90
    treatment, 90
Joints
    contractures, in Cockayne syndrome,
        319
    disease, degenerative, and
        alkaptonuria, 193
    hyperextensible, in Ehlers-Danlos
        syndrome, 97
    interphalangeal (*see* Interphalangeal
        joints)
    in rheumatoid arthritis, juvenile, 144

K

Kala-azar: and urticaria, 7
Kasabach-Merritt syndrome, 286–287
    surgical risk in, 287
    treatment, 287
Kawasaki disease, 45–55, 145
    arthralgia in, 52
    arthritis in, 52
    cardiac effects of, 51–52
    clinical manifestations, 46–53
    clinical phases of, 46
    conjunctiva in, 47, 48
    contrasted with periarteritis nodosa,
        46
    desquamation in, 50
    diagnosis, 53
        principal criteria, 47–53
    erythematous rash in, 47
    etiology, 45–46
    exanthem in, 48–49
    extremities in, 49–50
    feet in, 47, 50
    fever in, 47
    fingers in, 51
    fingertips in, 47

gastrointestinal manifestations of,
52–53
genetic susceptibility to, 46
hands in, 47, 50
histopathologic features, 49
laboratory studies, 53
lips in, 47
lymph nodes in, histopathologic
examination, 51
lymphadenopathy in, 47, 50–51
management, 53–55
outline for, 54
mouth in, 47, 48
pyuria in, 53
urticarial rash in, 49
Kayser-Fleischer rings: in
hepatolenticular degeneration,
190, 195
Keloid lesions: in dominant dystrophic
epidermolysis bullosa, 263
Keratitis
in porphyria, erythropoietic, 327
in tyrosine metabolism disorders, 201
in tyrosinemia II, 201
in xeroderma pigmentosum, 314
Keratoconjunctivitis
in biotin deficiency, 199
in hypoparathyroidism, 172
sicca, 146
in sarcoidosis, 355
Keratoderma: palmaris et plantaris in
mycosis fungoides, 359
Keratopathy: band, in
hyperparathyroidism, 170–171
Ketoconazole: in candidiasis, systemic,
86–87
17-Ketosteroids: in adrenogenital
syndrome, 179
Kidney
disease
in angiokeratoma corporis
diffusum, 296
in Cockayne syndrome, 318
in Henoch-Schönlein purpura, 39
lupus erythematosus and, 128
in mixed connective tissue disease,
150
failure
in angiokeratoma corporis
diffusum, 296

chronic, hyperparathyroidism
secondary to, 170
in toxic shock syndrome, 69
hamartoma, in tuberous sclerosis,
232
involvement
in Behcet's syndrome, 60
in Henoch-Schönlein purpura, 38
in lupus erythematosus, 124
transplant, and lupus erythematosus,
128
Klein-Waardenburg syndrome, 239
Klippel-Trenaunay-Parkes-Weber
syndrome, 289–290
in Riley-Smith syndrome, 293
Knees
in epidermolysis bullosa, dominant
dystrophic, 263
scars in Ehlers-Danlos syndrome, 97
xanthoma on, eruptive, 205
Kveim test: in sarcoidosis, 356
Kwashiorkor, 323–325
clinical manifestations, 324
"red children" in, 324
treatment, 324–325

L

LAMB syndrome, 241–242
Langerhans granules
in eosinophilic granuloma, 341
in histiocytosis X, 336
Laryngeal involvement: in xanthoma
disseminatum, 343
Laser
argon, in Sturge-Weber syndrome,
289
photocoagulation in pseudoxanthoma
elasticum, 113
La(SSB), 129
LATS, 163
in hyperthyroidism, 164
Leg (see Extremities, lower)
Leishmaniasis: in erythema nodosum,
18
Lens
dislocation
in homocystinuria, 193
in Marfan syndrome, 193
subluxation in homocystinuria, 192

Lentigine(s)
in LAMB syndrome, 242
multiple (*see* Multiple lentigines
syndrome)
Leopard syndrome (*see* Multiple
lentigines syndrome)
Leprosy: in erythema nodosum, 18
Lesch-Nyhan syndrome, 197–198
clinical manifestations, 197–198
diagnosis, 198
treatment, 198
Letterer-Siwe disease, 336, 337–339
benign form, 337
clinical features, 337–339
cutaneous form, 337
purpuric nodules in, 337
as bad prognostic sign, 337
remissions in, spontaneous, 339
Leukemia
in ataxia telangiectasia, 305
as hazard in urticaria pigmentosa,
351
livedo reticularis in, 122, 299
mast cell, 347, 351
monomyelocytic, 345
neurofibromatosis and, 227
Sweet's syndrome and, 41
urticaria and, 7
Leukocytoclastic angiitis, 35
palpable purpura as hallmark of, 36
Leukocytoclastic vasculitis, 39
in lupus erythematosus, 122
Leukoderma
in neurofibromatosis, 223
speckled, in tuberous sclerosis, 231
Leukodystrophy: Austin type of, 216
Leukokeratosis: in dyskeratosis
congenita, 270
Leukopenia: in lupus erythematosus,
124
Leukoplasia: in dyskeratosis congenita,
270, 271, 272
L'homme rouge: in mycosis fungoides,
359
Limbs (*see* Extremities)
Lip(s)
enlarged, diffusely, in multiple
endocrine adenomatosis
syndrome, 167
fleshy, protuberant, in multiple

mucosal neuroma syndrome, 168
in Kawasaki disease, 47
in lupus erythematosus, 120, 121
in telangiectasia, hereditary
hemorrhagic, 302
thick, in hypothyroidism, 159
acquired, 160
upper, cupid's bow-like, in Menkes'
kinky hair syndrome, 196
Lipemia retinalis: in type IV
hyperlipoproteinemia, 208
Lipoid proteinosis, 101–103
cause, 101
clinical manifestations, 101–102
diagnosis, 102
treatment, 103
Lipoma: in basal cell nevus syndrome,
243
Lipoprotein
alpha-lipoproteins, 203
beta-lipoproteins, 203
chylomicrons, 203
clearance disturbance in type III
hyperlipoproteinemia, 208
deficiency, familial high density (*see*
Tangier disease)
prebeta-lipoproteins, 203
Lipoproteinemia
familial, 206
type II, 206
type III, 205, 206
type IV, 206
Lisch nodules, 220, 221, 225
in neurofibromatosis, 226
Livedo reticularis, 299
etiology, 299
in lupus erythematosus, 122
in mixed connective tissue disease,
149
in periarteritis nodosa, adult, 56
with ulcer, 299
Livedo vasculitis, 299
Liver
abnormalities in toxic shock
syndrome, 69
biopsy in erythropoietic
protoporphyria, 328
complications in diffuse neonatal
hemangiomatosis, 292
disease

hyperlipoproteinemia and, type
   III, 208
   xanthoma and, 205
dysfunction
   in hepatolenticular degeneration,
      190
   in Kawasaki disease, 47
function abnormality in Gianotti-
   Crosti syndrome, 77
hemangioma, 293
in hepatolenticular degeneration, 195
porphyria and (*see* Porphyria,
   hepatic)
toxicity after ketoconazole, 87
in xanthogranuloma, juvenile, 344
"Lobster-claw" deformities: in focal
   dermal hypoplasia, 103
Lofenalac: in phenylketonuria, 191
Louis-Bar syndrome (*see* Ataxia
   telangiectasia)
Louse-born typhus fever, 81
Lung
   fibrosis in Sjögren's syndrome, 147
   honeycombing, in tuberous sclerosis,
      232
   infection in ataxia telangiectasia, 305
   involvement
      in Hand-Schüller-Christian
         disease, 340
      in sarcoidosis, 355
   lesions in eosinophilic granuloma,
      341
   in xanthogranuloma, juvenile, 344
Lunula
   absence in hyperpituitarism, 180
   in hypopituitarism, 180
Lupus band test, 126
Lupus erythematosus, 3, 119–131, 312
   cells, 150
   classic changes of, 122
   clinical manifestations, 120–128
   diagnosis, 124–127
      criteria for, 124
   discoid, 119
      disseminated, 119
   discoid lesion of, 121
   face in, 120, 121
   fingers in, 123
   genetic component, 119
   hospitalization in, 128

laboratory features, 126
lips in, 120, 121
livedo reticularis and, 299
in mothers, lupus erythematosus in
   newborn of, 128
mucous membrane lesions in, 122
neonatal, 128–131
   clinical features, 129–131
   diagnosis, 131
   discoid lesions of, scaly atrophic,
      129
   etiology, 129
   face in, 130
   forehead in, 130
   scalp in, 130
   treatment, 131
palate in, 121
palms in, 123
panniculitis, 123
pathogenesis, 119
photosensitivity of, 127
plugging in, 122
prognosis, 127
sex incidence, 120
skin lesions of, in mixed connective
   tissue disease, 149
subacute, 119–120
systemic, 119, 138
   classification, criteria for, 125
   contrasted with mixed connective
      tissue disease, 148–149
   manifestations of, 124
   Sjögren's syndrome and, 146
   urticaria and, 7
   treatment, 127–128
Lupus nephritis, 124
Lupus pernio, 356
Lupus profundus, 123
Lyell's disease, 20, 26
Lyme arthritis, 73
Lyme disease, 14, 72–75
   clinical features, 72–75
   diagnosis, 75
   mechanism of, 74
   neurologic signs and symptoms in, 74
   systemic features, 73
   treatment, 75
Lymph nodes
   hilar, enlargement in sarcoidosis, 355
   histopathology examination in

Lymph nodes *(cont.)*
   Kawasaki disease, 51
   mucocutaneous lymph node
     syndrome *(see* Kawasaki disease)
Lymphadenitis: in Gianotti-Crosti
   syndrome, 77
Lymphadenopathy
   in Gianotti-Crosti syndrome, 75, 76,
     77
   in infectious mononucleosis, 79
   in Kawasaki disease, 47, 50–51
   in lupus erythematosus, 124
   in Lyme disease, 73
Lymphangioma: in Maffucci's
   syndrome, 291
Lymphocyte defense system: defects in
   candidiasis, chronic
   mucocutaneous, 87
Lymphoma
   malignant, and mycosis fungoides,
     358
   mast cell, 351
Lymphomatoid granulomatosis, 42,
   44–45
   contrasted with Wegener's
     granulomatosis, 44–45
Lymphoreticular cancer: in ataxia
   telangiectasia, 303, 305
Lysosomal bone disease: and
   fucosidosis, 298
Lysyl
   hydroxylase, 100
   oxidase, 99
     in cutis laxa, 108

M

Macrocephaly: in Riley-Smith
   syndrome, 293
Macrogenitosomia praecox, 179
Macroglossia
   in hyperpituitarism, 180
   in hypothyroidism, 159
Maffucci's syndrome, 291
Malar
   flush in homocystinuria, 190, 192
   region, pigment in alkaptonuria, 190
Malignancy *(see* Cancer)
Malnutrition: in Hartnup disease, 320
"Maltese crosses:" in angiokeratoma
   corporis diffusum, 296

Mandible: in Hand-Schüller-Christian
   disease, 340
Marfan syndrome, 106–108
   blue sclerae in, 105
   clinical manifestations, 106–107
   contrasted with homocystinuria, 193
   diagnosis, 107
   elastosis perforans serpiginosa in, 113
   etiology, 106
   skin changes in, 107
   treatment, 107–108
Marfanoid appearance
   in multiple endocrine adenomatosis
     syndrome, 167
   in multiple mucosal neuroma
     syndrome, 168
Marfanoid build: in basal cell nevus
   syndrome, 243
Maroteaux-Lamy syndrome, 214
Mast cell
   on back on mastocytosis, 346
   degranulation, and mastocytosis, 348
   leukemia, 347, 351
   lymphoma, 351
   metachromatic granules in, 353
   proliferation in skin in uremia, 171
Mastocytoma, solitary, 345, 348, 349
   bullous, 346, 347, 349
Mastocytosis, 345–348
   adult varieties, 347
   bullous, 347, 352
   bullous variants, 347
   childhood varieties, 347
   classification, 347
   clinical spectrum, 345, 348
   diagnosis, 348
   diffuse cutaneous, 345, 347, 351,
     352–354
     diagnosis, 352–353
     erythrodermic, 347
     prognosis, 352
     scotch-grained, leather-like
       appearance in, 352
     treatment, 353–354
   erythrodermic, 351, 352–354
     diagnosis, 352–353
     diffuse, 352
     treatment, 353–354
   genetic pedigrees in, 345
   inherited basis for, 345
   prognosis, 347–348

screening for, 353
solitary, 347, 348–349
    clinical manifestations, 349
systemic, 345, 351
variant of, 346
vesicular variants, 347
MEA (*see* Multiple endocrine
        adenomatosis syndromes, MEA)
Measles: and purpura fulminans, 306
Medication (*see* Drugs)
Mediterranean fever, familial, 275–277
    clinical manifestations, 275–276
    diagnosis, 276–277
    treatment, 277
    type I, 275
Medulloblastoma
    in ataxia telangiectasia, 305
    in basal cell nevus syndrome, 243
Melanin
    hyperpigmentation in Addison's
        disease, 174
    ochromotic pigment differentiated
        from, 194
Melanocytes
    dopa-positive, 222–223
    in sclerosis, tuberous, 231
    -stimulating hormone (*see* MSH)
Melanoma
    dark urine in, 194
    malignant, and xeroderma
        pigmentosum, 313
    urticaria and, 7
Melanosis: and porphyria cutanea
        tarda, 330
Melanosomes: in tuberous sclerosis,
        231
Melena: in Peutz-Jeghers syndrome,
        269
MEN (*see* Multiple endocrine
        neoplasia)
Meninges
    angiomatosis in Sturge-Weber
        syndrome, 287
    in Sturge-Weber syndrome, 287
    in xanthogranuloma, juvenile, 344
Meningitis: aseptic, in Kawasaki
        disease, 47, 52
Meningococcal septicemia: and purpura
        fulminans, 306
Meningoencephalitis: in Lyme disease,
        73, 74

Menkes' kinky hair syndrome, 196–197
    clinical features, 196
    diagnosis, 196–197
    prenatal diagnosis, 197
    treatment, 197
Mental changes
    in acrodermatitis enteropathica, 252
    in Kwashiokor, 324
Mental deficiency
    in tuberous sclerosis, 227
    in xeroderma pigmentosum, 313
Mental deficit: progressive, in
        Cockayne syndrome, 319
Mental retardation
    in Cockayne syndrome, 318
    in fucosidosis, 297
    in Hartnup disease, 320
    in homocystinuria, 190
    in Lesch-Nyhan syndrome, 198
    in mucolipidosis III, 216
    in neurofibromatosis, 226
    in nevi achromicus, 239
    in phenylketonuria, 189, 190
    in sclerosis, tuberous, 231, 232
    in Sturge-Weber syndrome, 287, 288
    in tyrosine metabolism disorders, 201
    in tyrosinemia II, 201
Metabolism, errors of, 189–219
    inborn, porphyria cutanea tarda as,
        330
Metacarpals
    growth failure in
        pseudohypoparathyroidims, 173
    shortened in basal cell nevus
        syndrome, 243
Metastases: in skin calcification, 170
Metatarsals: growth failure in
        pseudohypoparathyroidism, 173
Methemoboglobinemia: side effect of
        dapsone, 256
Mice: ectoparasites of, 82
Microabscesses
    Pautrier, in mycosis fungoides, 360
    subepidermal, in dermatitis
        herpetiformis, 255
Microangiopathy: in diabetic
        dermopathy, 183
Microcephaly
    in phenylketonuria, 190
    in xeroderma pigmentosum, 313
Microscopy (*see* Electron microscopy)

Milia
  on face in basal cell nevus syndrome,
    243
  in porphyria
    cutanea tarda, 330
    variegata, 332
Milk: breast, and zinc, 251
Mitral
  floppy mitral valve syndrome, 98,
    100, 106
  prolapse, 112
Mixed connective tissue disease (see
    Connective tissue, disease,
    mixed)
ML (see Mucolipidosis)
Monilethrix: in Menkes' kinky hair
    syndrome, 196
Moniliasis
  (See also Candidiasis)
  severe, 252
Mononucleosis (see Infectious
    mononucleosis)
Mono-spot test, 80
"Moon" facies: in Cushing's syndrome,
    176, 177
Morning stiffness: in juvenile
    rheumatoid arthritis, 144
Morphea, 136
  elastosis perforans serpiginosa in, 113
  fasciitis as variant of, eosinophilic,
    141
  relationship with systemic
    scleroderma, 137
Morquio syndrome, 214
Mortality: in sarcoidosis, 357
Mouth (see Oral)
MPS (see Mucopolysaccharidosis)
MPS 1 (see Hurler syndrome)
MSH, 170
  in hyperpigmentation
    in adrenogenital syndrome, 79
    in hyperpituitarism, 180
Mucinosis: follicular, in mycosis
    fungoides, 359
Mucocutaneous lymph node syndrome
    (see Kawasaki disease)
Mucolipidosis, 215–216
  differentiated from
    mucopolysaccharidosis, 211
  I, 215

cherry red spot-myoclonus
    syndrome and, 215
  diagnosis, 215
  II, 215–216
    distinguished from Hurler
      syndrome, 216
    fishmouth appearance in, 215
    prenatal diagnosis, 216
  III, 216
Mucopolysaccharide(s)
  acid, in hyperthyroidism, 164
  metabolism and "stiff skin"
    syndrome, 217
Mucopolysaccharidosis, 209–214
  biochemical defect in, 210
  clinical features, 211
  distinguishing features of, 210
  IV, 214
  I-S, 212–213
  VI, 214
  "stiff skin" syndrome and, 216
  III, 213–214
  II, 213
    (See also Hunter syndrome)
    pathognomonic lesions in, 213
Mucous membranes
  in Addison's disease, 174
  in dyskeratosis congenita, 271
  in epidermolysis bullosa, dominant
    dystrophic, 262, 263
  oral (see Oral, mucous membranes)
  in sarcoidosis, 356
  in telangiectasia, hereditary
    hemorrhagic, 301
Mulberry cells: in angiokeratoma
    corporis diffusum, 296
Multiple endocrine adenomatosis
    syndrome, 166–169
  clinical manifestations, 166–169
  MEA I, 167
  MEA II, 167
  MEA III, 167
Multiple endocrine neoplasia
  type 1, 166, 167, 170
  type 2, 166
  type 2a, 167
  type 3, 166
Multiple lentigines syndrome, 222,
    240–241
  clinical manifestations, 241

formes frustes, 241
Multiple mucosal neuroma syndrome,
    168
Muscle
  anomalies in hypomelanosis of Ito,
      237–238
  calcification, 170
  mass increase in adrenogenital
      syndrome, 179
  spinal, atrophy in ataxia
      telangiectasia, 305
  striated, in dermatomyositis, 132
Musculoskeletal anomalies: in basal cell
    nevus syndrome, 242
Mus musculus, 82
Mutations: in tuberous sclerosis, 227
Mutilation: self-mutilating behavior in
    Lesch-Nyhan syndrome, 198
Mycoplasma infections: and Stevens-
    Johnson syndrome, 23
Mycosis cell, 358
Mycosis fungoides, 357–360
  cutaneous manifestations, 358
  diagnosis, 360
  erythematous stage, 358
  etiology, 357
  face tumor in, 359
  histopathology, 360
  mycotic phase, 358
  plaque phase, 358
  poikilodermatous, 359
  premycotic state, 358
  treatment, 360
  tumor stage, 358
Myeloma
  multiple, and urticaria, 7
  xanthoma and, 205
Myocarditis: in rickettsial disease, 85
Myoglobinuria: dark urine in, 194
Myopia: in homocystinuria, 190
Myxedema
  in hypopituitarism, 180
  hypothyroidism and, 158, 162
    acquired, 160
  pretibial, in hyperthyroidism, 164,
      165
Myxoma
  atrial, in NAME syndrome, 242
  mucocutaneous, in LAMB syndrome,
      242

N

Nail
  brittle, in hypothyroidism, 162
  in candidiasis, 172
  changes in Rothmund-Thomson
      syndrome, 317
  defects in Rothmund-Thomson
      syndrome, 317
  deformity in acrodermatitis
      enteropathica, 252
  in dyskeratosis congenita, 270, 271
  dystrophy (*see* Dystrophy, nail)
  in epidermolysis bullosa
    dominant dystrophic, 262
    generalized atrophic, 260
    junctional, 260
  fragile slow-growing, in
      hypopituitarism, 180
  in hypoparathyroidism, 172
  Plummer's, in hyperthyroidism, 164
  purple bands in fucosidosis, 298
  in toxic shock syndrome, 69
NAME syndrome, 241–242
Nasal (*see* Nose)
NBT: in chronic granulomatous disease
    of childhood, 88, 89
Neck
  papillomatous lesions in xeroderma
      pigmentosum, 314
  verrucous lesions in xeroderma
      pigmentosum, 314
Necrobiosis lipoidica diabeticorum,
    181–182
  diagnosis, 181
  etiology, 181
  plaques in, yellowish-red oval
      atrophic, 182
  treatment, 181–182
Necrolysis (*see* Toxic epidermal
    necrolysis)
Necrosis
  in Hand-Schüller-Christian disease,
      340
  ischemic, of bone, 124
  of skin in purpura fulminans,
      307
Necrotizing vasculitis, 42
Nelson syndrome, 178
Neonatal (*see* Newborn)

Neoplasia
  (*See also* Tumors)
  endocrine (*see* Multiple endocrine
    neoplasia)
Nephritis, 128
Nephrocalcinosis: in hyperthyroidism,
  169
Nephrotic syndrome: in familial
    Mediterranean fever, 276
Nerve
  fifth, in Sturge-Weber syndrome,
    287, 288
  optic, glioma of, in
    neurofibromatosis, 225
  trigeminal, in Sturge-Weber
    syndrome, 287, 288
Nervous system
  autonomic, in neurofibromatosis, 226
  central (*see* Central nervous system)
  involvement in periarteritis nodosa,
    adult, 57
Neurocutaneous disorders, 220–249
Neurofibroma, 221, 223–225
  "buttonholing" in, 224
  on iris, 225
  myxoid, in NAME syndrome, 242
  of skin, 220, 226
Neurofibromatosis, 110, 220–227
  blue-red macules in, 221, 225
  clinical manifestations, 220–225
  diagnosis, 226–227
  genetic counseling in, 227
  lesions resembling coast of
      California, 223
  neurologic disease in, 226
  osseous defects associated with, 226
  pseudoatrophic macules in, 221, 225
  "six spot" criterion of, 221
  systemic manifestations, 221,
    225–226
  treatment, 227
  variants of, 220
  with xanthogranuloma, juvenile, 345
Neurofibrosarcoma, 224–225
  surgery of, 225
Neurologic complications: in
    angiokeratoma corporis
    diffusum, 296
Neurologic deficit: in diffuse neonatal
    hemangiomatosis, 292

Neurologic disorders: and livedo
    reticularis, 299
Neurologic dysfunction: in
    hepatolenticular degeneration,
    190
Neuroma
  acoustic, 220
  of conjunctiva, 168
  of eyelids, 168
  lingual
    in multiple endocrine
      adenomatosis syndromes, 167
    in multiple mucosa neuroma
      syndrome, 168
  mucosal neuroma syndrome, 166,
    168
  plexiform, 224
Neuropathy
  in Lyme disease, 73
  peripheral, in ataxia telangiectasia,
    305
Neutrophilic dermatosis, febrile (*see*
    Sweet's syndrome)
Nevi
  achromicus, 238–239
    hemihypertrophy in, 239
    in hypomelanosis of Ito, 237
    mental retardation in, 239
    as variant of hypomelanosis of Ito,
      238
  angiomatous, with osteolysis, 293
  basal cell (*see* Basal cell nevus
    syndrome)
  blue, in LAMB syndrome, 242
  blue rubber-bleb nevus syndrome
    (*see* Blue rubber-bleb nevus
    syndrome)
  epidermal nevus syndrome (*see*
    Epidermal nevus syndrome)
  flammeus (*see* Port-wine stains)
  lipomatosus cutaneous superficialis,
      of Hoffman and Zurhelle, 104
  in NAME syndrome, 242
  sebaceous
    of Jadassohn, 244
    linear nevus sebaceous syndrome,
      244
  spilus, 222
  strawberry, 283
  unius lateris, 244

in boy, 245
vascular, incidence, 284
vasculosus hypertrophicus, 289–290
wooly nevus syndrome, 236
Nevoxanthoendothelioma, 343–345
Nevus (see Nevi)
Newborn
    abdomen, in epidermolysis bullosa,
        recessive dystrophic, 261
    biotin deficiency of, 199, 200
    hemangiomatosis of (see
        Hemangiomatosis, diffuse
        neonatal)
    hyperthyroidism of, transient, 163
    Letterer-Siwe disease of,
        manifestations on face and chest,
        339
    lupus erythematosus (see Lupus
        erythematosus, neonatal)
    pemphigus of, 65
    screening for hypothyroidism, 159
    thyrotoxicosis, 163
    tyrosinemia of, 200–201
Niacin deficiency: in pellagra, 321
Nicotinamide
    in Hartnup disease, 321
    in pellagra, 323
Nicotinic acid
    in pellagra, 321, 323
    synthesis decrease in Hartnup
        disease, 319, 320, 321
Niemann-Pick disease, 211
Nifedipine: in scleroderma, 140
Nikolsky sign, 27
    in staphylococcal scalded skin
        syndrome, 67
Nitro-blue tetrazolium test: in chronic
    granulomatous disease of
    childhood, 88, 89
Nitrogen mustard: in mycosis
    fungoides, 360
Nizoral: in candidiasis, systemic, 86–87
Nose
    in alkaptonuria, 194
    angiofibroma on, 229
    bridge depression in hypothyroidism,
        158, 159
    mucosa, angiokeratoma corporis
        diffusum of, 295
    pigment in alkaptonuria, 190

puffiness in hypothyroidism, 160
    in scleroderma, 139
    triangular-shaped, in
        hyperpituitarism, 180
    of werewolves, 327
Nuclear antigen: extractable, 148, 150
Nursing care: in epidermolysis bullosa,
    268
Nutrition
    parenteral, long-term, causing
        acrodermatitis enteropathica,
        251
    poor
        in acrodermatitis enteropathica,
            251
        in epidermolysis bullosa, recessive
            dystrophic, 261
Nystagmus: in Hartnup disease, 320
Nystatin: in systemic candidiasis, 86

O

Obesity
    in Cushing's syndrome, 176
    truncal, in Cushing's syndrome, 177
Ochronosis (see Alkaptonuria)
Ochronotic pigment: differentiated
    from melanin, 194
Ocular (see Eye)
Oldfield's syndrome, 274
Oligophrenia, phenylpyruvic (see
    Phenylketonuria)
Onychogryphosis: in epidermolysis
    bullosa simplex, 260
Onycholysis: in hyperthyroidism, 164
Ophthalmic (see Eye)
Optic
    atrophy in Cockayne syndrome, 319
    nerve, glioma in neurofibromatosis,
        225
Oral
    cavity changes in Kawasaki disease,
        48
    involvement
        in epidermolysis bullosa,
            junctional, 260
        in Kawasaki disease, 47, 48
    mucosa
        in dyskeratosis congenita, 270

Oral (cont.)
  in epidermolysis bullosa, recessive
    dystrophic, 261
  mucous membranes
    in Addison's disease, 175
    in Hand-Schüller-Christian
      disease, 339, 340
  xanthomatous deposits, 342
Orange-peel surface: in tuberous
  sclerosis, 229
Osler-Rendu-Weber disease (see
  Telangiectasia, hereditary
  hemorrhagic)
Osseous involvement: in sarcoidosis,
  355
Ossification centers: in hypothyroidism,
  161
Osteogenesis imperfecta, 104–106
  clinical groups, 104
  diagnosis, 106
  elastosis perforans serpiginosa, 113
  systemic manifestations, 104–106
  treatment, 106
Osteolysis: with angiomatous nevi, 293
Osteolytic defects: in Hand-Schüller-
  Christian disease, 339, 340
Osteoma: in Gardner's syndrome, 274
Osteopathia striata, 104
Osteoporosis
  in Cushing's syndrome, 177
  in Marfan syndrome, 193
  Menkes' kinky hair syndrome and,
    196
Otitis media, chronic
  in Hand-Schüller-Christian disease,
    339, 340
  in Letterer-Siwe disease, 377
Ovaries
  dysgerminoma in ataxia
    telangiectasia, 305
  hypoplastic, in multiple lentigines
    syndrome, 241

P

Pacemakers: and neonatal lupus
  erythematosus, 131
Pain
  abdomen
    in hyperlipoproteinemia, type I,
      206
    in hyperlipoproteinemia, type IV,
      208
    in Mediterranean fever, familial,
      275
    in Peutz-Jeghers syndrome, 269
    in porphyria, acute intermittent,
      329
    in sarcoidosis, 355
  articular, in Mediterranean fever,
    familial, 275
  attacks in angiokeratoma corporis
    diffusum, 295
  in eosinophilic granuloma, 340
Palate: in lupus erythematosus, 121
Pallor: in hypopituitarism, 180
Palms
  in dyskeratosis congenita, 270
  edema in toxic shock syndrome, 70
  hyperkeratosis in epidermolysis
    bullosa, 260
    generalized atrophic, 260
  in Letterer-Siwe disease, 337
  in lupus erythematosus, 123
  peeling in toxic shock syndrome, 69,
    70
  pits in basal cell nevus syndrome,
    242, 243
  in rickettsial disease, 83
Palsy
  Bell's, in Lyme disease, 73
  cerebral, spastic, in Lesch-Nyhan
    syndrome, 198
Panarteritis: and Sjögren's syndrome,
  146–147
Pancreatitis, 38
  in hyperlipoproteinemia, type I, 207
Pancytopenia: in dyskeratosis
  congenita, 272
Panhypopituitarism, 180
Papulovesicular acrolocalized
  syndrome, 77–78
Paralysis: in angiokeratoma corporis
  diffusum, 296
Parapsoriasis en plaque, 359
Parathyroid
  abnormalities in hyperthyroidism,
    169
  disorders and skin, 169–174
  hyperplasia, 169
  removal, and hypoparathyroidism,
    172

Parenteral
nutrition, long-term, causing
acrodermatitis enteropathica,
251
therapy, biotin-deficient, 199
Paresthesias: in angiokeratoma corporis
diffusum, 295
Parotid enlargement
in sarcoidosis, 355
in Sjögren's syndrome, 147
Paul-Bunnell test, 80
Pautrier microabscesses: in mycosis
fungoides, 360
PCT (see Porphyria, cutanea tarda)
Peau d'orange, 111
in hyperthyroidism, 164
in mastocytosis, solitary, 349
in sclerosis, tuberous, 229
Pediculosis humanus, 81
Pellagra, 321–323
Casal's necklace in, 322
clinical features, 321–323
diagnosis, 323
differential, 194
Hartnup disease and, 320
-like skin eruption in Hartnup
disease, 319
-like skin lesions in Kwashiorkor, 324
neurologic manifestations, 323
secondary infection in, 322
sun exposure and, 322
treatment, 321, 323
Pemphigoid: bullous, contrasted with
dermatitis herpetiformis, 255
Pemphigus neonatorum, 65
Penicillamine
elastosis performans serpiginosa and,
113, 114
hepatolenticular degeneration and,
195
Peptic ulcer: and urticaria pigmentosa,
350
Periactin: in mastocytosis, 353
Periadenitis mucosa necrotica
recurrence, 59
Periarteritis nodosa, 44, 55–57
adult, 46, 55, 56–57
bullae in, 56
diagnosis, 57
treatment, 57
benign cutaneous, 57

cause, 55
contrasted with Kawasaki disease, 46
infantile, 55–56
livedo reticularis in, 122, 299
Pericardium: in xanthogranuloma,
juvenile, 344
Periosteal thickening: in tuberous
sclerosis, 232
Peritonitis
benign paroxysmal (see
Mediterranean fever, familial)
familial paroxysmal (see
Mediterranean fever, familial)
Perniosis, 123
Perspiration
absence in Sjögren's syndrome, 147
in alkaptonuria, 194
Pertrichosis: delayed, in
hypothyroidism, 160
Petechiae
in Letterer-Siwe disease, 337
in toxic shock syndrome, 69, 70
Peutz-Jeghers syndrome, 268–270
clinical manifestations, 268–269
diagnosis, 269
symptoms, 269
treatment, 269–270
Phakoma: in tuberous sclerosis, 232
Phenistix: in phenylketonuria, 190,
191
Phenylalanine hydroxylase defect:
causing phenylketonuria, 189,
190
Phenylketonuria, 189–192
clinical manifestations, 189
diagnosis, 189–191
musty odor in, 189, 190
treatment, 191–192
Pheochromocytoma
in hyperthyroidism, 169
neurofibromatosis and, 226
Phlebectasia
congenital generalized, 299–301
etiology, 300
diffuse, 300
in Klippel-Trenaunay-Parkes-Weber
syndrome, 290
in Maffucci's syndrome, 291
Phlebotomy in porphyria
cutanea tarda, 331
variegata, 332

Photocoagulation: laser, in pseudoxanthoma elasticum, 113
Photophobia, 313
  in acrodermatitis enteropathica, 251
  in hypoparathyroidism, 172
Photosensitivity
  in Bloom syndrome, 315
  in Cockayne syndrome, 318, 319
  as decrease of ability to repair DNA, 312
  disorders, 312–335
  in Hartnup disease, 320
  in Kwashiorkos, 324
  in lupus erythematosus, 120, 121, 127
  in mixed connective tissue disease, 149
  in pellagra, 321
  in phenylketonuria, 189, 190
  in porphyria, erythropoietic, 325
  in Rothmund-Thomson syndrome, 317
Phototherapy: in hyperparathyroidism, 171
Physical activity: strenuous, and eosinophilic fasciitis, 140, 141, 142
Physiotherapy: in epidermolysis bullosa, 268
Pigment
  giant pigment granules in neurofibromatosis, 222
  in incontinentia pigmenti, 235
  ochronotic, differentiated from melanin, 194
Pigmentation
  Addisonian, in hyperthyroidism, 164
  in alkaptonuria, 194
  bluish, after atabrine and chloroquine, 194
  in dyskeratosis congenita, 272
  giant granules, in neurofibromatosis, 226
  increase in xeroderma pigmentosum, 313
  mottled
    in Bloom syndrome, 315
    in Cockayne syndrome, 319
  mucocutaneous, in Peutz-Jeghers syndrome, 268

in pellagra, 322
  retina, in Cockayne syndrome, 319
  in urticaria pigmentosa, 350
Pili torti: in Menkes' kinky hair syndrome, 196
Pitressin
  for diabetes insipidus in eosinophilic granuloma, 341
  xanthoma disseminatum and, 343
Pituitary disorders, 179–180
PKU (*see* Phenylketonuria)
Plantar pits: in basal cell nevus syndrome, 242, 243
Plasma: frozen, in purpura fulminans, 307
Plasmapheresis: in lupus erythematosus, 128
Plastic surgery: in epidermolysis bullosa, 268
Platyspondyly: in homocystinuria, 192
Pleura: in Hand-Schüller-Christian disease, 340
Pleurisy: in lupus erythematosus, 124
Pleuritis: in Mediterranean fever, familial, 275, 276
Plummer's nails: in hyperthyroidism, 164
Pneumonitis: and Q fever, 82
Poikiloderma congenitale (*see* Rothmund-Thomson syndrome)
Poliosis
  in Alezzandrini syndrome, 240
  sclerosis and, tuberous, 229
  in Vogt-Koyanagi-Harada syndrome, 240
Polyarteritis nodosa, 44, 55
Polyarthritis
  in lupus erythematosus, 124
  in scleroderma, 140
Polymyositis, 131
  contrasted with mixed connective tissue disease, 148–149
  diagnosis, 135
  in scleroderma, 139
Polyp(s)
  gastrointestinal, in Peutz-Jeghers syndrome, 269
  intestinal, in Gardner's syndrome, 274–275

Polyposis
  gastrointestinal, in Peutz-Jeghers syndrome, 268
  intestinal, in Gardner's syndrome, 274
Polyseritis, recurrent (*see* Mediterranean fever, familial)
Porphyria
  acute intermittent, 329–330
    neuropsychiatric symptoms of, 329
    psychologic manifestations, 329
    treatment, 329–330
  classification, 325, 326
  cutanea tarda, 330–331
    diagnosis, 330–331
    as inborn error of metabolism, 330
    treatment, 331
  dark urine in, 194
  diagnosis, differential, 194
  in epidermolysis bullosa, dominant dystrophic, 263
  erythropoietic, 325–328
    biochemical disturbance in, 325
    clinical manifestations, 325–327
    diagnosis, 327
    treatment, 327–328
    werewolves and, 327
  hepatic, 325, 329–332
    congenital cutaneous, 331
  -like symptoms in tyrosinemia I, 201
  variegata, 331–332
    weather-beaten appearance in, 332
Porphyrin fluorescence: and erythropoietic porphyria, 327
Port-wine stains, 283, 284–285
  in Cobb syndrome, 294
  in Sturge-Weber syndrome, 287, 288
  telangiectasia resembling, 290
Potassium iodide: in Sweet's syndrome, 41
Pot-belly appearance: in Kwashiorkor, 324
Prebetalipoproteinemia (*see* Hyperlipoproteinemia, type III)
Prebeta-lipoproteins, 203
Precocious puberty
  paradoxical, in acquired hypothyroidism, 160
  pseudoprecocious puberty, 178
Precosity, sexual (*see* Sexual precosity)

Premature aging: of skin, 312
Premature sexual development: in boys in adrenogenital syndrome, 179
Prematurity
  acrodermatitis enteropathica and, 251
  Ehlers-Danlos syndrome and, 96
  in Menkes' kinky hair syndrome, 196
  in tyrosinemia, 200
Prenatal diagnosis
  of angiokeratoma corporis diffusum, 296
  in ataxia telangiectasia, 305
  of Cockayne syndrome, 319
  of epidermolysis bullosa, recessive dystrophic, 262
  of Hurler syndrome, 212
  of Menkes' kinky hair syndrome, 197
  of mucolipidosis II, 216
Protein
  fetal, 304
  inadequate intake in Kwashiorkor, 324
Proteinosis (*see* Lipid proteinosis)
Proteinuria: in angiokeratoma corporis diffusum, 296
Proteus OX-19, 81, 82
Protoporphyria, erythropoietic, 328–329
  clinical manifestations, 328–329
  diagnosis, 329
  ferrochelatase deficiency in, 328
  treatment, 329
Protoporphyrin, 328
Pruritus
  in dermatitis herpetiformis, 254
  in hyperparathyroidism, 170
  in hyperthyroidism, 164
  uremic, 171
Pseudohermaphroditism, 178
Pseudo-Hurler polydystrophy, 216
Pseudohypoparathyroidism, 173
  in basal cell nevus syndrome, 243
  treatment, 174
Pseudoprecocious puberty, 178
Pseudo-pseudohypoparathyroidism, 173
Pseudosyndactyly: in recessive dystrophic epidermolysis bullosa, 261
Pseudotumors: in Ehlers-Danlos syndrome, 97

Pseudoxanthoma elasticum, 110–113
  clinical manifestations, 111–112
  diagnosis, 112–113
  elastosis perforans serpiginosa in, 113
  Marfanoid appearance in, 112
  pathogenesis, 111
  treatment, 113
  varieties of, 112
Psoralen: in mastocytosis, 353
Psoriasis: pustular, 252
Psychomotor regression: in fucosidosis,
  298
Psychomotor retardation: in Menkes'
  kinky hair syndrome, 197
Psychosis: frank, in Hartnup disease,
  320
Puberty
  delayed, in hypothyroidism, 160
  precocious (*see* Precocious puberty)
Pulmonary
  arteriovenous fistulae in hereditary
    hemorrhagic telangiectasia, 302
  stenosis, in multiple lentigines
    syndrome, 240
Purpura
  anaphylactoid (*see* Henoch-Schönlein
    purpura)
  fulminans, 306–308
    (*See also* Coagulation,
      disseminated intravascular)
    clinical features, 306–307
    diagnosis, 307
    treatment, 307–308
  in Hand-Schüller-Christian disease,
    340
  Henoch-Schönlein (*see* Henoch-
    Schönlein purpura)
  in hypothyroidism, 158, 162
  in Kwashiorkor, 324
  palpable, 36, 37
  in periarteritis nodosa, adult, 56
  in rickettsial disease, 83, 85
  in Rocky Mountain spotted fever, 84
  in Sjögren's syndrome, 147
  thrombocytopenic, thrombotic, and
    livedo reticularis, 299
PUVA
  in mastocytosis, 353
  in mycosis fungoides, 360
Pyelography: IV, in tuberous sclerosis,
  232

Pyloric atresia: in epidermolysis
  bullosa, 261
Pyoderma: in Cushing's syndrome, 177
Pyoderma gangrenosum, 272–274
  cause of, 273
  clinical manifestations, 273
  diagnosis, 273
  systemic disorders in, 272
  treatment, 273–274
    topical, 273
Pyridoxine phosphate: in
  homocystinuria, 193
Pyuria: in Kawasaki disease, 53

Q

Q fever, 81, 82–83
Quincke's edema, 2

R

Radiculoneuritis: in Lyme disease, 74
Radiography: of skull in Sturge-Weber
  syndrome, 288
Radioimmunoassay: in
  hyperthyroidism, 165
Radiotherapy
  in eosinophilic granuloma, 341
  in Kasabach-Merritt syndrome, 287
  in mycosis fungoides, 360
Rat
  flea, 82
  mite, 82
Raynaud's phenomenon, 7, 133
  absence in scleroderma, 137
  fasciitis and, eosinophilic, 140
  in lupus erythematosus, 122
  in mixed connective tissue disease,
    150
  in periarteritis nodosa, adult, 56
  in scleroderma, systemic, 138, 139
  in Sjögren's syndrome, 147
Rectum: biopsy in familial
  Mediterranean fever, 276
"Red children," in Kwashiorkor, 324
Reddish skin: in Kwashiorkor, 324
Reflux: gastroesophageal, 139
Renal (*see* Kidney)
Rendu-Osler-Weber syndrome, 139

Rendu-Osler-Weber syndrome
(*See also* Telangiectasia, hereditary
hemorrhagic)
Respiratory
difficulty in xanthoma disseminatum,
342
disease, before dermatomyositis, 134
involvement in Henoch-Schönlein
purpura, 38
stridor in epidermolysis bullosa, 261
tract
infection, in Bloom syndrome, 316
infection, recurrent, in ataxia
telangiectasia, 303
obstruction in diffuse neonatal
hemangiomatosis, 292
xanthomatous deposits, 342
retardation, mental (*see* Mental
retardation)
Reticuloendothelial
disorders, 336–363
system, 336
Reticulosis: histiocytic medullary, 343
Retina
atrophy in Cockayne syndrome, 318,
319
pigmentation in Cockayne syndrome,
319
Rhabdomyoma: in tuberous sclerosis,
232
Rheumatic fever, 12–14
acute, 3
livedo reticularis in, 122, 299
subcutaneous nodules in, 13
Rheumatoid arthritis
contrasted with mixed connective
tissue disease, 148
juvenile, 3, 12, 142–146
age of onset, 142
clinical manifestations, 143–145
course, 145
diagnosis, 145–146
etiology, 142, 143
mixed connective tissue disease
mimicking, 150
rash in, 143
subcutaneous nodules in, 142, 145
treatment, 146
livedo reticularis in, 122, 299
maternal, lupus erythematosus in
newborn in, 128

Sjögren's syndrome and, 146
telangiectasia in, cuticular, 123
Rheumatoid factor, 150
Rheumatoid nodules: in granuloma
annulare, 184
Ribonucleoprotein, 150
Ribs: bifid, in basal cell nevus
syndrome, 242, 243
Richner-Hanhart syndrome, 200
(*See also* Tyrosinemia II)
Rickets: vitamin D-resistant, and
tyrosinemia I, 201
Rickettsia
akuri, 82
mooseri, 82
prowazekii, 81
Rickettsial disease, 81–85
clinical manifestations, 83
diagnosis, 83–84
purpura fulminans and, 306
treatment, 84–85
Rickettsialpox, 81, 82
diagnosis, 82
Riley-Smith syndrome, 293
Ritter's disease, 65
Rocky Mountain spotted fever, 81, 83
purpura in, 84
fulminans, 306
Rodent (*see* Rat)
Ro(SSA), 129
Rothmund-Thomson syndrome,
317–318
clinical features, 317–318
elastosis perforans serpiginosa in, 113
life span in, normal, 317
treatment, 318
Rupture: of Achilles tendon in
alkaptonuria, 190

S

Saline: isotonic, in
hyperparathyroidism, 171
Salivary gland: enlargement in
Sjögren's syndrome, 147
Sanfilippo syndrome, 213–214
"Sarcoid belt," 354
Sarcoidosis, 354–357
in Addison's disease, 176
clinical manifestations, 355

Sarcoidosis *(cont.)*
  cutaneous features, 355–356
    "apple-jelly" color, 356
    Darier-Roussy type, 356
  diagnosis, 356–357
  in erythema nodosum, 18
  erythrodermic, 356
  etiology unknown, 354
  host response abnormality in, 354
  hypercalcemia secondary to, 170
  treatment, 357
Sarcoma
  angiosarcoma in Maffucci's
    syndrome, 291
  chondrosarcoma in Maffucci's
    syndrome, 291
Scalded skin *(see* Staphylococcal
    scalded skin syndrome)
Scalp
  in Letterer-Siwe disease, 338
  in lupus erythematosus, neonatal,
    130
  seborrhea of, in hypothyroidism, 158
  seborrhea-like eruption, in Letterer-
    Siwe disease, 337
Scanning: bone for mastocytosis
    screening, 353
Scarlatiniform rash: in toxic shock
    syndrome, 69
Scarlet fever: staphylococcal, 68
Scars
  atrophy in epidermolysis bullosa, 261
  in Bloom syndrome, 315
  after candidiasis, chronic
    mucocutaneous, 87
  hypopigmented, in dermatitis
    herpetiformis, 255
  papyraceous, of knee, in Ehlers-
    Danlos syndrome, 97
  in porphyria, erythropoietic, 325
Scheie syndrome, 212–213
Schirmer's test, 148
Scholastic performance: poor, in
    hypothyroidism, 162
Schwann cell, 223
Schwannoma: malignant, 225
Schwartzman-like phenomenon: in
    purpura fulminans, 307
Scintigraphy: in Sjögren's syndrome,
    148

Sclera
  in alkaptonuria, 190
  blue *(see* Blue sclerae)
Sclerodactyly, 137, 138
  in mixed connective tissue disease,
    149
  in scleroderma, systemic, 139
Scleroderma, 136–140
  in ataxia telangiectasia, 304
  clinical manifestations, 137–139
  diagnosis, 139–140
  diffuse, 137
  etiology, 137
  face in, 139
  fasciitis as variant of, eosinophilic,
    140, 141
  histologic differentiation, 140
  -like changes in eosinophilic fasciitis,
    141
  -like plaques in porphyria variegata,
    332
  linear, 137
  livedo reticularis in, 122
  nose in, 139
  systemic, 138
    relationship with morphea, 137
  treatment, 140
Sclerosis
  cutaneous, 138
  systemic
    clinical features, 137
    progressive, 137
Sclerosis, tuberous, 227–233
  ash-leaf-shaped hypopigmented
    macules in, 230
  clinical manifestations, 228–232
  diagnosis, 232
  family members at risk for, 233
  leg in, 230
  management, 232–233
  mutations in, 227, 233
  osseous manifestations, 232
  pathogenesis of, 228
  systemic lesions of, 231–232
  systemic manifestations, 228
  "tubers" in, 232
  white macules in, 229
  white spots in, 230
Sclerotic calcification: in brain in
    tuberous sclerosis, 232

Scoliosis: tuberous, formes frustes of, 232, 233
Scrotum
angiokeratoma of, 294
hemorrhage in Henoch-Schönlein purpura, 38
Seborrhea
-like rash in Letterer-Siwe disease, 337
of scalp in hypothyroidism, 158
Seborrheic rash: in Menkes' kinky hair syndrome, 196
Seizures
in fucosidosis, 298
in homocystinuria, 190, 192
in hypomelanosis of Ito, 238
in phenylketonuria, 189
salaam, in tuberous sclerosis, 231
in sclerosis, tuberous, 227, 231
in Sturge-Weber syndrome, 287, 288
Self-destructive biting: compulsive, in Lesch-Nyhan syndrome, 198
Sella turcica: enlargement in hypothyroidism, 161
"Senile" appearance: in childhood, in Cockayne syndrome, 318
Sepsis: in dermatomyositis, 136
Septicemia: in purpura fulminans, 306
Serum injections: hypersensitivity to, 3
Serum sickness, 8–9
clinical manifestations, 8–9
treatment, 9
Sex incidence: of lupus erythematosus, 120
Sexual development
premature, in boys in adrenogenital syndrome, 179
in xeroderma pigmentosum, 313
Sexual precocity
neurofibromatosis and, 226
with polyostotic fibrous dysplasia, in girls, 223
Sézary syndrome: in mycosis fungoides, 359
Shagreen patches: in tuberous sclerosis, 227, 228, 229
Sharp's syndrome (see Connective tissue, disease, mixed)
Sheehan's syndrome, 180

Shock
severe prolonged, in toxic shock syndrome, 69
toxic (see Toxic shock syndrome)
Short stature
in hypothyroidism, 162
in phenylketonuria, 190
in Rothmund-Thomson syndrome, 317
Shoulder
in dermatomyositis, 133
in Hunter syndrome, 214
Shunt: arteriovenous, and diffuse neonatal hemangiomatosis, 293
Sialography: in Sjögren's syndrome, 148
Simmond's disease, 180
Sinopulmonary infections: recurrent in ataxia telangiectasia, 304
Sipple syndrome, 166, 167
Sjögren's syndrome, 146–148
clinical manifestations, 147
contrasted with mixed connective tissue disease, 148
diagnosis, 147–148
ocular manifestations, 147
sarcoidosis and, 355
treatment, 148
Skeleton
aberrations, in multiple lentigines syndrome, 241
abnormalities, in Maffucci's syndrome, 291
anomalies
in epidermal nevus syndrome, 244
in hypomelanosis of Iro, 237–238
changes in phenylketonuria, 189
defects in multiple endocrine adenomatosis syndrome, 167
deformities
in nevus unius lateris, 245
in Waardenburg syndrome, 239
lesions in eosinophilic granuloma, 340, 341
malformations in incontinentia pigmenti, 236
manifestations of incontinentia pigmenti, 234
muscle in dermatomyositis, 132

Skeleton *(cont.)*
  system in epidermal nevus
      syndrome, 244
Skin
  aging, premature, 312
  anomalies in hypomelanosis of Ito,
      238
  in ataxia telangiectasia, 303
  atrophy *(see* Atrophy, skin)
  biopsy in mastocytosis, diffuse
      cutaneous, 352–353
  bronzing in neurofibromatosis, 223
  calcification, 170
      metastatic, 170
  calcinosis and dermatomyositis, 132
  cancer *(see* Cancer, skin)
  in candidiasis, 172
  changes
      in Hunter syndrome, 213
      in mucopolysaccharidoses, 211
  cobblestone appearance in
      erythropoietic protoporphyria,
      328
  coffee-colored, in Kwashiorkor, 324
  "cracked," in Kwashiorkor, 324
  dryness
      in biotin deficiency, 199
      in Sjögren's syndrome, 147
  erythematous blotches, in
      homocystinuria, 192
  in fasciitis, eosinophilic, 140
  fibrils, anchoring, absence of, in
      epidermolysis bullosa, recessive
      dystrophic, 261
  form of Letterer-Siwe disease, 337
  fragility in Ehlers-Danlos syndrome,
      96
  gastrointestinal tract and, 250–282
  graying of, diffuse, in
      neurofibromatosis, 223
  hemangioma, 283–286
  in hypopituitarism, 180
  lesions
      in eosinophilic granuloma, 341
      in Hand-Schüller-Christian
          disease, 340
      in hyperthyroidism, 165
      in Mediterranean fever, familial,
          275, 276

  sclerodermatous, in
      phenylketonuria, 189
  livid mottling in cutis marmorata,
      299
  in mastocytosis *(see* Mastocytosis,
      diffuse cutaneous)
  necrosis, in purpura fulminans, 307
  neurocutaneous disorders, 220–249
  neurofibroma of, 220, 226
  pale thick cool, in hypothyroidism,
      160
  pallid, in Menkes' kinky hair
      syndrome, 196
  pallor, grayish, in biotin deficiency,
      199
  parathyroid disorders and, 169–174
  pellagra-like lesions
      in Hartnup disease, 319
      in Kwashiorkor, 324
  phases in incontinentia pigmenti *(see*
      Incontinentia pigmenti, phase)
  puckering in eosinophilic fasciitis,
      141
  reddish, in Kwashiorkor, 324
  in rheumatoid arthritis, juvenile,
      142
  rigid, in mucolipidosis II, 215
  rough dry, in hypothyroidism,
      acquired, 162
  in sarcoidosis, 354
  scalded *(see* Staphylococcal scalded
      skin syndrome)
  sclerosis, 138
  "stiff skin" syndrome, 216–217
  striae in Cockayne syndrome, 319
  telangiectases on, in hereditary
      hemorrhagic telangiectasia, 301
  thick, pale cool, in hypothyroidism,
      acquired, 162
  tumor in epidermolysis bullosa,
      recessive dystrophic, 261
  in uremia, 170, 171
  warm soft smooth, in
      hyperthyroidism, 164
  widepored, in homocystinuria, 192
Skull
  bones in Cockayne syndrome, 319
  radiography, in Sturge-Weber
      syndrome, 288

Sleep disturbances: in hyperthyroidism, 164
Sodium concentration: in rickettsial disease, 83
Soft tissue
  hypertrophy in Klippel-Trenaunay-Parkes-Weber syndrome, 290
  tenderness and swelling in eosinophilic granuloma, 340
Solar urticaria, 4, 6
Solatene
  in porphyria, erythropoietic, 328
  in protoporphyria, erythropoietic, 329
Soles
  in dyskeratosis congenita, 270
  hyperkeratosis in epidermolysis bullosa, 260
    generalized atrophic, 260
  in Letterer-Siwe disease, 337
  peeling in toxic shock syndrome, 69
  in rickettsial disease, 83
Spasms: infantile, in tuberous sclerosis, 231
Spasticity
  in fucosidosis, 297, 298
  in Lesch-Nyhan syndrome, 198
Spine
  angiography in Cobb syndrome, 294
  deformities
    in homocystinuria, 192
    in neurofibromatosis, 226
  muscle atrophy in ataxia telangiectasia, 305
Spirochete, 72
Spleen
  infarct in type I hyperlipoproteinemia, 207
  in xanthogranuloma, juvenile, 344
Splenomegaly
  in Gianotti-Crosti syndrome, 76
  hepatosplenomegaly in Letterer-Siwe disease, 337
  in porphyria, erythropoietic, 325, 327
  urticaria pigmentosa and, 351
Sporodic lesions: in pellagra, 322
Sprue: celiac, 254
Squirrels: flying, 81

Staining: of mast cells, 353
Staphylococcal scalded skin syndrome, 65–68
  clinical manifestations, 65–67
  diagnosis, 67–68
  differentiated from toxic epidermal necrolysis, 28, 65, 67
  epidermal split in, superficial, 27
  treatment, 68
Staphylococcal scarlet fever, 68
Staphylococcus aureus: phage-group-I, 68
Stature (*see* Short stature)
Stenosis
  aortic, calcific, in alkaptonuria, 190
  pulmonary, in multiple lentigines syndrome, 240
Steroid(s)
  (*See also* Corticosteroids)
  acne in Cushing's syndrome, 177
  in Behcet's syndrome, 60
  in dermatomyositis, 135
  in eosinophilic granuloma, 341
  intralesional, in pyoderma gangrenosum, 273
  in lupus erythematosus, 128
    complications, 128
  in mixed connective tissue disease, 151
  pulse, in lupus erythematosus, 128
  in Stevens-Johnson syndrome, 26
  systemic
    in eosinophilic fasciitis, 140
    in epidermolysis bullosa, 267
    in pyoderma gangrenosum, 273
  urticaria and, 4
Stevens-Johnson disease, 23–26
  antihistamines in, 25
  diagnosis, 24–25
  mycoplasma infections and, 23
  treatment, 25–26
"Stiff skin" syndrome, 216–217
Stiffness: morning, in juvenile rheumatoid arthritis, 144
Still's disease, 142
  (*See also* Rheumatoid arthritis, juvenile)
Strawberry hemangioma (*see* Hemangioma, strawberry)

Strawberry nevus, 283
Strawberry tongue: in Kawasaki
    disease, 47, 48
Streptococcal infection: and purpura
    fulminans, 306
Stress: and eosinophilic fasciitis, 140
Striatum palmare: in type III
    hyperlipoproteinemia, 208
Stridor: respiratory, in epidermolysis
    bullosa, 261
Sturge-Weber syndrome, 287–289
    in Riley-Smith syndrome, 293
    "tramlines" in, 289
    treatment, 289
Sulfapyridine
    in dermatitis herpetiformis, 254, 255
    side effects, 255
    toxicity, 255
Sulfatidosis: juvenile, 216
Sulfones: in dermatitis herpetiformis,
    254
Sun
    exposure
        in lupus erythematosus, neonatal,
        129
        pellagra and, 322
    sensitivity in porphyria variegata, 332
Sutton's disease, 59
Sutures: premature closure, in
    xeroderma pigmentosum, 313
Sweating: decrease in fucosidosis, 298
Sweet's syndrome, 39–41
    clinical manifestations, 40–41
    diagnosis, 41
    etiology, 39, 40
    leukemic state, 39
    preleukemic state, 39
    treatment, 41
Symblepharon: in xeroderma
    pigmentosum, 314
Syndactyly: in Bloom syndrome, 315
Synovitis: in Mediterranean fever,
    familial, 275
Systole: increase in hyperthyroidism,
    164

T

Tampons: in toxic shock syndrome, 69,
    70

Tan: decreased ability in
    hypopituitarism, 180
Tangier disease, 209
    defect in, as uncertain, 209
    maculopapular eruption over, 209
Teeth
    (See also Dental)
    brown-stained, in erythropoietic
        prophyria, 327
    tooth pits and tuberous sclerosis,
        228, 231
Telangiectasia, 123
    in angiokeratoma corporis diffusum,
        295
    ataxia (see Ataxia telangiectasia)
    in Bloom syndrome, 315, 316
    in Cockayne syndrome, 318, 319
    in Cushing's syndrome, 176–177
    cuticular
        in dermatomyositis, 123, 133, 134
        in lupus erythematosus, 123
        in rheumatoid arthritis, juvenile,
        145
        in scleroderma, 138
    in dyskeratosis congenita, 270
    hereditary hemorrhagic, 301–303
        diagnosis, 303
        mucocutaneous lesions of, 301
        telangiectases on skin and mucous
        membranes in, 301
        treatment, 303
    in Klippel-Trenaunay-Parkes-Weber
        syndrome, 290
    in lupus erythematosus, 121, 122
    in lupus erythematosus neonatal, 129
    macularis eruptiva perstans, 350
        mastocytosis and, 345
    malar, in mixed connective tissue
        disease, 149
    in necrobiosis lipoidica diabeticorum,
        182
    oculocutaneous, in ataxia
        telangiectasia, 303
    of palms and fingers in lupus
        erythematosus, 123
    in Rothmund-Thomson syndrome,
        317
    in scleroderma, 138, 139
        systemic, 139
    in sclerosis, systemic, 137

in Sjögren's syndrome, 147
in xeroderma pigmentosum, 314
Telangiectatic erythema, congenital (*see* Bloom syndrome)
Telogen effluvium: in toxic shock syndrome, 69
Temporoparietal bossing: in basal cell nevus syndrome, 243
TEN (*see* Toxic epidermal necrolysis)
Tendon
  Achilles, rupture in alkaptonuria, 190
  reflexes, deep, delayed in hypothyroidism, 160
  xanthoma, 206
    in hyperlipoproteinemia, type II, 207
Testes
  hemorrhage in Henoch-Schönlein purpura, 38
  in xanthogranuloma, juvenile, 344
Tetracycline
  in Behcet's syndrome, 60
  in Q fever, 83
  in rickettsialpox, 82
Thenar eminence: in juvenile rheumatoid arthritis, 144
Thigh
  angiokeratoma of, disseminated, in fucosidosis, 297
  lesion in juvenile xanthogranuloma, 345
Thrombocytopenia, 286–287
  with hemangioma, cavernous, 286
  in hemangiomatosis, diffuse neonatal, 292
  idiopathic, livedo reticularis in, 122, 299
  in Letterer-Siwe disease, 337
  in mixed connective tissue disease, 150
  in rickettsial disease, 83
  surgical risk in, 287
  in toxic shock syndrome, 70, 71
  treatment, 287
Thrombocytosis, 53
  in Kawasaki disease, 47
Thromboembolism: in homocystinuria, 192
Thrombosis: coronary, and Kawasaki disease, 47

Thymus: transplantation in DiGeorge syndrome, 174
Thyroid
  ablation, radioactive, causing hypothyroidism, 158
  acropachy in hyperthyroidism, 164, 165
  agenesis, 157
  cancer in hyperthyroidism, 163
  carcinoma, medullary, 166, 167
    in hyperthyroidism, 169
  disorders, 157–166
  dysgenesis, 157
    hypothyroidism due to, 158
  nodules, hyperfunctioning, in hyperthyroidism, 163
  stimulator, long-acting, 163
    in hyperthyroidism, 164, 165
Thyroidectomy
  in hyperthyroidism, 166
  hypoparathyroidism after, 172
  hypothyroidism due to, 158
Thyroiditis
  chronic lymphocytic
    in hyperthyroidism, 163
    in hypothyroidism, acquired, 159
  Hashimoto's
    in hyperthyroidism, 163
    in hypoparathyroidism, 172
    hypothyroidism due to, 158
    hypothyroidism due to, acquired, 159
  Sjögren's syndrome and, 146
Thyrotoxicosis (*see* Hyperthyroidism)
Thyrotropin (*see* TSH)
Tick
  bite causing erythema chronicum migrans, 72
  dog, 83
  wood, 83
Tinea corporis: differentiated from erythema chronicum migrans, 15
Toes: mitten-like deformities in epidermolysis bullosa, recessive dystrophic, 261
Toluidine blue test: in Hurler syndrome, 211
Tomography: computed, in tuberous sclerosis, 232

Tongue
  "black," in pellagra, 323
  in dyskeratosis congenita, 271
  pale, in biotin deficiency, 199
  strawberry, in Kawasaki disease, 47,
    48
  in telangiectasia, hereditary
    hemorrhagic, 302
  thickened, in hypothyroidism, 160
Tonsils: in Tangier disease, 209
Tooth (*see* Teeth)
Touton giant cells: in xanthoma
    disseminatum, 342
Toxic epidermal necrolysis, 20, 26–28
  biopsy in, cutaneous punch, 28
  clinical manifestations, 27
  corticosteroids in, systemic, 28
  diagnosis, 27–28
  differentiated from staphylococcal
    scalded skin syndrome, 28, 65,
    67
  pathogenesis, 27
  subepidermal bullae, 27
  treatment, 28
Toxic goiter, 163
Toxic shock syndrome, 68–71
  clinical features, 69–71
  desquamation in, 69, 70
  diagnosis, 70–71
    criteria for, 69
  mucous membranes in, 70
    hyperemia of, 71
  pathology, 70
  severe prolonged shock in, 69
  tampons in, 69, 70
  treatment, 71
Toxicity
  hepatic, after ketoconazole, 87
  sulfapyridine, 255
Toxin
  exfoliative, 65
  in toxic shock syndrome, 79
Tracheostomy: in xanthoma
    disseminatum, 343
"Tramlines:" in Sturge-Weber
    syndrome, 289
Transfusion
  in granuloma, eosinophilic, 341
  replacement, in angiokeratoma
    corporis diffusum, 297

Transplantation
  of colon, in epidermolysis bullosa,
    267
  of kidney, and lupus erythematosus,
    128
  thymus, in DiGeorge syndrome, 174
Trauma
  in Addison's disease, 176
  fasciitis and, eosinophilic, 140, 141,
    142
  mechanical, in epidermolysis bullosa
    simplex, 257
  in Mediterranean fever, familial, 276
Tremor: intension, in Hartnup disease,
    320
Trichopoliodystrophy (*see* Menkes'
    kinky hair syndrome)
Trichorrhexis nodosa: in Menkes' kinky
    hair syndrome, 196
Trigeminal nerve: in Sturge-Weber
    syndrome, 287, 288
Trihexosyl ceramide, 294
Trisomy 10 (*see* Cockayne syndrome)
Trunk
  Chinese figure-like
    hyperpigmentation in
    incontinentia pigmenti, 235
  in epidermolysis bullosa, dominant
    dystrophic, 264
Tryptophan
  in Hartnup disease, 319, 320
  in pellagra, 321
TSH in hyperthyroidism, 164
  hypersecretion, 163
Tuberous (*see* Sclerosis, tuberous)
Tumor(s)
  (*See also* Neoplasia)
  eye, in juvenile xanthogranuloma,
    344
  face, in mycosis fungoides, 359
  fibrous, in Gardner's syndrome, 274
  of gingiva in Hand-Schüller-Christian
    disease, 340
  increased predisposition to, in Bloom
    syndrome, 316
  in Peutz-Jeghers syndrome, 269
  skin, in epidermolysis bullosa,
    recessive dystrophic, 261
  stage of mycosis fungoides, 358
  xeroderma pigmentosum and, 313

Typhus fever
  endemic, 81–82
  epidemic, 81
    diagnosis, 81
    treatment, 81
  flea-borne, 81–82
  louse-borne, 81
  murine, 81–82
Tyrosine aminotransferase, 200
  deficiency in tyrosinemia II, 201–202
Tyrosine metabolism disorders,
    200–203
  cabbage-like odor in, 201
  diagnosis, 202
  treatment, 203
Tyrosinemia
  in newborn, 200–201
  I, 200, 201
    cabbage-like odor in, 201
    cause of, 201
  II, 200, 201–202
    blisters in, 202
    erosions in, 202
    eye abnormalities in, 202
    neurologic features, 202
    tyrosine aminotransferase deficiency
      in, 201–202
Tyrosinosis (see Tyrosinemia, I)
  oculocutaneous (see Tyrosinemia, II)
Tzanck test: in toxic epidermal
    necrolysis, 28

U

Ulcer(s)
  aphthous, in pellagra, 323
  buccal, in Letterer-Siwe disease, 337
  in eosinophilic granuloma, 340
  of fingertips in dermatomyositis, 134
  genital, in Behcet's syndrome, 59
  gingival, in Letterer-Siwe disease,
    337
  in Hand-Schüller-Christian disease,
    340
  in inguinal region in histiocytosis X,
    338
  in Letterer-Siwe disease, 337
  with livedo reticularis, 299
  mutilating, in erythropoietic
    porphyria, 325

in necrobiosis lipoidica diabeticorum,
    181, 182
  in pellagra, 322
  peptic, and urticaria pigmentosa, 350
  in sclerosis, systemic, 137
  stasis, in angiokeratoma corporis
    diffusum, 296
Ulcerative colitis: in erythema
    nodosum, 18
Ultrasound: in tuberous sclerosis, 232
Ultrastructure: in epidermolysis
    bullosa, acquired, 265
Ultraviolet light: in mastocytosis, 353
Ultraviolet radiation: damaging skin,
    photosensitivity after, 312
Uremia
  hypercalcemia secondary to, 170
  with pruritus, 171
  skin in, 170, 171
Uric acid: in Lesch-Nyhan syndrome,
    198
Urine
  black, 194
  dark, in alkaptonuria, 190, 194
  darkening on standing, in acute
    intermittent porphyria, 329
  fluorescence in porphyria cutanea
    tarda, 331
  in porphyria, erythropoietic, 327
  red, in erythropoietic porphyria, 325
Uroporphyrin I: elevation in
    erythropoietic porphyria, 327
Urticaria, 1–7
  aquagenic, 4, 5–6
  cholinergic, 4
    treatment, 5
  clinical manifestations, 1–3
  cold, 4, 6–7
  contrasted with Henoch-Schönlein
    purpura, 36
  in dermatitis herpetiformis, 254
  diagnosis, 3
    differential, 3
  etiology, 1, 3
  factitious, 4
  giant, 2
  in hyperthyroidism, 164
  in lupus erythematosus, 121, 122
  in Mediterranean fever, familial, 276
  micropapular, 4–5

Urticaria *(cont.)*
  in periarteritis nodosa, adult, 56
  physical, 4–7
  pigmentosa, 347, 349–351
    adult form, 350, 351
    bullous, 346, 347
    clinical manifestations, 349–350
    mastocytosis, 345, 346
    peptic ulcer and, 350
    prognosis, 350–351
    symptoms, 351
    with systemic disease, 351
    systemic involvement in, 351
  pressure, 4
  psychogenic factors in, 3
  rash of, in Kawasaki disease, 49
  solar, 4, 6
  treatment, 3–4
Uveitis
  bilateral, in Vogt-Koyanagi-Harada
    syndrome, 239
  in sarcoidosis, 355
Uveoparotid fever: in sarcoidosis, 355

V

Vaccinia: and purpura fulminans, 306
Valvulitis: in alkaptonuria, 190
Varicosities: in Klippel-Trenaunay-
    Parkes-Weber syndrome, 290
Vascular *(see* Vessels)
Vasculitic syndromes, 35–64
Vasculitis, 2
  leukocytoclastic, 39
  necrotizing, 42
  in Rocky Mountain spotted fever, 85
Vasopressin
  for diabetes insipidus in eosinophilic
    granuloma, 341
  xanthoma disseminatum and, 343
Vein *(see* Arteriovenous)
Verrucous lesion: in incontinentia
    pigmenti, 234
Vertebra
  anomalies in basal cell nevus
    syndrome, 242
  body break in hypothyroidism, 161
Vesicles
  in dermatitis herpetiformis, 254
  in Letterer-Siwe disease, 337

Vesicular lesions: on arm in
    incontinentia pigmenti, 234
Vesiculation: in pellagra, 322
Vessels
  abnormalities in alkaptonuria, 193
  atherosclerotic, complicating type III
    hyperlipoproteinemia, 208
  cerebral *(see* Cerebrovascular)
  changes in pseudoxanthoma
    elasticum, 112
  collagen disorders, 119–156
  of conjunctiva, tortuosity in
    angiokeratoma corporis
    diffusum, 296
  dilatation, disorders associated with,
    299–306
  disease
    alkaptonuria complicated by, 194
    atheromatous, in Cockayne
      syndrome, 318, 319
    involvement in Behcet's syndrome,
      59
    lesions with systemic significance,
      283–311
    nevi, incidence, 284
    system in epidermal nevus
      syndrome, 244
    telangiectatic, in necrobiosis lipoidica
      diabeticorum, 182
Virilism: and adrenogenital syndrome,
    178, 179
Virus(es)
  Epstein-Barr, 78
  in Vogt-Koyanagi-Harada syndrome,
    240
Visceral involvement: absence in
    eosinophilic fasciitis, 140
Vistaril: in mastocytosis, 353
Vitamin
  B_6 in homocystinuria, 193
  D intoxication, hypercalcemia
    secondary to, 170
  D-resistant rickets, and tyrosinemia
    I, 201
  E, oral, in epidermolysis bullosa, 266
Vitiligo
  in Addison's disease, 176
  in Alezzandrini syndrome, 240
  in candidiasis, chronic
    mucocutaneous, 87

differentiated from tuberous
sclerosis, 230
in hyperthyroidism, 164
hypoparathyroidism and, 172
hypopigmentation in, 231
in Vogt-Koyanagi-Harada syndrome,
240
Vogt-Koyanagi-Harada syndrome,
239–240
as autoimmune disorder, 239
clinical course, 240
encephalitic symptoms, 240
meningeal symptoms, 240
Vogt-Koyanagi syndrome (see Vogt-
Koyanagi-Harada syndrome)
Voice: deepening, in adrenogenital
syndrome, 179
von Recklinghausen disease (see
Neurofibromatosis)
Vulva: angiokeratoma of, 294

W

Waardenburg syndrome, 239
Warty lesion: in incontinentia
pigmenti, 234
Waterhouse-Friderichsen syndrome,
307
Watson-Schwartz test: in acute
intermittent porphyria, 329
Weakness: in fucosidosis, 297
Weaning: and acrodermatitis
enteropathica, 251
Wegener's granulomatosis, 42–43
contrasted with
Henoch-Schönlein purpura, 43
lymphomatoid granulomatosis, 44
etiology, 42
mucocutaneous involvement, 42
ophthalmologic findings in, 42
presenting features, 42
skin lesions of, 42
Weil-Felix agglutination reaction, 81,
82
in rickettsial disease, 83
Werewolves: and erythropoietic
porphyria, 327
Wermer's syndrome, 167
Wilson's disease (see Hepatolenticular
degeneration)

Wood's light
brown-stained teeth that fluoresce
under, in erythropoietic
porphyria, 327
in tuberous sclerosis, 229, 231
Wooly nevus syndrome, 236

X

Xanthelasma, 204
in hyperlipoproteinemia, type II, 207
xanthoma and, tendinous, 206
Xanthogranuloma, juvenile, 227,
343–345
with neurofibromatosis, 345
Xanthoma
clinical manifestations, 203–206
disseminatum, 342–343
lesions of, 342
eruptive, 203
in hyperlipoproteinemia, type I,
207
hyperlipoproteinemia and, type
III, 208
in knee, 205
with hyperlipoproteinemia, type II,
207
palpebrarum, 204
papuloeruptive, 203, 205
plane, 203, 204–205
striatum planum, 205
tendinous, 203, 206
in hyperlipoproteinemia, type II,
207
tuberous lesions and, 206
tendon, 206
in hyperlipoproteinemia, type II,
207
tuberous, 203, 206
Xenopsylla cheopis, 82
Xeroderma pigmentosum, 312–315
clinical features, 312–313
diagnosis, 313–314
malignant changes in, 313
neurologic complications of, 313
treatment, 314–315
Xerosis
hyperthyroidism and, 170
Kwashiokor and, 324

Xerostomia, 146
X-ray (*see* Radiography, Radiotherapy)

Z

Zinc
  -binding ligands, 250
  deficiency, syndromes of, 251
  deficient diet, and acrodermatitis
    enteropathica, 251
  gluconate in acrodermatitis
    enteropathica, 253
  level decrease in acrodermatitis
    enteropathica, 253
  malabsorption in acrodermatitis
    enteropathica, 250
  sulfate in acrodermatitis
    enteropathica, 253
  trapping of, 251